FRONTLINE WORKERS IN ASSISTED LIVING

Frontline Workers in Assisted Living

Edited by
MARY M. BALL
MOLLY M. PERKINS
CAROLE HOLLINGSWORTH
CANDACE L. KEMP

The Johns Hopkins University Press
Baltimore

The Johns Hopkins University Press
2715 North Charles Street
Baltimore, Maryland 21218-4363
www.press.jhu.edu

Library of Congress Cataloging-in-Publication Data
Frontline workers in assisted living / edited by Mary M. Ball . . .
[et al.].
 p. ; cm.
 Includes bibliographical references and index.
 ISBN-13: 978-0-8018-9493-0 (hardcover : alk. paper)
 ISBN-10: 0-8018-9493-X (hardcover : alk. paper)
 1. Congregate housing—United States—Employees. I. Ball,
Mary M.
 [DNLM: 1. Assisted Living Facilities—manpower—United
States. 2. Homes for the Aged—manpower—United States.
3. Caregivers—United States. 4. Personnel Management—
United States. WT 27 AA1 F935 2010]
 HV1454.2.U6F76 2010
 331.7'6136261—dc22   2009038862

A catalog record for this book is available from the
British Library.

*Special discounts are available for bulk purchases of this book. For
more information, please contact Special Sales at 410-516-6936 or
specialsales@press.jhu.edu.*

To the direct care workers who helped us understand their essential role in the lives of assisted living residents. They represent frontline workers everywhere.

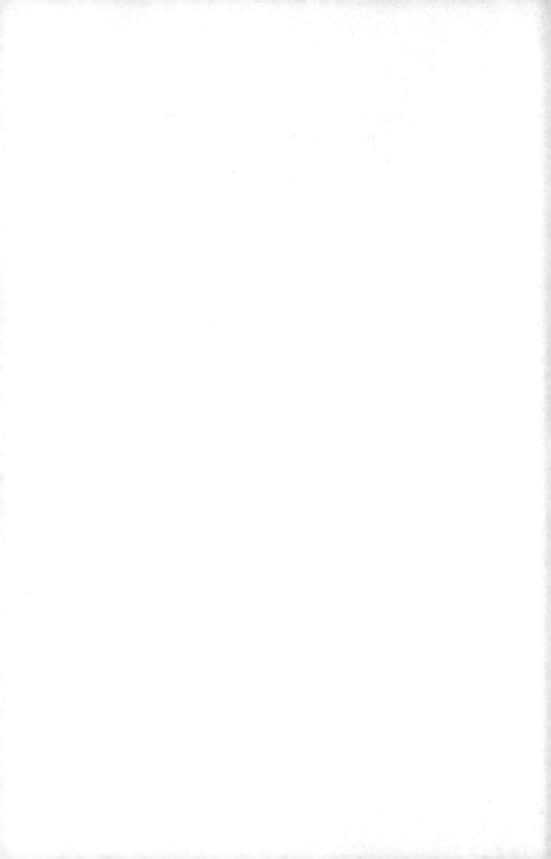

CONTENTS

CONTRIBUTORS

Robert M. Adelman, Ph.D., Assistant Professor, Department of Sociology, University of Buffalo, Buffalo, New York

Jim Baird, Ph.D., Instructor, Department of Sociology, Georgia State University, Atlanta, Georgia

Mary M. Ball, Ph.D., Associate Research Professor, Gerontology Institute, Georgia State University, Atlanta, Georgia

Carolyn Furlow, Ph.D., Statistician, SAIC, Office on Smoking and Health, Centers for Disease Control and Prevention, Atlanta, Georgia

Carole Hollingsworth, M.A., Research Coordinator, Gerontology Institute, Georgia State University, Atlanta, Georgia

Candace L. Kemp, Ph.D., Assistant Professor, Gerontology Institute, Georgia State University, Atlanta, Georgia

Michael J. Lepore, Ph.D., Postdoctoral Fellow, Center for Gerontology and Health Care Research, Brown University, Providence, Rhode Island

Guangya Liu, M.A., doctoral student, Department of Sociology and Anthropology, North Carolina State University, Raleigh, North Carolina

Molly M. Perkins, Ph.D., Senior Research Fellow and Adjunct Assistant Professor, Gerontology Institute, Georgia State University, Atlanta, Georgia

Larry Polivka, Ph.D., Scholar in Residence, The Claude Pepper Foundation, Inc., Tallahassee, Florida

Robyn I. Stone, Dr.P.H., Executive Director, Institute for the Future of Aging Services; Senior Vice President of Research, American Association of Homes and Services for the Aging, Washington, DC

W. Mark Sweatman, M.B.A., doctoral student, Department of Sociology, Georgia State University, Atlanta, Georgia

PREFACE

This book is about frontline workers in assisted living facilities (ALFs). They, like their counterparts in other long-term care settings, are the ones who provide the lion's share of care to residents. Most direct care workers (DCWs) are women and minorities, and they represent an especially vulnerable group of the working poor. This book puts a face on these DCWs and tells how and why they made their decisions to enter the field of caregiving. It explores their diverse work worlds and day-to-day jobs and considers how the relationships they have with other care staff, facility administrators, and residents affect their job experiences and attitudes. It examines predictors of job satisfaction and retention and reveals the strategies administrators use to hire, train, and reward their workers. Finally, this book offers recommendations for how ALFs and other long-term care facilities can improve the satisfaction and retention of DCWs.

The book derives from a study of 400 DCWs working in 45 ALFs in the state of Georgia carried out between the fall of 2005 and the summer of 2007. It employs both qualitative and quantitative methods, which allows for an understanding of *how* and *why* various factors influence job satisfaction and retention, as well as of the strength of relationships, and makes possible predictions to larger populations of ALFs. Assisted living (AL) in Georgia represents the broad spectrum of care settings included under this rubric in the United States. The goal of the study was to learn how to maximize the satisfaction and retention of DCWs in AL. The study was supported by the National Institute on Aging (Grant # 5R01AG21183).

The Plan for the Book

This book has 11 chapters divided into three parts. Part I, "Frontline Workers: The Long-Term Care Context," serves as the backdrop for the remainder of the book. In Chapter 1, Robyn Stone provides an overview of long-term care (LTC) workforce issues, identifies the most pressing problems, examines factors that contribute to these problems, and discusses existing LTC policy. Stone also describes the characteristics of DCWs in the United States, examines the forces that are driving the increasing diversity of workers, and discusses the implications of these changes for future workers, residents who depend on their care, and the LTC industry. Stone makes clear the quality, economic, and moral imperatives for improvement of the direct care workforce.

Chapter 2 narrows the LTC focus to AL. In this chapter, Larry Polivka provides a selective review of the research literature on AL and discusses the implication of research findings for key AL regulatory and affordability issues. A theme throughout his chapter is how best to ensure an adequate quality of care and quality of life for residents in AL. Polivka discusses implications of AL regulation and the various manifestations of the AL care environment for the direct care workforce and concludes with a suggested AL research agenda.

Part II, "Assisted Living Work and Workers," presents the major findings from the statewide study conducted in Georgia. In Chapter 3, Mary Ball and Molly Perkins describe the qualitative and quantitative methods used to collect and analyze data. They also present the characteristics of the participants and their work settings and place both within the national AL context.

In Chapter 4, Michael Lepore, Mary Ball, Molly Perkins, and Candace Kemp consider the personal characteristics, experiences, and values of DCWs that, together with external influences, lead them to choose caregiving, in the context of AL, as a career. They discuss the implication of workers' moral, material, and professional motives for the ability of the AL industry to attract and retain workers.

In Chapter 5, Mary Ball, Carole Hollingsworth, and Michael Lepore explore the universal nature of AL work and examine how DCWs' work experiences vary across facilities and workers. They discuss the multiple factors that influence the job design, including task configuration and workload, and consider how workers' job expectations compare with their job reality and how their experiences influence their attitudes toward their jobs.

In Chapter 6, Molly Perkins, Mark Sweatman, and Carole Hollingsworth use qualitative methods to examine co-worker relationships and the influence that these relationships have on satisfaction and retention of DCWs. They focus on staff-staff relationships as well as the relationships that DCWs have with their direct supervisors and facility administrators. Their findings show

how a myriad of factors influence these relationships and how these relationships influence workers' satisfaction, as well as their ability to find and maintain what they perceive to be a "good" job.

In Chapter 7, Candace Kemp, Mary Ball, Carole Hollingsworth, and Michael Lepore explore the quality and meaning of the relationships workers have with residents and the multilevel factors that affect relationship development, maintenance, and meaning. More than half of workers are black women caring for white residents, and the authors of this chapter pay special attention to the influence of race and culture on the quality of relationships and, ultimately, on worker satisfaction.

Chapter 8 addresses individual-level predictors of job satisfaction. Jim Baird, Robert Adelman, Mark Sweatman, Molly Perkins, Mary Ball, and Guangya Liu develop four empirical models analyzing the effects of sociodemographic, human capital, job content, and workplace experiences on workers' overall job satisfaction. In addition to other important findings, this analysis provides important new insights regarding the influence of race and racism on DCWs' overall job satisfaction.

Chapter 9 examines predictors of direct care staff turnover. Building on a conceptual model proposed by Kiyak and colleagues (1997) for nursing home staff and on other recent research, Molly Perkins, Robert Adelman, Carolyn Furlow, Mark Sweatman, and Jim Baird use hierarchical linear modeling (HLM) and structural equation modeling (SEM) techniques to explore the effects of individual, facility, and community characteristics on employee turnover. This is the first study in AL to use this analytic approach to simultaneously examine both macro- and micro-level influences on employee turnover.

Part III, "Lessons Learned," is devoted to informing LTC policy and practice. In Chapter 10, Mary Ball, Carole Hollingsworth, and Michael Lepore provide information about the hiring practices of this diverse group of homes and discuss the qualities that administrators most value in prospective DCWs. They then examine facility strategies for training workers and the attitudes of workers toward the training they receive. Finally, they discuss the adequacy and appropriateness of training in relation to hiring practices and discuss the implications of both for staff satisfaction and retention.

In Chapter 11, Mary Ball, Carole Hollingsworth, and Candace Kemp describe facilities' reward systems, including salaries, benefits, and other incentives. They examine DCWs' attitudes toward reward systems and the multilevel factors that influence their development and maintenance and discuss how these systems influence staff satisfaction and retention.

In the Conclusion, Mary Ball, Molly Perkins, Carole Hollingsworth, and Candace Kemp summarize the major findings of the study and confront their often contradictory implications for workers and facilities. They conclude with a set of specific recommendations for policy and practice based on the findings.

ACKNOWLEDGMENTS

The material presented in this book derives from the project "Job Satisfaction and Retention of Direct Care Staff in Assisted Living," which was funded by the National Institutes on Aging (1R01 AG021183). We are grateful for their support.

First we would like to thank the study participants—the facility owners and administrators and the direct care workers. Owners and administrators provided access to their homes and workers and information about facility operation and facilitated our data collection. DCWs shared information about themselves and their job experiences and attitudes. Without these two groups of key players our study and this book would not have been possible.

We also want to thank the following graduate students for their significant role in data collection and analysis: Davette Taylor Harris, Neela Lakatoo, Huali Qin, Zhiqui Li, Ramani Sambhara, April Ross, Staci Bolton, Karen Armstrong, Shanzhen Luo, Allie Glover, and Karuna Sharma. Mark Sweatman, Michael Lepore, and Guangya Liu, contributors to these chapters, also participated in data collection and analysis.

We acknowledge the support and advice of our research advisory committee, which helped guide our research objective and design. Members include representatives of the Georgia Long-Term Care Ombudsman Program, the Assisted Living Association of Georgia, the Georgia Chapter of the Assisted Living Federation of America, the Georgia Office of Regulatory Services, the Georgia Department of Labor, and administrators of local assisted living facilities.

Finally, we are indebted to Dr. Frank J. Whittington, former director of the Gerontology Institute, for his support and guidance throughout the conceptual development and conduct of the research on which this book is based.

FRONTLINE WORKERS IN ASSISTED LIVING

The Foundation for the Book

Mary M. Ball, Ph.D.
Molly M. Perkins, Ph.D.
Carole Hollingsworth, M.A.
Candace L. Kemp, Ph.D.

The Genesis of the Book

This book derives from a history of collaborative research on long-term care (LTC) by its coeditors. Our initial study (1996–1997), which focused on the experiences of elders living in assisted living (AL) communities, identified 11 components of quality of life as defined by the residents. This study highlighted the importance of holding on to independence and autonomy even in AL (Ball et al., 2000, 2004) and led to two in-depth qualitative investigations designed to learn how to maximize resident independence and autonomy in the AL environment. These latter studies further demonstrated the importance of achieving *goodness of fit* between the resident and the facility's social and physical environment in increasing residents' quality of life and ability to age in place in AL (Ball et al., 2004, 2005; Perkins, Ball, Whittington, & Combs, 2004).

Over the course of our resident-focused work, we became keenly aware of the key role that direct care workers (DCWs) play in the lives of residents in the AL setting. This knowledge, together with the fact that almost no research had addressed this topic in AL, led our research team to shift its focus to an exploration of how to improve the quality of the work experiences of the DCWs. We began with an in-depth study in two assisted living facilities (ALFs) with the goal of understanding how workplace relationships influence job satisfaction and retention (Ball et al., 2009). This initial study led to the larger, statewide study—titled "Job Satisfaction and Retention of Direct Care Staff in Assisted Living"—that forms the basis of this book.

Background for the Study

Evidence is convincing that a critical shortage of DCWs exists in nursing homes and residential care settings, and dramatic increases in numbers of older persons over the coming decades will compound these shortages. Low staff retention and high turnover rates produce staff shortages, and together these factors negatively impact the quality of residents' care, as well as their overall quality of life. High turnover also increases provider costs related to recruitment and training of new staff, overtime, and use of temporary staff (U.S. General Accounting Office [GAO], 2001). Turnover for DCWs is much higher than for the labor force in general (GAO, 2001), with annual turnover rates reported to range from 40 percent to more than 100 percent.

Over the past several decades, numerous studies have focused on variables that influence satisfaction and retention of DCWs in LTC settings. A review of literature on nurse aide turnover (Salmon et al., 1999) found that turnover may be attributed to three types of structural factors: (1) opportunity structure (unemployment rates and job opportunity); (2) organizational structure of the facility (ownership and size); and (3) control factors (a combination of extrinsic and intrinsic motivators). The literature shows that key extrinsic motivators are pay and benefits, whereas job satisfaction and job commitment are identified as primary intrinsic motivators. Findings show that turnover decisions are based on both wanting to leave (dissatisfaction) and having the opportunity to do so.

A study by Banaszak-Holl and Hines (1996) found that DCW turnover in nursing homes is significantly higher in counties with more beds and lower in counties with higher unemployment rates and higher per capita incomes, suggesting that turnover rates are higher in areas where aides have more employment opportunities. Recent research also shows that facility size is related to DCW turnover, indicating that smaller facilities tend to have lower rates of turnover, possibly reflecting the greater autonomy and more frequent rewards that are believed to exist among DCWs in smaller homes, compared with larger facilities (Castle & Engberg, 2006). Some studies have shown a relationship between ownership and turnover. For example, higher turnover rates have been found in proprietary nursing homes, probably due to lower salaries (Broughton & Golden, 1995; Castle & Engberg, 2006).

Numerous studies conducted in nursing homes have cited low wages and few benefits as factors contributing to DCW turnover (Close, Estes, Linkins, & Binney, 1994; Foner, 1994). The physical demands of the work, heavy workloads, staffing levels, and other aspects of the workplace environment also have been named as factors leading to turnover (GAO, 2001). Aides who developed strategies to organize their work to accomplish required tasks have been found to have lower turnover (Bowers & Becker, 1992).

Intrinsic motivators, primarily job satisfaction but also organizational commitment, also play a key role and operate along with extrinsic factors—but on different planes—to help explain DCWs' decisions to stay or leave (Salmon et al., 1999). Job satisfaction in turn is influenced by a variety of factors related to the environment, job design, and the employee's personality and other personal traits. According to Stamps (1997), like turnover, conceptualization and measurement of job satisfaction varies in the literature. Commonly it is used as both an independent variable (e.g., high levels of satisfaction are likely to result in high levels of performance or low levels of turnover) and a dependent variable.

A study of 283 DCWs in midwestern nursing homes found that the most important job satisfaction factors are personal growth and development, job security, and job challenge (Atchison, 1998). Atchison concluded that more job, social, and advancement opportunities at work are important incentives. Studies also have shown that job security is related to DCW turnover in nursing homes (Gaddy, 1995). Ramirez, Teresi, Holmes, and Fairchild (1998) examined multivariate relationships between job assignment and job satisfaction, burnout, and demoralization among nurse aides. They found that a heavier workload is significantly related to dissatisfaction. Their findings also showed that stress resulting from racial discrimination is significantly related to burnout and demoralization, often leading to turnover. Other studies have shown that heavy care responsibilities contribute to burnout and turnover (Smyer, Brannon, & Cohn, 1992). Consistently, previous studies have shown that job satisfaction, burnout, and stress are related, which in turn influence quality of care and absenteeism (Cohen-Mansfield & Noelker, 2000).

Studies in nursing homes have found that satisfied DCWs are those who are involved in decision making (e.g., care planning) (Caudill & Patrick, 1991;

Kruzich, 1995). Involvement in decision making also is related to turnover. In a study in 250 nursing homes, Banaszak-Holl and Hines (1996) found a significant reduction in turnover when aides were involved in care planning.

Research findings are mixed regarding the effect of training on job satisfaction. Findings from one study indicate that training must be linked to changes in job structure, increased work autonomy, and chance for advancement in order to increase satisfaction (Banaszak-Holl & Hines, 1996). Although Ramirez and colleagues (1998) found a negative relationship between hours of training and satisfaction, other research has shown that increased training in care of cognitively impaired residents reduces burnout and stress, both associated with satisfaction (Chappell & Novak, 1992; Ejaz, Noelker, Menne, & Bagaka, 2008).

Some evidence exists that social support affects satisfaction and turnover. Aides are most satisfied with aspects of their jobs that involve socializing with residents and are less likely to describe their job as stressful if they have personal relationships with care recipients (Ball et al., 2009; Cantor, 1988; Grieshaber, Parker, & Deering, 1995). Research has also shown that staff who are friendly with co-workers stay longer (Caudill & Patrick, 1989), that social support from residents' family and friends reduces burnout and stress (Chappell & Novak, 1992; Kemp, Ball, Hollingsworth, Perkins, & Lepore, 2009), and that supervisor supportiveness is extremely important for satisfaction and quality of life of staff (Feldman, Sapienza & Kane, 1990). Support groups for aides also improve retention and satisfaction and reduce burnout (Sherman, 1991; Widmer & Kuipers, 1991; Wilner, 1994).

Management style of supervisors, including how policies are put into effect, how employees are handled, and the amount of praise and respect given, has been shown to be associated with satisfaction and turnover (GAO, 2001; Salmon et al., 1999). Positive communication between aides and supervisors, including informal interactions, has also been found to be important to satisfaction (Acampora, 1993; LeSar, 1987). Waxman, Carner, and Berkenstock (1984) found that in facilities where certified nursing assistants (CNAs) perceive the environment as highly structured turnover is especially high. In facilities with low turnover, the facility is administratively decentralized and less rigidly controlled, indicating that turnover is influenced more by management style practiced by supervisors than by wages and benefits. Gaddy's (1995) findings are similar, showing that financial concerns are not as important in predicting turnover as personal/staff conflicts and personal satisfaction with resident care. Recent findings from a national study of DCWs employed in nursing homes, ALFs, and home care agencies show that staff relationships with supervisors are at least as important as pay (Kemper et al., 2008).

Some evidence exists for relationships between job satisfaction and DCWs' personal attributes. Kiyak, Namazi, and Kahana's (1997) study of job commitment and turnover among women working in nursing homes and community settings found that personal characteristics, such as age, length of employment, and type of agency, influence job satisfaction. These findings show that satisfaction is greater among DCWs who are older, married, have been at the job longer, and have a professional position. Feldman and colleagues (1990) found that black workers are more likely to perceive their jobs as monotonous, to be less closely bonded to clients, to perceive pay inequities, and to be less satisfied with their work than white workers. Others (Ramirez et al., 1998) also found that race is significantly related to job satisfaction, burnout, and demoralization, but in different directions for different racial groups. These findings show that Jamaican and African Caribbean aides are more likely to be dissatisfied, whereas being African American is not a predictor of job satisfaction.

Although findings are mixed on the relationship between income and job satisfaction, most studies show a positive relationship (Salmon et al., 1999). For many nurse aides, low pay is rated as the least satisfying part of the job (Grieshaber et al., 1995; Helmer, Olson, & Heim, 1993). In Hawes, Phillips, and Rose's (2000) study of AL, 55 percent of staff agree or strongly agree that their wages are inadequate.

The literature shows a number of factors that influence both turnover and job satisfaction, and considerable research has examined the link between satisfaction and turnover. Consistently, research has shown that high rates of turnover are related to high levels of *dissatisfaction* (Stamps, 1997). Kiyak and colleagues' (1997) nursing home study shows that the best predictor of turnover is intent to leave, which in turn is best predicted by job dissatisfaction. These findings show that younger dissatisfied employees are more likely to indicate intent to leave, especially paraprofessionals (not administrative staff). In this study, job satisfaction was less important in predicting actual turnover than was intent to leave. More recent research (Castle, Engberg, Anderson, & Men, 2007; Parsons, Simmons, Penn, & Furlough, 2003) has shown a direct relationship between job satisfaction and intent to leave, as well as turnover.

Other studies have shown no, or unexpected, relationships between DCW job satisfaction and turnover. Helmer and colleagues (1993) found that DCWs in nursing homes are particularly dissatisfied with their pay but that dissatisfaction with pay is not related to turnover. Grau, Chandler, Burton, and Kolditz's (1991) study found that none of the six dimensions of satisfaction they investigated were linked with turnover. Waxman and colleagues (1984) found that nursing homes with the highest turnover have staff with the highest level of job satisfaction. Results also have shown that higher-quality homes also have higher turnover. These researchers linked their paradoxical findings to union status (i.e., three facilities with lowest turnover included unionized staff, whereas four with highest turnover had nonunionized staff).

Comparatively little research exists that addresses the development and maintenance of a qualified paraprofessional workforce. Particularly lacking are studies of job satisfaction of DCWs in residential settings such as AL (Hawes, Phillips, & Rose, 2000). Further, little conclusive evidence exists that directly links job satisfaction and retention, especially in studies that simultaneously control for factors at multiple hierarchical levels (i.e., individual, facility, and community) that may influence these relationships.

The current study, which uses both qualitative methods and multilevel statistical modeling techniques, provides important new information regarding the interrelationships between multiple hierarchical factors that influence DCW satisfaction and turnover in AL, thus addressing some of the questions raised by previous research. This book, which provides the first comprehensive, in-depth information about the viewpoints and experiences of DCWs in AL, brings to life these workers and their work worlds. It offers valuable insights to LTC researchers, policy makers, and service providers by identifying factors that influence their job satisfaction and retention and provides important information about the characteristics and training of these workers. It also illuminates how workers' perspectives vary across racial and ethnic groups and AL settings.

Conceptual Framework

The current study builds on previous models of turnover proposed in the literature. Specifically, we build on a model first proposed by Price and Mueller (1981) and later adapted by Kiyak and colleagues (1997), as well as more recent research (see, for example, Castle & Engberg, 2006; Castle et al., 2007). In recognizing the complexity of disentangling the multilevel factors that influence staff satisfaction and retention in AL, we use a variety of methods to provide more comprehensive and representative findings than those shown in previous research.

This research also is informed by theory from our own previous research (Ball et al., 2004, 2005, 2009; Kemp et al., 2009; Perkins et al., 2004), as well as feminist theories on caregiving and women's work relationships (Benson, 1986; Foner, 1994; Kanter & Stein, 1979; Lamphere, 1985) and sociological theories on work, group culture, and labor force race relations (Braverman, 1974; Feagin, 1991; Hodson et al., 1993; Tuch & Martin, 1991). In addition to making an important contribution to existing literature on satisfaction and turnover in LTC, this study fills an important void in the growing literature on low-wage workers (Munger, 2002; Newman, 1999; Shipler, 2005; Shulman, 2005), most of which focuses on workers in urban settings and includes little information regarding the experiences of care workers.

The overall goal of this study is to learn how ALFs can create an environment that maximizes job satisfaction and retention of DCWs. The specific research aims are

1. to understand the meaning of job satisfaction for DCWs in ALFs;
2. to understand how individual, sociocultural, and environmental factors influence job satisfaction and retention of DCWs in ALFs and the relationship between these variables; and
3. to identify successful strategies of direct care, managerial, and administrative staff that support job satisfaction and retention of DCWs in ALFs.

REFERENCES

Acampora, A. 1993. Satisfaction on the job: The "value" factor. *Journal of Long Term Care Administration* 21, 17.

Atchison, J. 1998. Perceived job satisfaction factors of nursing assistants employed in Midwest nursing homes. *Geriatric Nursing* 19, 135–38.

Ball, M. M., Lepore, M. L., Perkins, M. M., Hollingsworth, C., & Sweatman, M. 2009. "They are the reason I come to work": The meaning of resident-staff relationships in assisted living. *Journal of Aging Studies* 23, 37–47.

Ball, M. M., Perkins, M. M., Whittington, F. J., Connell, B. R., Hollingsworth, C., & King, S. V. 2004. Managing decline in AL: The key to aging in place. *Journals of Gerontology: Social Sciences* 4, S202–12.

Ball, M. M., Perkins, M. M., Whittington, F. J., Hollingsworth, C., King, S. V., & Combs, B. L. 2005. *Communities of care: Assisted living for African American elders*. Baltimore: Johns Hopkins University Press.

Ball, M. M., Whittington, F. J., Perkins, M. M., Patterson, V., Hollingsworth, C., King, S. V., et al. 2000. Quality of life in assisted living facilities: Viewpoints of residents. *Journal of Applied Gerontology* 19, 304–25.

Banaszak-Holl, J., & Hines, M. 1996. Factors associated with nursing home turnover. *The Gerontologist* 36, 512–17.

Benson, S. P. 1986. *Counter culture: Saleswomen, managers, and customers in American department stores, 1890–1940.* Urbana: University of Illinois Press.

Bowers, B., & Becker, M. 1992. Nurse's aides in nursing homes: The relationship between organization and quality. *The Gerontologist* 32, 360–66.

Braverman, H. 1974. *Labor and monopoly capital: The degradation of work in the twentieth century.* New York: Monthly Review Press.

Broughton, W., & Golden, M. 1995. Profile of Pennsylvania nurse's aides. *Geriatric Nursing* 16, 117–20.

Cantor, M. 1988. *Factors related to strain among home care workers: A comparison of formal and informal caregivers.* Paper presented at the 41st Annual Scientific Meeting of the Gerontological Society of America, San Francisco, CA.

Castle, N. G., & Engberg, J. 2006. Organizational characteristics associated with staff turnover in nursing homes. *The Gerontologist* 46, 62–73.

Castle, N. G., Engberg, J., Anderson, R., & Men, A. 2007. Job satisfaction of nurse aides in nursing homes: Intent to leave and turnover. *The Gerontologist* 47, 192–204.

Caudill, M., & Patrick, M. 1989. Nursing assistant turnover in nursing homes and need satisfaction. *Journal of Gerontological Nursing* 15 (6), 24–30.

———. 1991. Turnover among nursing assistants: Why they leave and why they stay. *Journal of Long Term Care Administration* 19, 29–32.

Chappell, N., & Novak, M. 1992. The role of support in alleviating stress among nursing assistants. *The Gerontologist* 32, 351–59.

Close, L., Estes, C. L., Linkins, K. W., & Binney, E. A. 1994. Political economy perspective on frontline workers in long-term care. *Generations* 18 (3), 23–28.

Cohen-Mansfield, J., & Noelker, L. 2000. Nursing staff satisfaction in long-term care: An overview. In J. Cohen-Mansfield, F. K. Ejaz, & P. Werner (Eds.), *Satisfaction surveys in long-term care* (pp. 52–75). New York: Springer.

Ejaz, F. K., Noelker, L. S., Menne, H. L., & Bagaka, J. G. 2008. The impact of stress and support on direct care workers' job satisfaction. *The Gerontologist* 48, 60–70.

Feagin, J. 1991. The continuing significance of race: Antiblack discrimination in public places. *American Sociological Review* 56, 101–16.

Feldman, P., Sapienza, A., & Kane, N. 1990. *Who cares for them? Workers in the home care industry.* New York: Greenwood Press.

Foner, N. 1994. *The caregiving dilemma.* Berkeley: University of California Press.

Gaddy, T. 1995. Nonlicensed employee turnover in a long-term care facility. *Health Care Supervisor* 13 (4), 54–60.

Grau, L., Chandler, B., Burton, B., & Kolditz, D. 1991. Institutional loyalty and job satisfaction among nurse aides in nursing homes. *Journal of Aging and Health* 3, 47–65.

Grieshaber, L., Parker, P., & Deering, J. 1995. Job satisfaction of nursing assistants in long-term care. *Health Care Supervisor* 13 (4), 18–28.

Hawes, C., Phillips, C. D., & Rose, M. 2000. *High service or high privacy assisted living facilities, their residents and staff: Results from a national survey.* Washington, DC: U.S. Department of Health and Human Services.

Helmer, F., Olson, S., & Heim, R. 1993. Strategies for nurse aide job satisfaction. *Journal of Long Term Care Administration* 21, 10–14.

Hodson, R., Welsh, S., Rieble, S., Jamison, C. S., & Creighton, S. 1993. Is worker solidarity undermined by autonomy and participation? Patterns from the ethnography literature. *American Sociological Review* 58, 398–416.

Kanter, R. M., & Stein, B. (Eds.). 1979. *Life in organizations.* New York: Basic Books.

Kemp, C. L., Ball, M. M., Perkins, M. M., Hollingsworth, C., & Lepore, M. L. 2009. "I get along with most of them": Direct care workers' relationships with residents' families in assisted living. *The Gerontologist* 49, 224–35.

Kemper, P., Heier, B., Barry, T., Brannon, D., Angelelli, J., Vasey, J., et al. 2008. What do direct care workers say would improve their jobs? Differences across settings. *The Gerontologist* 48 (Special Issue 1), 17–25.

Kiyak, H., Namazi, K. H., & Kahana, E. F. 1997. Job commitment and turnover among women working in facilities serving older persons. *Research on Aging* 19, 223–46.

Kruzich, J. 1995. Empowering organizational contexts: Patterns and predictors of perceived decision-making influence among staff in nursing homes. *The Gerontologist* 35, 207–16.

Lamphere, L. 1985. Bringing the family to work: Culture on the shop floor. *Feminist Studies* 11, 519–40.

LeSar, K. 1987. Who provides for the nursing assistant? *Provider* 13 (4), 20–22.

Munger, F. (Ed.). 2002. *Laboring below the line: The new ethnography of poverty, low-wage work, and survival in a global economy.* New York: Russell Sage Foundation.

Newman, K. S. 1999. *No shame in my game.* New York: Random House.

Parsons, S. K., Simmons, W. P., Penn, K., & Furlough, M. 2003. Determinants of satisfaction and turnover among nursing assistants. *Journal of Gerontological Nursing* 3, 51–58.

Perkins, M. M., Ball, M. M., Whittington, F. J., & Combs, B. L. 2004. Managing the needs of low-income board and care residents: A process of negotiating risks. *Qualitative Health Research* 14, 478–95.

Price, J. I., & Mueller, C. W. 1981. A causal model of turnover for nurses. *Academy of Management Journal* 24, 543–65.

Ramirez, M., Teresi, J., Holmes, D., & Fairchild, S. 1998. Ethnic and racial conflict in relation to staff burnout, demoralization, and job satisfaction in SCUs and non-SCUs. *Journal of Mental Health and Aging* 4, 459–79.

Salmon, J., Crews, C., Reynolds-Scanlon, S., Jang, Y., Wever, S., & Oakley, M. 1999. *Nurse aide turnover: Literature review of research, policy and practice.* Florida Policy Exchange Center on Aging. University of South Florida, Tampa.

Sherman, E. 1991. Catastrophic shortage of caregivers. *Perspectives on Aging* 20, 39–41.

Shipler, D. K. 2005. *The working poor: Invisible in America.* New York: Vintage Books.

Shulman, B. 2005. *The betrayal of work: How low-wage jobs fail 30 million Americans.* New York: New Press.

Smyer, M., Brannon, D., & Cohn, M. 1992. Improving nursing home care through training and job redesign. *The Gerontologist* 32, 327–33.

Stamps, P. 1997. *Nurses and work satisfaction: An index for measurement.* Chicago: Health Administration Press.

Tuch, S., & Martin, J. 1991. Race in the workplace: Black/white differences in the sources of job satisfaction. *Sociological Quarterly* 32, 103–16.

U.S. General Accounting Office. 2001. Nursing Workforce: Recruitment and Retention of nurses and nurse aides is a growing concern. Testimony statement of William J. Scanlon, Director Health Care Issues.

Waxman, H., Carner, E., & Berkenstock, G. 1984. Job turnover and job satisfaction among nursing home aides. *The Gerontologist* 24, 503–9.

Widmer, L., & Kuipers, J. 1991. Tackling turnover: Support groups for nursing assistants. *Geriatric Nursing* 12, 252.

Wilner, M. A. 1994. Working it out: Support groups for nursing assistants. *Generations* 18 (3), 39–40.

Part I / Frontline Workers

The Long-Term Care Context

CHAPTER ONE

Direct Care Workers in Long-Term Care and Implications for Assisted Living

Robyn I. Stone, Dr.P.H.

Direct care workers (DCWs)—nursing assistants, home health and home care aides, personal care workers, and personal service attendants—form the center-piece of the formal long-term care (LTC) system (Institute of Medicine [IOM], 2008; Stone & Dawson, 2008). These so-called frontline caregivers provide hands-on care to millions of elderly and younger people with disabilities, in settings ranging from the nursing home, to assisted living and other residen-tial care options, to private homes. Eight out of every 10 hours of paid care received by a LTC consumer are provided by DCWs, who are often referred to as the "eyes and the ears" of the care system (Paraprofessional Healthcare Institute [PHI], 2009). In addition to helping with activities of daily living, such as bathing, dressing, using the toilet, and eating, these workers provide the "high touch" that is essential to quality of life, as well as quality of care, for elders and chronically disabled individuals.

This chapter provides an overview of the direct care workforce in LTC with a special emphasis on frontline caregivers employed in assisted living facili-ties (ALFs). Unfortunately, there are no national estimates of the size of this subpopulation of caregivers and little research on the characteristics of and workforce issues germane to the assisted living (AL) workforce. Most of the literature and policy and practice attention has been focused on the DCWs in nursing homes and, to a lesser extent, in home care. Much of the information presented in this chapter, therefore, is derived from analyses that have been conducted in these settings. To the extent that research has been conducted on workers in AL, this chapter has attempted to document the findings.

Who Are the Direct Care Workers?

In 2006, there were an estimated 1.4 million nursing aides employed in nursing home and residential care settings. Another 587,000 DCWs were home health aides, and 767,000 personal care/home care aides were employed in home- and community-based settings (PHI, 2009). As noted above, there are no national estimates of the number of direct care workers—nursing assistants, personal care workers, and other frontline caregivers—who are working specifically in ALFs.

A study of the demographic characteristics of DCWs using data from the 2000 census indicates that the median age of nursing home aides is 36 years. Home care aides are somewhat older, with a median age of 46 years (Montgomery, Holly, Deichert, & Kosloski, 2006). The vast majority of DCWs are female—91.3 percent of nursing home aides and 91.8 percent of home care aides. Three out of five nursing home aides and two-thirds of home care aides are not married. A little over one-quarter of those employed in nursing homes and one-third of those working in home care have not completed high school. Many of the female DCWs are likely to be single mothers who are supporting their families with one relatively low income while balancing their job (and sometimes more than one job) with child care and other family responsibilities. These conflicting pressures may contribute to absenteeism and affect the quality of the worker's job performance and commitment to the work.

There is much ethnic and racial diversity among DCWs. Although a little over half of nursing home and home care aides are white, 31 percent of those employed in nursing homes and 26 percent of those employed in home care settings are African American. Almost 8 percent of nursing home aides and 16 percent of home care aides are Hispanic. Fourteen percent of the nursing home aides and almost one out of four home care aides are foreign-born. The wide variation in ethnicity and cultures represented among staff in LTC settings has heightened the potential for tension, miscommunication, and conflict between caregivers and care recipients, between peers, and between supervisors and direct care workers (McDonald, 2007; Parker & Geron, 2007). This increased diversity underscores the need for improving the English language skills of many workers and building cultural competence knowledge and skills into formal and on-the-job training programs for direct care workers and managers.

The Emerging Interest in Direct Care Workers

Historically, concerns about DCWs in LTC have ebbed and flowed, with the issue gaining greater attention during relatively prosperous economic times, when employers compete for workers and thus staff—who might otherwise be employed by the LTC industry—find other, more attractive job options. During the late 1990s, such a period of low unemployment left many LTC employers of DCWs not only with high rates of turnover (which is typical in the industry) but also with high vacancy rates. The latter in particular caused both providers and policy makers to pay increased attention to how direct care jobs were failing to compete within a suddenly competitive job market— admittedly more out of concern for how these vacancies were impacting consumers and the providers themselves, but nonetheless resulting in a renewed interest in how to find and keep direct care workers.

A growing number of policy makers, practitioners, worker associations, and researchers have highlighted the need for a more systemic approach to developing and sustaining DCWs. The argument for this attention is based on the premise that, while the last spike in vacancy rates was indeed exacerbated by the full-employment economy, the underlying U.S. demographics of both LTC consumers (demand for services) and the health care workers (supply of labor) will combine in the future to make the resulting "care gap" not simply an episodic by-product of occasional strong economies but a permanent crisis for the future of caregiving (see, for example, the discussion in the U.S. Department of Health and Human Services [USDHHS] report to Congress [USDHHS, 2003]). Several key issues underlie this increased focus on a more long-term, systemic approach to developing and sustaining a qualified, committed direct care workforce.

Workforce Improvement as a Quality Issue in Long-Term Care

Over the past 20 years, there has been increasing interest in and concern about the quality of care being provided in nursing homes and other LTC settings (Noelker & Harel, 2001; Wunderlich & Kohler, 2001). However, before 2000, much of the policy, practice, and research activity focused on how to improve quality outcomes for residents and home care clients through a range of regulatory and, more recently, quality improvement activities. With the exception of entry-level certification requirements for nursing home and home health aides, the performance of the DCW usually had been an afterthought in those discussions of LTC quality (Stone & Dawson, 2008).

The 2001 IOM report identified workforce development as one of its nine guiding principles and acknowledged that quality of care depends largely on the performance of the caregiving workforce (Wunderlich & Kohler, 2001). Until recently, most of the discussion of workforce issues has focused on achieving minimum staffing levels for nurses and DCWs. A major nursing home staffing study indicated that, to maximize quality of care, a nursing home would need to provide 2.78 hours of nurse aide care per resident day, substantially more than the current average of 2.02 aide hours per day (Abt Associates, 2003). Unlike nursing home and home health care, there are no minimum staffing requirements in AL, and with the exception of several states (e.g., Connecticut, Kansas, New Jersey, Washington), there are few training or competency requirements either before the initial hire or on an ongoing basis (Carlson, 2005).

The 2001 IOM report also emphasized that an adequate staffing level is a necessary, but not sufficient, condition for positively affecting the quality of life and quality of care of consumers. A more recent IOM study (2008), focused specifically on creating a geriatric workforce for an aging America, emphasized that organizations must not only have adequate numbers of staff but must also create work environments that help retain all LTC professionals and DCWs. The study highlighted the importance of both orientation programs for newly hired staff and continuing education for existing staff. It is important to note that only 19 states require a certain minimum of training hours for DCWs in AL. Only 10 require 25 or more hours, significantly less than the number of training hours required for workers in nursing homes and home health care (PHI, 2006). This difference is particularly striking given the fact that a DCW in AL is much less likely than his or her peers in the nursing home or home care setting to have any consistent nurse oversight and often has a much more complex array of responsibilities that include doing the laundry and housekeeping as well as personal care and the monitoring of a resident's functional status (Sievers, 2006).

Across the country, LTC providers report significant DCW vacancies and high turnover rates. Nursing homes, AL and other residential care providers, home health agencies, community-based home care and adult day programs, and individuals and their families all indicate that they experience difficulties in recruiting and, more important, retaining frontline caregivers (PHI, 2009; Stone & Dawson, 2008). Nationally, data on turnover rates show wide variation, ranging from 40 to 100 percent annually (Decker et al., 2003; PHI, 2006). Staff turnover in AL settings ranges from 21 to 135 percent, with an average of 42 percent (Maas & Buckwalter, 2006).

High staff turnover and vacancies have negative effects on the major stakeholders within the LTC system—workers, consumers (including their families), LTC providers, and third-party payers, primarily the Medicaid and Medicare programs (Stone & Dawson, 2008). Turnover is expensive, although there is a dearth of studies that have attempted to quantify the per-worker costs of frontline turnover in different LTC settings. Seavey (2004) conducted a meta-analysis of the literature and concluded that a minimum direct cost of turnover per worker is at least $2,500. Most of the studies she reviewed estimated the costs of separation and vacancy, hiring, training, and increased worker injuries. Seavey noted, however, that the indirect costs of turnover (lost productivity until the replacement is trained, reduced service quality, lost revenues, lost clients to other agencies, deterioration in organizational culture and employee morale) may be substantial and tend to be overlooked because they are less visible and harder to measure.

In addition, turnover and vacancies are costly not only to providers but also consumers (through reduction in quality of care and life and care hours not received) and to the workers (through increased worker injuries, increased physical and emotional stress, and deterioration in working conditions and increase in the likelihood of quitting). Compromised care quality can result in deterioration of the resident/LTC client's health or functional condition, which in turn leads to increased transfers to more expensive, higher-acuity settings, unnecessary emergency visits and hospital stays, and even higher mortality (Kosel & Olivo, 2002; Seavey, 2004). Such adverse outcomes have a ripple effect and inevitably raise costs to third-party payers, primarily Medicaid and Medicare. These downstream medical costs ultimately are borne by citizens whose tax dollars support the public programs that finance LTC (Seavey, 2004).

A number of studies point to a relationship between high turnover among DCWs and poorer quality of the services delivered and the quality of life provided in nursing homes and AL and home-based settings (see the meta-analysis conducted by Bostick, Rantz, Flessner, & Riggs [2006]). Researchers involved in a national nursing home staffing study found a strong relationship between aide retention in California nursing homes and select quality outcomes (Kramer, Eilertsen, Lin, & Hutt, 2000). For short-stay nursing home residents, the study found a strong negative association between higher retention rates and both electrolyte imbalances and urinary tract infection rates. Aide retention rates also affected the functional status and pressure ulcer rates of long-stay residents.

Castle and Engberg (2005) found that increases in nurse aide turnover, especially those of moderate to high levels, result in a decrease in quality outcomes as measured by rates of physical restraint, catheter and psychoactive drug use, pressure ulcers, and quality-of-care deficiencies reported on state surveys. In a follow-up study, these researchers found that when one-year turnover rates of certified nursing assistants and LPNs were more than 50 percent, there was a negative relationship between turnover rates and quality outcomes (Castle & Engberg, 2007).

Other studies have highlighted the important role that an empowering organizational culture can play in attaining better DCW and care recipient outcomes. Eaton (2001) documented reductions in mortality and pharmaceutical use and increases in resident functioning after the introduction of innovative organizational programs that improved the work environment of nursing home aides. These models included the development of self-managed work teams, improved information sharing between nurses and direct care staff, and enhanced responsibilities for DCWs. In their evaluation of the Wellspring nursing home quality-improvement program, Stone and colleagues (2002) found that the empowerment of the DCWs, including their significant participation in care planning and care plan implementation, was associated with reduced turnover, a reduction in health-deficiency citations from state surveyors, and a decrease in incontinence rates. Findings from a study of direct care staff in 61 ALFs in Maryland highlight the importance of organizational structure to caregivers in this setting (Sikorska-Simmons, 2006). Positive perceptions of the facility's organizational culture were associated with higher job satisfaction levels and greater organizational commitment. Respondents highlighted the importance of teamwork, participation in decision making, and supportive relationships among staff.

Workforce Improvement as an Economic Development Issue

The second major issue driving this interest in the recruitment and retention of a quality, stable direct care workforce is the potential for these occupations to contribute to the economic development of communities across the country, assuming, of course, that the overall quality of these jobs—including wages, benefits, and career opportunities—is improved. Given the aging of the U.S. population over the next 40 years and increased longevity among younger people with disabilities, the LTC sector will undoubtedly be a growth industry. In 2000, approximately 13 million Americans needed LTC. By 2050, the number is expected to increase to 27 million; the population aged 85 or older—those most at risk for needing LTC—is expected to increase fivefold (USDHHS, 2003).

Although it is difficult to predict the level of family caregiving that will be available and relied on in the future, projections of wealth patterns among elderly Americans in 2015 and 2030 indicate that real income and liquid (non-housing) assets will increase greatly between 2000 and 2030 (Knickman et al., 2003). These estimates suggest that many individuals needing LTC will prefer and be able to pay for services. Furthermore, to the extent that more baby boomers are motivated to purchase LTC insurance, this is almost certain to stimulate increased demand for paid services—especially at home and in residential alternatives to nursing homes.

The Bureau of Labor Statistics (BLS) (2006) estimated that employment of DCWs in LTC settings in the next 10 years will grow faster than health care employment in general and three times as fast as all industries. During the coming decade, there will be an increase of 35 percent in jobs for nursing assistants, home health and home care aides, and personal care workers. Including both new jobs and replacement jobs for retiring workers and those who leave the occupation, the BLS projects that *almost 1 million* new DCWs will be needed between 2004 and 2014 (Hecker, 2004). The demand for DCWs in home- and community-based settings—including assisted living—is projected to grow even higher than that for nursing homes: the BLS projects a 41 percent increase in the demand for home care and personal care aides and a 56 percent increase in demand for home health aides over the 10-year period (BLS, 2006; Hecker, 2004).

Although the projections farther out into the future are more equivocal, the demographic trends suggest that the demands on the LTC sector will create many job opportunities, particularly in communities that are becoming disproportionately elderly because younger people have moved out (e.g., in many rural areas), substantial numbers of elderly have aged in place (e.g., in many inner cities), or elderly individuals have migrated to retirement destinations. Workforce improvement efforts that help to create more valuable, attractive jobs for young people as well as older people looking for second careers can positively affect the economic health of many communities and regions across the country.

Workforce Improvement as a Moral Imperative

While quality and economic development are important motivators, ethical concerns about the status of the DCW have also been a driver in raising these issues to a priority level. A recent white paper, for example, developed by the American Association of Homes and Services for the Aging Commission on Ethics in Aging Services (2007) outlined the providers' moral imperative in creating an ethical workplace that specifically addresses the needs of the DCW. Despite the critical role that DCWs play in the LTC system, they are among the lowest wage earners in the United States. In 2007 the median hourly wage for DCWs was $10.48 (PHI, 2009). Inflation-adjusted wages for these workers show that, over the past eight years, while nursing assistants have experienced a modest increase in their real hourly wages to just over $9.00 (measured in 1999 dollars), real wages for home health aides and personal care/home care aides have both declined and are under $8.00 an hour (PHI, 2009). A report by the National Center for Assisted Living (2004) reported the median hourly wage for a DCW employed in assisted living facilities in 2003 was $8.61.

These low wages may encourage DCWs to leave the LTC or health care field. One study in North Carolina found that nursing aides who had left jobs in the health sector were better off financially than those who remained in the field (Konrad, 2003). The study compared North Carolina workers trained as nursing aides who remained certified as an aide with those who did not remain certified. Among those who had not been certified as an aide since 1990, the median 1998 wage was $14,425, compared with $11,358 for actively certified nursing aides. The median wage of those no longer certified rose to $17,359 in 2001, while the comparable wage for currently certified aides increased to $12,877. While wages increased slightly in North Carolina over the four-year period, median wages remained substantially lower for those still certified compared with those who had left the field.

This financially disadvantaged status is exacerbated by the lack of health coverage experienced by a large portion of these caregivers. One in every four nursing assistants and more than one-third of home care workers lack health insurance coverage (PHI, 2009). DCWs are uninsured at a rate that is 50 percent higher than that for the general population under age 65, and nursing home workers are twice as likely to be uninsured than hospital workers (Case, Himmelstein, & Woolhandler, 2002). Co-insurance premiums for workers in LTC, furthermore, can be as much as 50 percent of the total premium (Michigan Assisted Living Association, 2001). For low-wage workers, such high co-pays make offering health coverage meaningless because it is unaffordable.

These workers also face strenuous physical demands and high job-related injury rates compared with other health- and non-health-related industries. Car accidents pose the greatest danger for home care workers (PHI, 2009). A recent study on the mental health status of various occupations found that DCWs have the highest depression rates among all occupational categories (Substance Abuse and Mental Health Services Administration, 2007).

In addition to this disadvantaged status, these workers—who provide up to three-quarters of all LTC—have few opportunities for job advancement and upgrading their skills. There is, furthermore, often a stigma associated with being a DCW, particularly a home care aide or personal care attendant, jobs in which one is frequently referred to as a "girl" or viewed as a simply a domestic worker—"the maid" (PHI, 2003).

Given the low quality of and value attributed to these jobs, Friedland (2004, p. 7) notes that "it could reasonably be argued that our long-term care system—paid primarily by public tax dollars—has an obligation to create jobs that provide a livable wage; that our publicly funded health system has a responsibility, at the very least, to provide its own workers with health insurance." Friedland goes on to lament that moral persuasion alone has failed to offer significant improvements in the quality of direct care jobs. The author of this chapter agree with this sentiment and believe that there is a moral imperative to improve the recruitment and retention of DCWs in LTC by supporting public policies and educational and provider practices that help to elevate these jobs to recognized, valued professions.

The Long-Term Outlook

As noted earlier, the unprecedented increase in the size and proportion of the elderly population and the growth in the nonelderly disabled population will increase the demand for DCWs across all LTC settings. There is, however, serious concern about the availability of these caregivers in the future. In the coming decades, as baby boomers enter old age and begin to require assistance, the pool of workers available to provide basic LTC services will fail to keep up with demand (Harahan & Stone, 2009; PHI, 2009). That is, the number of potential entry-level workers who traditionally fill DCW jobs—women aged 25 to 54 in the civilian workforce—is projected to increase by only 3.2 percent during the next seven years (BLS, 2006). This tightening of the traditional labor pool is caused by the baby boom generation having passed through this age range and the slowed rate of increased participation of women in the workplace. One study has calculated that to maintain the current ratio of paid LTC personnel to the oldest old (those over age 85) would require the LTC workforce to grow by 2 percent a year from now until 2050 and to add more than 4 million personnel (Friedland, 2004).

The number of older adults in nursing homes declined from 4.2 percent to 3.6 percent between 1985 and 2004. One recent study found that the declines were steepest among adults aged 85 and older—the population most likely to be disabled and in need of LTC (Alexcih, 2006). During this time period, alternatives to nursing homes have rapidly emerged—particularly AL and home- and community-based services. The shift to these settings will influence the number and types of caregivers that will be needed in the future, as well as the regulatory requirements regarding credentialing and ongoing training.

The future impact of new technology on the supply and demand for personnel is promising but uncertain. The introduction of labor-saving technology may reduce paperwork burdens and rates of injury and improve worker efficiency, allowing fewer personnel to do more with less. A recent study that examined the potential of retirees to be retrained as DCWs found that both elderly respondents and employers were interested in this possibility but were concerned about the physical demands that are placed on this workforce

(Hwalek, Straub, & Kosniewski, 2008). Technology could play a role in miti-gating this concern and expanding the labor pool of older workers in LTC.

Labor growth between 2000 and 2020 will rely on immigrants and people aged 55 and older. Immigrants are a particularly important source of labor in the home- and community-based service sector. They may be more willing than those born in the United States to work in caregiving occupations with lower wages. In addition, there are numerous examples of immigrants trained as nurses, pharmacists, and other professions in their country of origin (e.g., the Philippines, Eastern European countries) who have not been able get their credentials in a timely fashion in the United States and who have been em-ployed as DCWs in LTC. This trend will probably continue or even increase over time. It is important, therefore, to recognize the impact that immigration policy, and any changes in the laws, may have on the supply of workers today and in the future.

Implications for Assisted Living

This chapter has underscored the important role that the DCW plays in de-termining the quality of care and quality of life of consumers of LTC services. The demand for AL options will continue to grow as baby boomers seek out alternatives to nursing homes and as states continue to use their resources—both Medicaid and state dollars—to encourage the development of AL for lower-income older adults. It is imperative, therefore, that we have a better understanding of the current direct care workforce in AL and the factors that are going to create and sustain a quality workforce in this sector.

First, we must gather data at the state and federal levels that provide esti-mates of the number of workers and the characteristics of those who provide direct care and services in ALFs. We also need to understand how the need for this workforce and the supply vary by size, ownership patterns, and other fac-tors (e.g., whether the facility is freestanding or part of a system). In addition, we need to document the wages and benefits for this part of the direct care workforce as well as the working conditions and career opportunities, in both absolute terms and how they compare with those in the nursing home and home care sectors.

Given the fact that training—both initial and ongoing—has been demon-strated to affect the quality of the job and quality outcomes in the nursing home and home care settings, it is essential that we explore the current status of training for DCWs in AL, including what should be required to enter the field and to grow in the field. In their national study of AL, Hawes and colleagues (2003) found that 80 percent of the staff believed that confusion and urinary incontinence were normal aspects of the aging process and had serious difficulties working with residents who had dementia. Maas and Buckwalter (2006) recommend that DCWs in non-dementia-specific facilities have 55 hours of training before they are hired and 6 hours of continuing education annually. These numbers increase to 90 and 12, respectively, for those employed in dementia-specific units or facilities. Maas and Buckwalter also identify a range of topics that should be addressed, including the concept and philosophy of AL, normal aging, maintaining health and functioning, person-centered care, end-of-life care, relationships with families, and a specific emphasis on dementia.

One area of expertise and training that deserves special attention is medication management. AL residents take, on average, between 3.8 and 6.2 medications a day on a regular basis, and there is a significant lack of consistency in the delivery and monitoring of medications in this setting. A recent study of medication management in AL found that 22 states permit nurses to delegate medication management/administration to aides and other DCWs (Reinhard, Young, Kane, & Quinn, 2006). There is, however, great variation in the extent and content of training, the degree of responsibility, and the amount of oversight. Researchers who examined the role of medication aides in two states found that DCWs in Illinois were responsible for medication assistance, remedies, and follow-up as well as reporting of resident changes. In New Jersey, the responsibilities were broader, including quality discovery and reporting of medication errors and monitoring for medication changes and side effects (Miller, 2007). The study author indicated that the DCW's success in this arena requires consistent training, ongoing communication with the supervisory nurse and clear expectations. She also found that multiple demands on a DCW's time increase the risk of error and that the involvement of a pharmacist helps to ensure safe outcomes.

Conclusion

As AL options proliferate across the country, policy makers, providers, consumers, and researchers must pay attention to the development and sustainability of a quality frontline workforce in this setting. Efforts to ensure the delivery of appropriate services and quality-of-care/quality-of-life outcomes for residents will be impossible without this focus and increased investments.

REFERENCES

Abt Associates. 2003. Staffing patterns and quality. *HealthWatch* 6, 2.

Alexcih, L. 2006. *Nursing home use by "oldest old" sharply declines.* Presented at the National Press Club, Washington, DC, November 21. Retrieved November 5, 2007, from www.lewin.org.

American Association of Homes and Services for the Aging Commission on Ethics in Aging Services. 2007. *Our moral imperative: Creating an ethical workplace.* White paper prepared for AAHSA, Washington, DC.

Bostick, J. E., Rantz, M. J., Flessner, M. K., & Riggs, C. J. 2006. Systematic review of studies of staffing and quality in nursing homes. *Journal of the American Medical Directors Association* 7, 366–76.

Carlson, E. M. 2005. *Critical issues in assisted living: Who's in, who's out, and who's providing the care.* Report prepared by the National Senior Citizens Law Center with support from the Harry and Jeanette Weinberg Foundation, Inc., Washington, DC.

Case, B., Himmelstein, D., & Woolhandler, S. 2002. No care for the caregivers: Declining health insurance coverage for health care personnel and their children. *American Journal of Public Health* 92, 404–8.

Castle, N. G., & Engberg, J. 2005. Staff turnover and quality of care in nursing homes. *Medical Care* 43, 616–26.

———. 2007. The influence of staffing characteristics on quality of care in nursing homes. *Health Services Research* 42, 1822–26.

Decker, F. H., Kruhn, L., Mathews-Martin, L., Dollard, K. J., Tucker, A. M., & Bizette, L. 2003. *Results of the 2002 AHCA Survey of Nursing Staff Vacancy and Turnover Rates in Nursing Homes.* Washington, DC: American Health Care Association.

Eaton, S. 2001. What a difference management makes! Nursing staff turnover variation within a single labor market. In *Appropriateness of minimum nurse staffing ratios in nursing homes, phase 2 final report.* Prepared by Abt Associates, Cambridge, MA.

Friedland, R. 2004. *Caregivers and long-term care needs in the 21st century: Will public policy meet the challenge?* Washington, DC: Georgetown University Long Term Care Financing Project.

Harahan, M. F., & Stone, R. I. 2009. Who will care? Building the geriatric long-term care labor force. In R. B. Hudson (Ed.), *Boomer bust? The boomers and their future* (Vol. 2, pp. 233–53). Westport, CT: Praeger Perspectives.

Hawes, C., Philips, C. D., Rose, M., Holan, S., & Sherman, M. 2003. A national study of assisted living facilities. *The Gerontologist* 43 (6), 875–82.

Hecker, D. 2004. Occupational employment projections to 2012. *Monthly Labor Review* 127, 80–105.

Hwalek, M., Sraub, V., & Kosniewski, K. 2008. Older workers: An opportunity to expand the long-term care/direct care labor force. *The Gerontologist* 40 (Special Issue 1), 90–103.

Institute of Medicine. 2008. *Retooling for an aging America: Building the health care work-*

force. Committee on the Future Health Care Workforce for Older Americans. Washington, DC: National Academies Press.

Knickman, J. R., Hunt, K. A., Snell, E. K., Alexcih, L. M., & Kennell, D. L. 2003. Wealth patterns among elderly Americans: Implications for health care affordability. *Health Affairs* 22, 168–74.

Konrad, T. R. 2003. *Where have all the nurse aides gone? Part 3.* Report prepared for the North Carolina Division of Facility Services and the Kate B. Reynolds Charitable Trust. North Carolina Institute on Aging. Retrieved from www.aging.unc.edu/research/winatepup/reports/aidespart3.pdf.

Kosel, K., & Olivo, T. 2002. *The business case for work force stability.* VHA Research Series, Vol. 7. Irving, TX: VHA Inc. Retrieved from www.vha.com/research/public/stability.pdf.

Kramer, A., Eilertsen, T., Lin, M., & Hutt, E. 2000. Effects of nurse staffing on hospital transfer quality measures for new admissions. In Health Care Financing Administration Report to Congress, *Appropriateness of minimum nurse staffing ratios in nursing homes.* Washington, DC.

Maas, M. L., & Buckwalter, K. C. 2006. Providing quality care in assisted living facilities: Recommendations for staffing and staff training. *Journal of Gerontological Nursing* 32 (11), 14–22.

McDonald, I. J. 2007. *Respectful relationships: The heart of better jobs better care.* Issue Brief no. 7. Washington, DC: Better Jobs Better Care National Program Office.

Michigan Assisted Living Association. 2001. *Mental health provider 2001 wage and benefit survey.* Lansing, MI: Michigan Assisted Living Association.

Miller, J. 2007. *Identification of clinician and staff roles related to medication management and safety in assisted living facilities in two states.* Presentation at the School of Nursing, University of Washington, Seattle, WA.

Montgomery, R. J., Holley, L., Deichert, J., & Kosloski, K. 2006. A profile of home care personnel from the 2000 census: How it changes and what we know. *The Gerontologist* 45, 593–600.

National Center for Assisted Living. 2004. *Facts and trends: Assisted living sourcebook.* Washington, DC: National Center for Assisted Living.

Noelker, L. S., & Harel, Z. 2001. *Linking quality of long-term care and quality of life.* New York: Springer.

Paraprofessional Healthcare Institute. 2003. *Long-term care financing and the long-term care workforce crisis: Causes and solutions.* Report prepared for the Citizens for Long-Term Care Coalition, Washington, DC.

———. 2006. *Who are direct care workers?* Fact Sheet, November 2006, of the PHI National Clearinghouse on the Direct Care Workforce. Retrieved from www.directcareclearinghouse.org.

———. 2009. Who are the direct care workers? *Facts 3*, Bronx, NY.

Parker, V. A., & Geron, S. M. 2007. Cultural competence in nursing homes: Issues and implications for education. *Gerontology and Geriatrics Education* 28, 37–54.

Reinhard, S. C., Young, H. M., Kane, R. A., & Quinn, W. V. 2006. Nurse delegation of medication administration for older adults in assisted living. *Nursing Outlook* 54, 74–80.

Seavey, D. 2004. *The cost of frontline turnover in long-term care.* A Better Jobs Better Care practice and policy report. Washington, DC.

Sievers, L. 2006. *Assisted living that few can afford*. Report presented to the Adult Day Care Facilities and Assisted Living Residences Task Force in New York, prepared for the Empire State Association of Assisted Living, May.

Sikorska-Simmons, E. 2006. Organizational culture and work-related attitudes among staff in assisted living. *Journal of Gerontological Nursing* 32 (2), 19–27.

Stone, R. I., & Dawson, S. L. 2008. The origins of Better Jobs Better Care. *The Gerontologist* 48 (Special Issue 1), 5–13.

Stone, R. I., Reinhard, S. C., Bowers, B., Zimmerman, D., Phillips, C., Hawes, C., et al. 2002. *Evaluation of the Wellspring model for improving nursing home quality.* New York: Commonwealth Fund.

Substance Abuse and Mental Health Services Administration. 2007. Depression among adults employed full-time, by occupational category. *The National Survey on Drug Use and Health Report.* October.

U.S. Bureau of Labor Statistics. 2006. *Occupational outlook handbook, 2006-07 edition.* Retrieved from www.bls.gov/oco/home.htm.

U.S. Department of Health and Human Services. 2003. *The future supply of long-term care personnel in relation to the aging baby boom generation.* Report to Congress. Washington, DC.

Wunderlich, G. S., & Kohler, P. O. 2001. *Improving the quality of long-term care.* Institute of Medicine. Washington, DC: National Academy Press.

CHAPTER TWO

Research and Regulation in Assisted Living

Achieving the Vision

Larry Polivka, Ph.D.

This book is about frontline workers in assisted living (AL), a residential care setting that is not easy to define. The concept of AL covers a wide range of congregate living arrangements that vary by facility size, service provision, regulatory standards, funding sources, and resident characteristics. This variation has made it difficult to generate a broad consensus in support of a common definition of AL, which could be used for organizing research or developing a universally acceptable regulatory framework. The range of difference within AL is probably just as great as the difference between AL and the other long-term care settings, home care and nursing homes. In fact, the difference between AL and nursing homes may have begun to shrink in that some AL facilities (ALFs) now have highly impaired (cognitively and physically) residents who meet nursing eligibility criteria and some nursing homes have begun to adopt some of the "homelike" features of the AL model as advocated by Eden Alternative and Green House supporters and the Nursing Home Pioneers (Pioneer Network, 2007) group. These trends have important implications for hiring, training, and retaining a quality workforce.

Although a rigorously precise definition of AL has yet to emerge, most states have regulatory standards that require ALFs to provide or arrange for personal and supportive services 24 hours a day, meals, social activities, some level of health care, and housing in a group residential setting. The states vary considerably, however:

> The intensity of services, the range of disabilities for which services are pro-
> vided, the type of living arrangements, and many other aspects vary a great
> deal, often within as well as between states. Most AL residences provide pri-
> vate rooms or apartments, a communal dining area, and common areas for
> socialization and activities. Although most residences have from 11 to 50 beds,
> two-thirds of residents live in larger residences (those with more than 50 beds).
> The majority of AL residences (55%) are free-standing. The remainder share a
> campus with some other type of residential setting, such as a nursing home,
> rehabilitation center, board and care home, independent living apartments, or
> continuing care retirement community. About half are non-profit, and about
> half are for-profit; very few are government-run. (Wright, 2004, pp. 3–4)

Most states now have AL definitions and regulatory standards that include provisions designed to emphasize the significance of such quality-of-life values as resident choice, autonomy, dignity, and the protection of privacy. The role of these values also is beginning to be addressed in the regulation of nursing homes.

Because of differences in how AL is defined, it is difficult to pinpoint the number of residents living in these types of facilities. According to a recent report (Mollica, Sims-Kastelein, & O'Keeffe, 2007), based on information from 50 states and the District of Columbia, currently approximately 38,000 licensed residential care facilities with about 975,000 units/beds in the United States fall under the rubric of AL. Monthly costs for AL care vary considerably by geographic location, type of accommodation (private versus shared room), and number and types of services and amenities provided. Data from a recent national marketing survey of 1,518 ALFs located in both metropolitan and nonmetropolitan areas in the United States (ranging in size from 3 to 344 beds, with an average size of 60 beds) show that, based on state averages, monthly base rates per resident range from approximately $1,980 to $4,700, with a national average of $3,000 (Metlife Mature Market Institute, 2008). Residents and their families cover most (86%) of AL costs, and only about 8 percent receive Medicaid payments, compared with approximately 69 percent of nursing home residents who receive this support (Redfoot, 2007).

This review of the literature on AL is selective in that I focus on the research that, in terms of scope and findings, I think is most relevant to the debate over how these programs should be regulated in order to provide adequate quality of care and life for residents, which includes developing and maintaining a quality workforce. Many gaps exist in the research literature on these programs, and substantial methodological limitations, especially in the scope and size of resident and facility samples, are evident in most of the completed research. Nevertheless, enough findings of sufficient scientific quality are available to justify their use in offering provisional assessments of the relative merits of alternative regulatory policies and funding strategies.

The rapid growth of the AL population over the past decade is clear evidence of the appeal of this long-term care option and of what the industry describes as its core values of privacy, autonomy, dignity, and a homelike environment. However, the AL industry also has received intermittently negative media attention over the past several years. Most of this attention has focused on the quality of care received by some residents. A report prepared by the U.S. General Accounting Office (1999) found that many facilities do not provide residents, or potential residents, with enough information about costs, services, and retention policies, and some facilities may not be accurately representing their services and facility rules in their advertising.

Although such reports are not evidence of extensive quality-of-care problems in the industry, they have sparked discussions in some quarters about the possible need to regulate AL more stringently. This emerging discussion in turn has raised concern within the AL industry about potential political support for a regulatory approach based on current nursing home regulation. Some policy analysts and consumer advocates argue that as the population of more seriously impaired residents and those with acute medical conditions in ALFs grows, the regulatory scheme should become medically oriented and more stringent in terms of who is allowed to enter and remain, what kinds of services can be delivered and by whom, qualifications needed for staff, and how the quality of services will be defined and monitored. The potential for significant regulatory changes makes it imperative that policy analysts, policy makers, and advocates gain a clear understanding of the currently available research findings on AL and pay careful attention to the results of research as they are reported over the next several years.

This chapter is divided into three sections. The first section includes a selective review of the research literature on AL, including research on small family-model homes, which are referred to in the literature by a variety of names (e.g., adult foster care, board and care, and domiciliary care homes) and typically house 16 or fewer residents. The second section discusses the implications of the findings from this research for several regulatory issues and alternative approaches to providing adequate quality of care and quality of life for residents in AL, including ensuring a quality workforce. The third section presents concluding comments and a suggested AL research agenda.

What Do We Know about Community-Residential Care?

The research on AL has grown along with the industry over the past 10 years, with the most extensive and significant findings becoming available since 2000. Before the publication of this book, few studies have focused specifically on staffing in AL. Although major gaps in our knowledge of AL still exist and important questions remain largely unanswered, we now have a good deal of information that can help us think constructively about the future of the AL industry.

The research of Hawes, Rose, and Phillips (1999) provides among the most important early AL information. Their study, which used a national sample of ALFs estimated to be about 40 percent (4,300) of all ALFs across the country in the mid-1990s, was the first to provide a relatively comprehensive, empirically oriented view of AL. This study included homes with more than 10 beds and that served a primarily elderly population and self-identified as AL or offered basic services such as activities of daily living (ADL) assistance, meals, and 24-hour oversight. Close to two-thirds (70%) of facilities surveyed had either a full-time or part-time RN on staff, and close to half (40%) had a full-time RN.

In a subsequent report based on a subset (41%) of the larger sample composed of 300 facilities designated as either "high service" or "high privacy" that included 1,500 residents and 569 staff members, Hawes, Phillips, and Rose (2000) reported several findings that are especially relevant to regulatory and other policy issues in AL. With regard to resident admission, discharge, and retention, findings showed that during a 12-month period, 19 percent of the residents in the sample facilities were discharged; only 8 percent were discharged to nursing homes and almost 4 percent to other ALFs. Overall, 60 percent of those who moved did so to receive a higher level of care. Only 12 percent of those who moved indicated, through proxy respondents (family members), dissatisfaction with the care they had received in the facility they left. A decline in cognitive status was the only resident variable that significantly increased the likelihood of entering a nursing home. The researchers also found that when facilities had a full-time RN involved in direct care, residents were half as likely to move to a nursing home. The vast majority (85%) of residents reported that their top two priorities on entering the ALF were the availability of a private bath (#1) and private bedroom. Among those who had left an ALF (19% over 12 months), a majority (65%) continued to identify these same privacy-oriented priorities.

Hawes and colleagues (2000) also found that resident assessments of their facilities were generally positive, with a majority of residents reporting that they were treated with affection (60%) and dignity (80%). Twenty-six percent of residents, however, indicated that they needed more help with toileting activities, and 90 percent thought they could stay in their facility as long as they wanted to remain, although most were uninformed about policies governing retention and discharge from their facility. Other major concerns reported by residents (and their family members) were inadequate staffing levels and staff turnover.

Hawes and colleagues' (2000) study also provided the first extensive data on AL staff. Findings showed that staff were predominately female (97%), more than half (68%) were white, and most (85%) had completed high school. Only 61 percent worked full-time, and half had worked in the facility for two or more years. Slightly over half (51%) were resident care assistants, and 20 percent were licensed professionals. The median ratio of direct care staff to residents was 1:14. Overall, staff reported positive views regarding their work environment, although more than half (55%) indicated dissatisfaction with pay and 70 percent reported that they did not have good opportunities for advancement. Assessments of staff knowledge and training showed that, overall, staff had inadequate understanding regarding various health conditions and what constituted normal aging. Although 80 percent of the staff had received training in dementia care, most (88%) believed that symptoms (e.g., memory loss and confusion) were a normal part of aging.

Earlier research conducted in Oregon that included a sample of ALFs and nursing homes found that both types of facilities achieved comparable outcomes in terms of ADL trajectories, pain and discomfort levels, and psychological well-being after controlling for differences in baseline conditions (Kane, Baker, Salmon, & Veazie, 1998). Although nursing home residents were substantially more impaired than those in ALFs, these findings are encouraging in terms of the capacity of ALFs to accommodate "aging in place" by providing necessary health care services (Frytak et al., 2001). It should be recognized that Oregon has a relatively mature AL industry, regulatory policies and public funding strategies designed to maximize the nursing home diversion potential of ALFs, and the opportunity for AL residents to exercise choice, including the decision to "age in place."

In a more recent study of quality of life in nursing homes, ALFs, and in-home long-term care programs in Florida, Salmon (2001) found that the major predictor of quality of life was the degree of personal control the respondent experienced. Respondents in ALFs expressed the greatest satisfaction with their quality of life and the level of personal control they experienced. Respondents in the home care programs expressed a clear preference for home care over nursing homes, but they also reported less satisfaction with both their quality of life and personal control than the AL respondents did. Another recent study of community-based programs in Florida found that AL residency reduced nursing home use by 47 percent compared with the other in-home services programs (Andel, Hyer, & Slack, 2007).

A study of the Veterans Administration Assisted Living Pilot Program (ALPP) (Hedrick et al., 2007) found that adult family homes enrolled residents with greater ADL care needs than those admitted to the larger AL and residential care facilities, which tended to employ more staff with professional health training. The researchers described several potential benefits for residents of small facilities, such as the family-like environment, where residents may receive more individualized care, and potentially lower costs, which could allow for program expansion.

Zimmerman and colleagues (Zimmerman, Sloane, & Eckert, 2001; Zimmerman et al., 2005) have conducted extensive survey research in ALFs and nursing homes in New Jersey, North Carolina, Florida, and Maryland. Their sample included 233 facilities stratified into three types: small (under 16 residents), traditional (16 and over residents and built before 1987), and new-model facilities (16 and over residents, built in or after 1987, and having two or more private-pay rates, at least 20% of residents needing transfer assistance, at least 25% of residents with incontinence, or an RN or LPN on duty at all times). Among their more interesting policy-relevant findings was that type of facility made no difference with regard to likelihood of resident discharge based on functional status. Variables found to affect discharge included the state in which the facility was located and facility profit status and age. Findings also showed that new-model facilities scored higher on policy choice, privacy, and policy clarity than did the other facility types and that traditional and new-model types provided more health and social services compared with small facilities. Zimmerman and colleagues (2005) also found that facilities in continuing care environments or those that had an RN or LPN on staff were more likely to transfer residents to nursing homes. However, residents were less often hospitalized when facilities provided more RN care. In addition, Zimmerman and colleagues (2005) found that small facilities (average 8.9 beds) fared as well as new-model properties with respect to medical outcomes and nursing home transfers and better in terms of functional and social decline and social withdrawal.

These findings indicate that the larger and newer ALFs are better able to provide services and meet the privacy and autonomy desires of residents. It should be noted that privacy is often a necessary, if not always sufficient, condition for the effective exercise of personal control and autonomy and for maintaining interpersonal relations (Polivka & Salmon, 2003). Small facilities, however, may provide more familial, homelike settings that many impaired elders seem to prefer, despite fewer opportunities for privacy and autonomy. Many elders may also prefer to age in place in small facilities, even in the absence of privacy and some of the health services offered by larger facilities. The major point is that potential residents should have an array of facility types, including small, less sophisticated facilities, from which to choose. Other studies have found that small or midsize facilities frequently are less expensive than larger facilities and are often more willing to accept Medicaid and Supplemental Security Income (SSI)–supported residents than are larger properties (Ball et al., 2005; Salmon, 2003; Stearns & Morgan, 2001), a finding that has major implications for state long-term care policy and the use of Medicaid-waiver funds to expand community-based alternatives to nursing homes. A significant factor affecting operation of these homes is their ability to pay for quality staff (Perkins, Ball, Whittington, & Combs, 2004).

Morgan, Eckert, Gruber-Baldini, and Zimmerman (2002) suggest that researchers, policy makers, and regulators exercise caution in defining and comparing facilities for purposes of descriptive and evaluative analysis and for regulating the range of facilities that may be described as AL. Small facilities, for example, may not be able to offer the same level of control and autonomy or service as larger, purpose-built facilities, but residents, as noted above, may well find them more homelike, more affordable, and accommodating enough in terms of autonomy and control, especially in comparison with nursing homes or even their own homes. In sum, the advantages and shortcomings of the whole range of AL options should be recognized without claiming that one style of AL is necessarily superior to another or better designed to meet everyone's needs, preferences, or ability to pay. As this book will show, staffing issues and the experiences of frontline workers vary across facility size and type.

Findings from Morgan, Eckert, and Lyon's (1995) study of small board and care homes in Baltimore and Cleveland also support the view that small facilities have the capacity to serve a wide range of residents, including those with serious impairments. The authors point out, however, that the popularity of small facilities could increase the perception among policy makers that they need to be more rigorously and conventionally regulated, which eventually could lead to their extinction or at least substantially reduce their affordability and overall appeal.

The importance of small facilities from a quality-of-life perspective is evident in findings from a qualitative study by Ball and colleagues (2005) of both large and small facilities in Georgia. The researchers found that the quality of internal social relationships, including those between residents and staff, was commonly better for residents in the small, family-model facilities, especially for those without routine contact with family members. The importance of internal social relationships is supported by the results of a study by Street, Burge, Quadagno, and Barrett (2007), who found that they were the major predictor of the overall quality of life for residents.

Community-residential care is not for everyone requiring long-term care assistance, especially for those who develop extensive and complex medical care needs. For many AL residents, however, a substantial amount of "aging in place" is already occurring in ALFs, and the number of residents who "age in place" without ever entering a nursing home is likely to increase in the future as AL providers become more confident of their ability to accommodate the changing needs of residents in a relatively flexible regulatory environment. Findings from a study by Ball, Perkins, Whittington, Connell, and colleagues (2004) demonstrate the complex and often idiosyncratic nature of "aging in place" in ALFs: there may be as many ways of "aging in place" as there are AL residents, and overly precise regulations specifying the terms of retention are likely to end up displacing many residents whose quality of life is largely dependent on remaining in their ALF. Ball, Perkins, Whittington, Connell, and colleagues (2004) conclude that residents' ability to age in place is a "balancing act" that is influenced by multiple community-, facility-, and individual-level factors that are complex, dynamic, and interactive. Of key importance is the "fit" between the capacity of the facility and that of the resident to manage resident decline. Obviously, staff qualifications and staffing levels are key factors affecting aging in place.

These are important "facts on the ground" that have major implications for the future of AL regulation and the role of AL in the long-term care system. Although many of these studies are based on relatively small samples and much more research is needed, we can speculate about the significance of their findings for long-term care policy generally and regulation specifically. For example, to the extent that personal control and autonomy are important determinants of quality of life in long-term care, AL may be the optimal setting of care, including for many now receiving care in their own homes. That is, AL may be for many frail elderly persons the best setting for achieving an effective balance between autonomy and supportive services, including health care and more human interaction to combat loneliness.

ALFs can offer the kinds of resources, especially staff services, transportation, and social activities, necessary to make the achievement of personal control and autonomy a far more practical matter than may be possible in many in-home environments, where achieving the same level of opportunity to exercise personal control is beyond the financial means of most individuals or the public sector to provide, or too great a burden on the individual's informal care providers. These possibilities should be kept firmly in mind as we think about AL regulation and how to achieve the full potential of AL as a long-term care program.

Policies, funding, and regulatory strategies should reflect our awareness of and support for the different forms of AL and the need to provide consumers with as many options as possible, as long as they are consistent with the basic values of the AL philosophy and basic safety requirements. This means that small facilities should not be held to precisely the same standards, which they are not likely to meet, as the larger, purpose-built, new-paradigm ALFs. Other researchers note that if regulation and funding turn on adherence to the new paradigm's parameters, it may mean the demise of the smaller facilities (Ball et al., 2005; Perkins et al., 2004; Zimmerman et al., 2002). This perspective will undoubtedly complicate the way AL is regulated, but if it results in maintaining or supporting the expansion of the range of community-residential options available to consumers of housing with services, then it should be considered worth the additional complexity.

The findings reviewed here indicate that, overall, AL is often an optimal environment for residents as they age in place, including many residents who have cognitive impairment and medical needs. There is a danger, however, that, as a consequence of serving an increasing number of cognitively and physically impaired residents, states will impose restrictive regulations that will unnecessarily limit the potential of AL to serve this population (Chapin & Dobbs-Kepper, 2001).

Implications for Assisted Living

The vast majority of older people and their families strongly prefer home- and community-based alternatives to nursing home care (Ball, Perkins, Whittington, Connell, et al., 2004; Mollica, 2009). The primary reasons for this strong preference are the desire to maintain a modicum of personal control and to preserve their privacy and dignity to the maximum extent possible (Ball, Perkins, Whittington, Hollingsworth, et al., 2004; Ball et al., 2005). This consumer preference is the fundamental rationale for creating a far better balanced system of long-term care than is currently available to frail elderly people, particularly those dependent on public support. Both AL and home care should be vastly expanded in response to the deep preference among elderly people for alternatives to nursing homes. At this point, however, AL is probably the most underdeveloped alternative program in the public sector. Most of the AL growth since 1990 has occurred in the private sector, and states, on the whole, are just beginning to develop and expand their AL programs, primarily through Medicaid-waiver initiatives. Home and Community-Based Services (HCBS) Medicaid-waiver programs, authorized under Section 1915(c) of the Social Security Act, enable states to waive certain Medicaid requirements in order to cover home- and community-based services, such as AL, and may include case management and skilled nursing services. Despite growth in funding for HCBS, expenditures for nursing homes remain considerably higher than those for home- and community-based services. In 2007, Medicaid spent $47 billion on nursing homes versus $17 billion on HCBS-waiver programs for older people and adults with physical disabilities, although expenditures for HCBS vary considerably by state, ranging from 1 to 61 percent (Houser, Fox-Grage, & Gibson, 2009).

The pervasive preference among elderly people for alternatives, including AL, to nursing homes should not be frustrated by excessive or inappropriate regulation. AL has demonstrated the capacity to serve seriously impaired residents effectively, and regulations should be designed to maximize this potential through the use of flexible, inclusive admission and retention criteria. Providers can help maximize this potential by providing necessary care, including nursing care, for residents with health care conditions that require continuing care. The preservation and enhancement of AL's core values should be the top priority in the development of AL regulations.

As noted earlier, for many frail elders, AL is a more propitious setting for achieving these values than their own homes. The only sure outcome of imposing a nursing home mode of regulation on AL would be precisely what we have achieved in nursing homes—a rigid, institutional environment that restricts consumer direction, resident autonomy, and privacy. We should pay more attention to reversing these outcomes in nursing homes and avoid creating a regulatory framework that could have the same results in AL.

The wide variance in AL regulation across the states represents a natural laboratory, and every effort should be made over the next 5–10 years to determine the relative costs and benefits of their regulatory strategies. We need this information before we prematurely decide to move to a single national regulatory framework. Researchers already are building a useful body of knowledge for developing reasonable regulations over the next decade. Anecdotal accounts in the media should not lead to a "rush to judgment" and the implementation of conventionally stringent regulations that could kill the very thing we should be most committed to preserving: the fundamental values of AL.

Serious consideration, however, should be given to Hawes, Phillips, and Rose's (2000) findings concerning the impact of cognitive decline and the role of RN care in preventing movement to a nursing home or in facilitating aging in place. Providers should be prepared to use this information in the development and deployment of their services, and policy makers and regulators should monitor these areas carefully and consult closely with providers and advocates before deciding how they should be interpreted from a regulatory perspective. Clearly, however, the provision of sound dementia care and skilled nursing care is an essential component of any efforts to maximize the aging-in-place potential of AL. In addition, better training is needed for direct care staff in a variety of areas, and interventions are required to improve staff satisfaction and increase retention, which has a direct effect on the quality and continuity of resident care.

We also could enhance the quality of care by requiring that residents taking more than four medications have their medication regimen evaluated by a consultant pharmacist at least annually. Pharmacists often are more knowledgeable than physicians or nurses about medications, and physicians usually are willing to listen to pharmacists and adjust prescriptions accordingly. As pointed out in Chapter 5 of this volume, direct care staff often are the ones who assist residents with medications, a fact that has implication for staff training.

Management of medications is closely related to the issue of nurse delegation, which refers to training and permitting unlicensed personnel to administer medications with ongoing RN oversight and supervision (Reinhard, Young, Kane, & Quinn, 2003). Nurse delegation can play an important role in making AL more affordable by limiting the cost of health care–related services. Three-fifths of states provide for some form of delegated nurse supervision of unlicensed staff or the use of trained aides to administer oral medications in AL, and some also allow these staff to administer injections. Most informants from state boards of nursing report few consumer complaints in regard to nurse delegation, although no formal mechanisms for reporting errors exist (Reinhard et al., 2003).

Sikma and Young (2001) found considerable enthusiasm among RNs for supervised delegation. However, the fact that many AL residents who have serious chronic conditions have been found to be undermedicated or not to be receiving appropriate medications (Sloane et al., 2004) indicates a need for better medical assessments and medication management protocols. Regulation should address such concerns, which also arise in nursing home and home care settings (Munroe, 2003), including mandating periodic (e.g., quarterly) evaluations by pharmacists or physicians for certain residents. The Assisted Living Workgroup (2003) developed several medication management recommendations, most of which focus on the roles, training, and monitoring of medication management assistants working under the supervision of a nurse according to the provisions of nurse delegation acts.

Every effort should be made to develop a greater quality-of-life focus in the regulation of ALFs—a focus designed to achieve the original vision for AL, especially the emphasis on resident choice, dignity, privacy, and a homelike environment conducive to the formation of close social relationships among residents and with staff members. For Ball and colleagues (2005), making quality of life a central feature of AL regulations will require training AL workers to provide the kind of personalized care that preserves the personality, identity, and will of the resident. This training would prepare workers to focus "much more attention on the socioemotional state of residents and concern itself with the person's definition of quality of life" (p. 266). The authors believe that requiring training that is focused on quality of life would help redefine the work of AL staff as "professional and important and allow for a realignment of values" (p. 266).

Several other workforce-related issues will become increasingly important, from the regulatory and funding perspectives, as the number of ALFs grows and AL populations become more diverse in terms of health and functional assistance needs and socioeconomic characteristics. Administrative and caregiving staff will need to receive gradually more extensive pre- and in-service training in the areas of physical health and dementia care. Pre-employment qualifications also may need to be enhanced, which will raise the costs of staff turnover, which is now relatively high in many communities and set to increase further with demography-driven (population aging) tightening of long-term care labor markets over the next several years. We can develop more efficient methods of delivering training, but retraining experienced and dedicated staff will require higher salaries, better benefits, and improved work environments designed to empower workers, unleash creativity, and inspire a sense that caregiving is a highly valued career with a promising opportunity horizon. These workforce enhancements will be unavoidably expensive, which will make sensitivity to the cost and affordability implications of regulatory interventions in AL an increasingly important issue.

Finally, as Ball and colleagues (2005) noted, regulatory policy should recognize the unique value and challenges of small facilities. Regulations, thus, should not be allowed to drive small facilities into extinction. Rather, the authors suggest that older persons of limited means are far better served by adjusting standards to fit the available resources than by raising expectations beyond the ability of that market to reach them.

States should continue to take a cautious approach to AL regulation. We need to learn more about the effects of the different regulatory schemes across the states, the impact of Medicaid-waiver funding on the demographics of

AL, and a wide range of outcomes, including the extent of AL's capacity to substitute for nursing home care and the capacity of AL to provide specialty care, especially dementia care. The already valuable body of research findings will grow substantially over the next few years and help us make far more informed decisions about regulation than we are prepared to make now.

Conclusion

The best available information indicates that the AL industry, with the support of policy makers and the regulatory community, has built a sound foundation for continuing success. The industry is not perfect, and some course corrections are in order. I am impressed, however, by the extent of progress achieved over the past 15 years. As head of the Florida State Aging Agency in 1989, I felt that the biggest gap in the long-term care system was the absence of a congregate care program that would allow the frail elderly to "age in place" and offer them the same freedom (personal control, privacy) and level of service that had been made available in their own homes through home care programs since the late 1970s. This kind of community residential care has been achieved primarily through the growth of the AL industry for private-pay residents and is arguably the most positive development in long-term care in the past decade.

The biggest problem in AL at this point is not insufficient regulation. The major problem confronting policy makers and people in need of long-term care is the relatively meager number of AL beds available to the less affluent elderly people who require public support, have limited access to community resources, and want to avoid ending up in a nursing home. For many of these people, AL offers the optimal long-term care setting not only for receiving the physical care they need but also for achieving a quality of life (e.g., autonomy and privacy) that may not be available in their own homes. Our primary goals for AL should be to expand access for publicly supported residents and avoid regulatory schemes that would undermine the quality-of-life features that constitute the fundamental appeal of AL as a long-term care program.

Medicaid waivers are essential to long-term care financing, as demonstrated by the way they have been used to transform care for the developmentally disabled over the past 20 years and long-term care for the elderly in Oregon, Washington, and Arizona over the past decade. These examples indicate the capacity of waivers to change the fundamental nature of long-term care on a permanent basis and help address the fiscal crisis by containing overall long-term care costs. Most states need to make much more expansive use of Medicaid waivers to fund systemic long-term care changes, including increased availability of AL for impaired older people who are dependent on publicly supported services. Few states have adopted the Oregon and Washington approach to funding the growth of affordable AL through the Medicaid program. Policy makers, AL providers, and residents will continue to struggle for the foreseeable future with "a number of issues that require reconciliation of what appears to be inherently contradictory goals" (O'Keeffe & Wiener, 2005, p. 4).

At this point, I think the available research indicates that most of the state regulatory standards governing "quality of care" (standards setting minimally acceptable quality) and "aging in place" (standards allowing flexibility in terms of facilities deciding whom they will admit and retain) are generally sound but that disclosure standards need to be more fully developed. We also need far more research on quality of life and investigations—such as the one presented in this book—that examine workforce issues, which will be used to inform regulatory policy and prepare providers to care for an increasingly impaired AL population. The financing issues will remain problematic in terms of both funding levels and reimbursement rates and restrictions (no room and board coverage) until federal and state policy makers decide to make AL as available as institutional care in the publicly funded long-term care system.

AL is a relatively fragile form of housing and long-term care that is largely sustained by the fact that many older people much prefer it to nursing home care and may, in many cases, find it preferable to in-home care. It would not take the application of many nursing home–style regulations, however, to make AL substantially less affordable *and* far less attractive than it has proven to be over the past ten years. Every effort should be made to contain these risks by always assuming the perspective (needs and preferences) of the consumer and by supporting rigorous research, the results of which can be used to guide policy and dilute the distorting influence of purely anecdotal accounts of bad *or* good outcomes.

Clearly, frontline workers in AL and other long-term care settings are principal players in whether or not residents are able to realize the core AL values of autonomy, privacy, dignity, and the ability to age in place in the least restrictive environment. They must be trained in the importance of these values and how to incorporate them into their care regimens, and facility administrators must use staffing levels and policies that give direct care workers the time and freedom to respond to residents' individual needs and preferences. Findings presented in this book will provide valuable information to guide policy and practice regarding how best to incorporate frontline workers into the AL care mission and support them in their roles.

REFERENCES

Andel, R., Hyer, K., & Slack, A. 2007. Risk factors for nursing home placement in older adults with and without dementia. *Journal of Aging and Health* 19, 213–28.

Assisted Living Workgroup. 2003. *Assuring quality in assisted living: Guidelines for federal and state policy, state regulation, and operations.* A report to the U.S. Senate Special Committee on Aging. Washington, DC.

Ball, M. M., Perkins, M. M., Whittington, F. J., Connell, B. R., Hollingsworth, C., & King, S. V. 2004. Managing decline in assisted living: The key to aging in place. *Journals of Gerontology: Social Sciences* 4, S202–12.

Ball, M., Perkins, M., Whittington, F., Hollingsworth, C., King, S., & Combs, B. 2004. Independence in assisted living. *Journal of Aging Studies* 18, 467–83.

———. 2005. *Communities of care: Assisted living for African American elders.* Baltimore: Johns Hopkins University Press.

Chapin, R., & Dobbs-Kepper, D. 2001. Aging in place in assisted living: Philosophy versus policy. *The Gerontologist* 1, 43–50.

Frytak, J. R., Kane, R. A., Finch, M. D., Kane, R. L., & Maude-Griffin, R. 2001. Outcome trajectories for AL and nursing facility residents in Oregon. *Health Services Research* 1, 91–111.

Hawes, C., Phillips, C. D., & Rose, M. 2000. *High service or high privacy assisted living facilities, their residents and staff: Results from a national survey.* Washington, DC: U.S. Department of Health and Human Services.

Hawes, C., Rose, M., & Phillips, C. D. 1999. *A national study of assisted living for the frail elderly: Results of a national survey of facilities.* Beachwood, OH: Myers Research Institute.

Hedrick, S. C., Guihan, M., Chapko, M., Manheim, L., Sullivan, J. H., Thomas, M., et al. 2007. Characteristics of residents and providers in the assisted living pilot program. *The Gerontologist* 3, 365–77.

Houser, A., Fox-Grage, W., & Gibson, M. J. 2009. *Across the states: Profiles of long-term care and independent living* (8th ed.). Washington, DC: AARP Public Policy Institute. Retrieved June 1, 2009, from http://assets.aarp.org/rgcenter/il/d19105_2008_ats.pdf.

Kane, R. A., Baker, M. O., Salmon, J., & Veazie, W. 1998. *Consumer perspectives on private versus shared accommodations in assisted living settings* (Report 9807). Washington, DC: American Association of Retired Persons.

Metlife Mature Market Institute. 2008. *The Metlife market survey of nursing home and assisted living costs.* Westport, CT: Metlife Mature Market Institute. Retrieved June 1, 2009, from www.metlife.com/assets/cao/mmi/publications/studies/mmi-studies-2008-nhal-costs.pdf.

Mollica, R. L. 2009. *Taking the long view: Investing in Medicaid home and community-based services is cost effective* (AARP Public Policy Institute Insight on the Issues I26). Washington, DC: AARP Public Policy Institute. Retrieved June 1, 2009, from http://assets .aarp.org/rgcenter/il/i26_hcbs.pdf.

Mollica, R., Sims-Kastelein, K., & O'Keeffe, J. 2007. *Residential care and assisted living compendium.* Washington, DC: U.S. Department of Health and Human Services. Retrieved June 1, 2009, from http://aspe.hhs.gov/daltcp/reports/2007/07alcom.htm.

Morgan, L., Eckert, K., Gruber-Baldini, A., & Zimmerman, S. 2002. *The methodologic imperative for small assisted living facilities.* Presentation at the 55th Gerontological Society of America Meeting, Boston, MA.

Morgan, L., Eckert, K., & Lyon, S. 1995. *Small board-and-care homes: Residential care in transition.* Baltimore: Johns Hopkins University Press.

Munroe, D. 2003. Assisted living issues for nursing practice. *Geriatric Nursing* 2, 99–105.

O'Keeffe, J., & Wiener, J. 2005. Public funding for long-term care services for older people in residential care settings. *Journal of Housing for the Elderly* 3/4, 51–79.

Perkins, M., Ball, M. M., Whittington, F. J., & Combs, B. L. 2004. Managing the needs of low-income board and care home residents: A process of negotiating risks. *Qualitative Health Research* 14, 478–95.

Pioneer Network. 2007. Who we are: Our history. Retrieved September 27, 2007, from www.pioneernetwork.net/who-we-are/our-history.php.

Polivka, L., & Salmon, J. R. 2003. Autonomy and personal empowerment: Making quality-of-life the organizing principle for long-term care policy. In J. L. Ronch & J. A. Goldfield (Eds.), *Mental wellness in aging: Strengths-based approaches* (pp. 15–31). Baltimore: Health Professions Press.

Redfoot, D. 2007. *How do residents in assisted living and nursing homes compare?* Washington, DC: Center for Excellence in Assisted Living. Retrieved June 1, 2009, from www .theceal.org/column.php?ID=16.

Reinhard, S., Young, H., Kane, R., & Quinn, W. 2003. *Nurse delegation of medication administration for elders in assisted living.* New Brunswick, NJ: Rutgers Center for State Health Policy.

Salmon, J. R. 2001. *The contribution of personal control and personal meaning to quality of life in home care, assisted living facilities, and nursing home settings.* Unpublished doctoral dissertation, University of South Florida.

———. 2003. *The diversity of assisted living: One size does not fit all.* Presentation at the Gerontological Society of America Annual Meeting, San Diego, CA.

Sikma, S., & Young, H. 2001. Balancing freedom with risks: The experience of nursing task delegation in community-based residential care settings. *Nursing Outlook* 49, 193–201.

Sloane, P. D., Gruber-Baldini, A. L., Zimmerman, S., Roth, M., Watson, L., Boustani, M., et al. 2004. Medication undertreatment in assisted living settings. *Archives of Internal Medicine* 18, 2031–37.

Stearns, S., & Morgan, L. A. 2001. Economics and financing. In S. Zimmerman, P. Sloane, & J. Eckert (Eds.), *Assisted living: Needs, practices and policies in residential care for the elderly* (pp. 271–91). Baltimore: Johns Hopkins University Press.

Street, D., Burge, S., Quadagno, J., & Barrett, A. 2007. The salience of social relationships for resident well-being in assisted living. *Journals of Gerontology: Social Sciences* 62, S129–34.

U.S. General Accounting Office. 1999. *Assisted living: Quality of care and consumer protection issues* (Publication GAO/T-HEHS-99-111). Washington, DC: Government Printing Office.

Wright, B. 2004. *In brief: An overview of assisted living: 2004.* Washington, DC: AARP Public Policy Institute. Retrieved February 18, 2008, from www.aarp.org/research/housing-mobility/assistedliving/aresearch-import-924-INB88.html.

Zimmerman, S., Eckert, J. K., Morgan, L., Gruber-Baldini, A. L., Mitchell, C. M., & Reed, P. S. 2002. *Promising directions in assisted living research,* Presentation at the 55th Annual Gerontological Society of America Meeting, Boston, MA.

Zimmerman, S., Sloane, P., & Eckert, J. K. 2001. Emerging issues in residential care/assisted living. In S. Zimmerman, P. Sloane, & J. Eckert (Eds.), *Assisted living: Needs, practices and policies in residential care for the elderly* (pp. 317–32). Baltimore: Johns Hopkins University Press.

Zimmerman, S., Sloane, P., Eckert, J. K., Gruber-Baldini, A. L., Morgan, L., & Hebel, J. R. 2005. How good is assisted living? Findings and implications from an outcomes study. *Journals of Gerontology: Social Sciences* 60, S195–204.

Part II / Assisted Living Work and Workers

CHAPTER THREE

Overview of Research

Mary M. Ball, Ph.D.
Molly M. Perkins, Ph.D.

The overall goal of this study is to learn how assisted living facilities (ALFs) can create an environment that maximizes job satisfaction and retention of direct care workers (DCWs). Our specific research aims are

1. to understand the meaning of job satisfaction for DCWs in ALFs;
2. to understand how individual, sociocultural, and environmental factors influence job satisfaction and retention of direct care staff in ALFs and the relationship between these variables; and
3. to identify successful strategies of direct care, managerial, and administrative staff that support job satisfaction and retention of DCWs in ALFs.

In this chapter, we describe in detail the qualitative and quantitative methods we used to collect and analyze our data. We also present the characteristics of the participants and their work settings, and we place both within the national context of assisted living (AL).

The Research Setting

This study was set in Georgia, where ALFs are designated "personal care homes" and include a wide range of facilities. Georgia has 2,359 licensed ALFs with 28,512 beds (Georgia Office of Regulatory Services, 2007). The majority of ALFs have six or fewer beds. Like 18 other states, Georgia does not have an *assisted living* licensing category (Mollica & Johnson-Lamarche, 2005). Medicaid funding is available only in small homes (2–24 residents) through Georgia's Home and Community-Based Services (HCBS) Medicaid-waiver program. Available data suggest that Georgia AL residents resemble the national profile of an increasingly impaired and majority white and female population (Ball et al., 2000, 2005; Georgia State Health Planning Agency, 1993; Hawes, Rose, & Phillips, 1999).

Georgia's AL regulations require that all persons who provide direct care to residents be at least 18 years of age. Regulations also specify training requirements, which include current certification in emergency first aid and CPR and completion of at least 16 hours of continuing education annually in courses approved by the state regulatory agency (see Chapter 10, this volume, for details). In addition, regulations require that homes maintain numbers of staff adequate to protect the health, safety, and welfare of the residents. The minimum staff-to-resident ratio is 1:15 in the daytime (similar to the national median of 1:14) and 1:25 at night. Like most states, regulations prohibit medication administration or provision of skilled services by facility staff. National data indicate that Georgia resembles a majority of other states on a number of staffing issues, including minimum staffing levels, training requirements, job content, and pay (Ball et al., 2000; Hawes, Phillips, & Rose, 2000; Mollica & Johnson-Lamarche, 2005).

Research Design and Methods
Qualitative and Quantitative Study Approaches

In this study we use both qualitative and quantitative methods. A number of researchers have discussed the motivations and strategies for combining qualitative and quantitative methods (Creswell, 2003; Groger & Straker, 2002; Morgan, 1998; Wenger, 1999). Motivations typically revolve around a complementary of methods that yields enhanced understanding of the phenomenon under study (Morgan, 1998). Combining methods requires decisions about sequence, priority, and at what stage in the research process integration will occur (Creswell, 2003). Most commonly, methods are used sequentially, usually with qualitative methods used first to discover key issues for subsequent quantitative study. Less frequently, the order is reversed (Morgan, 1998). Typically one method is given priority, but the two approaches sometimes have equal weight and are used simultaneously. We use qualitative and quantitative methods simultaneously with equal priority, which allowed for a shorter data-collection period compared with a sequential approach. Integration of methods occurs primarily at the interpretation stage.

Our research aims and questions lend themselves to this dual approach. Because relatively little is known about the views of DCWs in ALFs or about their work experiences, questions about the meaning of job satisfaction within the AL context (research aim 1) are best answered with qualitative methodology (Sankar & Gubrium, 1994). Qualitative study also is appropriate for understanding *how* and *why* individual, sociocultural, and environmental factors influence job satisfaction and retention (research aim 2), for identifying strategies that support satisfaction and retention (research aim 3), and for discovering how job satisfaction and retention can be maximized in the AL environment in ways that respect the cultural values, beliefs, and practices of all staff (overall study goal). Quantitative methods allow us to test the strength of relationships and to investigate both the direct and indirect effects of multiple factors, including individual-, facility-, and community-level characteristics, on staff turnover. Because of the complexity of the many factors that influence long-term care (LTC), this combination of methods is especially appropriate and enhances the overall value of the study.

Research Sample
Selection of Facilities

The sample frame for this study was all ALFs in Georgia with 16 beds or more that served a primarily elderly population and were located within 150 miles of Atlanta (N=301). Within this radius are included medium- and small-sized metropolitan service areas (MSAs), numerous small towns, and rural areas. By expanding the geographic area beyond metro Atlanta, we were able to include facilities located in places of all sizes and economic conditions. We eliminated homes with 15 or fewer residents because our previous studies indicate that they are substantially different from larger facilities regarding both issues of recruitment and retention and experiences of direct care staff.

We selected 45 ALFs by systematic random sampling within strata. The sample was roughly proportional to the total number of ALFs in each geographic area and represented approximately 12 percent of the sample pool. In selecting our sample, we first created a comprehensive list of ALFs meeting the stated parameters of the sample pool and then stratified homes according to size and geographic area. We used three categories to stratify by size: 16–25 beds, 26–50 beds, and 51+ beds. Geographic strata were based on Georgia's 12 planning and service areas (PSAs), 9 of which are located within a 150-mile radius of Atlanta. To increase the number of ALFs in the more rural parts of the state, we combined these 9 PSAs into three strata. Geographic contiguity, number of facilities, and anticipated cultural characteristics of residents were the basis for the specified combinations. Area 1 includes the 10-county Atlanta region and has 135 ALFs in the sample pool. Area 2, located south, southwest, southeast, and east of Atlanta, includes three medium-sized MSAs and has 81 ALFs. Area 3, located northeast, northwest, and north of Atlanta, includes the mountain areas and two small-sized MSAs and has 85 ALFs in the facility pool. These three areas varied in racial composition (ranging from 10% black in area 3 to 32% black in area 1) and population density (ranging from 2,484 persons per square mile in one county of area 1 to 11 persons per square mile in one county of area 2) (U.S. Census Bureau, 2000).

To solicit facility participation, we first sent a letter explaining the project to the owner or executive director and then followed up with a phone call, and in a few cases a visit, to allow potential participants to ask questions and address concerns before making decisions. Refusals were replaced with the next home on the list within the appropriate size category and area. Out of a total of 94 facilities contacted, 49 refused (52% refusal rate). The most common reason for refusal was the anticipated time commitment. For about half of refusals, no reason was given.

Selection of Participants

We selected administrative staff based on their knowledge of each ALF's organizational structure and operation. Although for the most part we selected one administrator per home, when multiple sample ALFs had a single owner and contiguous locations (three small homes), we selected only one administrator. In one of the large (51+) homes, we selected an additional administrator whose primary responsibility was hiring and managing direct care staff. Our total administrator sample was 44.

The strategy for sampling DCWs was guided by how the data from each type of interview would be analyzed. For type 1 interviews, which collected data to be analyzed both quantitatively and qualitatively, we randomly selected 370 participants stratified by shift and employment status (full- or part-time). DCWs who refused were replaced by the next available person on the list. We selected approximately 4–6 staff from each home in the 16–25 size category; 8–10 from homes in the 26–50 category; and 12–14 from homes in the 51+ category. This sampling strategy resulted in 79 staff from homes with 16–25 residents; 103 from homes with 26–50 residents; and 188 from homes with 51+ residents.

For type 2 interviews, which were in-depth in nature and analyzed only qualitatively, we used purposive sampling (Patton, 2002) to choose workers who represented conceptual dimensions relevant to our research aims. The final sample of 41 participants varied according to race, ethnicity, nativity, age, education, training, gender, marital status, dependent care responsibilities, tenure, shift, full- or part-time status, and job experience. Eleven of these participants were selected previously for type 1 interviews, yielding a combined total sample size of 400. Pseudonyms are used throughout for facilities and participants.

Statistical Power

Because no data regarding staff satisfaction and retention in AL were available when this study was designed, we calculated an a priori power analysis assuming no aggregate-level data and adjusted this estimate to take aggregate data into account once approximately two-thirds of the data were collected. We used Cohen's (1988) general guidelines for the a priori power analysis and the Optimal Design program (Spybrook, Raudenbush, Liu, & Congdon, 2006), a software program for estimating power for longitudinal and multilevel research designs, for the post hoc analyses. Intent to leave, a continuous outcome variable in the conceptual model (see Figure 9.1), was used as the dependent variable in these analyses.

Based on an alpha level of .05, 26 predictor variables, and an estimated medium population effect size, an a priori power analysis showed that a minimum of 226 participants were needed to ensure statistical power of .90. The proposed sample of 308 participants substantially exceeded the required number. After completing 207 type 1 interviews in 27 facilities, an ad hoc power analysis based on an alpha of .05, the harmonic mean of the within-group sample size equal to 6, and an intraclass correlation (ICC) of .13 showed that at least 45 homes were needed for statistical power of .80 to detect an effect size of .30, a value that falls within the moderate range according to Cohen (1988). A second ad hoc power analysis conducted after completing data collection in 45 homes based an alpha of .05, the harmonic mean of the within-group sample size equal to 6, and an ICC of .09 showed that we had power of .80 to detect a moderate effect size (Cohen, 1988) of 42.

Data Collection

The primary methods of data collection were (1) face-to-face interviews with administrative and direct care staff; (2) limited participant observation; and (3) review of facility documents. Three research teams with a total of 12 researchers participated in data collection over a 16-month period.

On our initial visit to each site, we toured the facility and conducted an in-depth interview with the manager or director. We also made an effort to meet direct care staff and posted fliers describing the project around the facility. In subsequent visits, we typically met formally with staff to explain project goals, the potential risks and benefits of participation, and research procedures, including the consent process, sample selection, confidentiality, and length of the interview. Most staff welcomed the chance to participate. Our refusal rate for interviews was only 9 percent; refusals generally related to scheduling conflicts. All participants were paid $25 for a completed interview.

Interviewing

We conducted in-depth qualitative interviews with 44 administrators. These interviews lasted approximately 1½ hours and addressed the facility's organizational structure, policies and procedures, and the administrator's knowledge regarding DCWs' experiences and attitudes. We also asked administrators about their own education and training, employment histories, and job motivations. All administrator interviews were tape-recorded and transcribed verbatim. In addition, administrators provided information about the personal characteristics and care needs of residents, employee pay levels and benefits, direct care staff turnover during the previous year, and staffing ratios and patterns. We also collected facility marketing materials and documents containing personnel policies and procedures.

We conducted type 1 quantitative interviews with 370 workers, using a guide constructed specifically for this study, based on the study aims and findings from our previous research. This instrument consisted of 112 open- and closed-ended questions and included two standardized job satisfaction scales (see "Quantitative Measures," below). Questions focused on workers' personal characteristics; experiences and attitudes about their jobs; quality of relationships with residents, co-workers, administrators, and residents' families; and views about the work environment. Type 1 interviews lasted on average 47 minutes. After completion of the interviews, respondents self-administered the satisfactions scales. The scales took participants an average of 9 minutes to complete.

We conducted in-depth, qualitative type 2 interviews lasting approximately 1½ hours with 41 workers. Researchers employed a detailed guide, which covered work routines, social relationships, attitudes toward work and individuals in the work setting, and personal information. In cases of staff who participated in both type 1 and 2 interviews (N=11), type 1 interviews were conducted first to avoid any potential bias from having first participated in an in-depth interview. Throughout data collection, theoretical sampling of information guided questioning in the subsequent interviews and homes and sampling of participants. All type 2 interviews were tape-recorded and transcribed verbatim.

Participant Observation

Researchers conducted observations of DCWs as they performed tasks and during staff meetings, training sessions, and break time. Observations were recorded through detailed field notes, which included what was going on, who was involved, what people did and said, where activities occurred and when they took place, and how participants reacted to what was going on. Researchers also recorded detailed information about each facility's physical environment and collected diagrams of the facility layout when available. The average observation time was approximately 8 hours in the small homes, 15 hours in the medium homes, and 22 hours in the large homes, for a total of 657 hours during 369 visits. Participation by researchers was minimal and included attending meetings and assisting with meal service and activities. These activities helped to build rapport with staff. Researchers conducted informal interviews during observations, which increased understanding of the meaning of what was observed and added to overall knowledge about DCWs' job attitudes and work experience.

Quantitative Measures

Actual turnover, intent to leave, and job satisfaction are the primary outcome measures used in this study. Independent variables include individual-level characteristics (e.g., staff sociodemographic characteristics and job attributes), facility-level characteristics (e.g., facility size and ownership type), and community-level characteristics (e.g., facility geographic location and county unemployment rate).

Actual turnover (respondent terminated the job versus respondent did not terminate the job) was assessed through a one-year follow-up of the staff who completed type 1 interviews. These data were collected from administrators at each facility and included information regarding staff members' departure dates and reasons for leaving.

We assessed *intent to leave* by asking DCWs to indicate on a scale of 1 to 10, where 1 is "very unlikely" and 10 is "very likely," the likelihood of leaving within one year. This single-item measure was adapted from a measure used in other studies that has shown to be valid measure of intention to leave a job (Kiyak, Namazi, & Kahana, 1997; Lambert, Hogan, & Barton, 2001).

We measured *job satisfaction* using the 18-item Job in General (JIG) scale and a revised version of the 72-item Job Descriptive Index (JDI) (Balzer et al., 1997, 2000). The JDI measures five principal dimensions of job satisfaction: (1) satisfaction with the job itself; (2) opportunities for promotion; (3) relationship with co-workers; (4) satisfaction with pay; and (5) relationship with supervisors. The JIG, which is used in the analyses reported in this book, measures general feelings about the job and was designed to provide a global and long-term assessment of the job as a whole. Internal reliability analyses of each scale have consistently yielded alpha coefficients ranging from .86 to .90 and above (Balzer et al., 2000; Johnson & Johnson, 2000). In this sample, internal consistency coefficients for the five subscales of the JDI ranged from .75 to .90. The JIG also demonstrated good reliability (Cronbach's alpha = .88).

Individual-level characteristics include sociodemographic characteristics, employment history, and job characteristics of DCWs and administrators. Data collected from DCWs include age, gender, race, ethnicity, educational attainment, marital status, number of dependents residing in the household, job status, average number of weekly hours worked, shift, job tenure in months, specialized training in resident care, perceived workload, and job content.

Data on *facility-level characteristics* were collected from facility administrators and include the range of fees charged by a facility, facility size, facility ownership, sociodemographic characteristics describing the residents and DCW population in each home, and residents' health problems and functional status.

Community-level characteristics include measures of local economic conditions where each home is located and serve as proxies for alternative employment opportunities. These variables are measured at the county level and include county unemployment rates, per capita income, the combined number of AL and nursing home beds in each of the 25 counties represented, and facilities' geographic location (rural versus urban). Sources of these data include the U.S. Census Bureau (2000), Georgia Department of Labor (2006), and Georgia Office of Regulatory Services (2006).

Quantitative Data Analysis

The 370 staff members in our sample are nested within 45 ALFs. In Chapter 9, which focuses on individual- and facility-level factors that predict staff turnover, we use hierarchical linear modeling (HLM), a statistical procedure that allows the simultaneous modeling of group- and individual-level variances. In Chapter 8, which focuses on individual-level predictors of staff satisfaction, we use a simpler and more straightforward regression-based technique in Stata 10.0 (StataCorp, 2007) referred to as the Huber-White Sandwich estimator, which takes into account the correlation of error terms between residents within the same facility to obtain robust standard errors (Rogers, 1993; Williams, 2000). Both techniques avoid violating the assumption of independence of observations, a violation that traditional regression techniques commit in analyzing hierarchical data (Kreft & De Leeuw, 2006). Quantitative analysis also includes standard descriptive statistical procedures (i.e., frequencies, measures of central tendency, variability, and bivariate correlation).

Qualitative Data Analysis

We used the *grounded theory* approach (Charmaz, 2006; Strauss, 1987; Strauss & Corbin, 1998) to analyze all types of qualitative data—type 2 interview transcripts, open-ended responses from type 1 interviews, and field notes from participant observation. This approach consists of a constant comparative method of inquiry whereby data collection, hypothesis generation, and analysis occur simultaneously. Thus, throughout the project, collection of interview and observation data was informed by concepts and hypotheses generated from ongoing analysis. A major advantage of grounded theory analysis is its flexibility to address new findings and modify assumptions made a priori by the investigators. This process involves two analytic procedures: coding and memoing.

Analytic codes are similar to subject areas on which the study participants elaborate. In the first stage of coding, data were examined for emergent themes or concepts based on both questions asked by the investigators and issues raised by the informants, an analytic process called *open coding.* As concepts were identified, they were grouped into categories in terms of their properties and dimensions. Many of these initial codes were closely linked to our three research aims. For example, when referring to the meaning of job satisfaction, codes that emerged were quality of workplace relationships, task configuration, and workload levels. As new themes emerged, codes were modified, collapsed, or dropped.

In the next stage of coding—*axial coding*—we related initial categories to other categories, or *subcategories,* through what Strauss and Corbin (1998) refer to as a *paradigm model.* This model links categories in a set of relationships denoting causal conditions, context, intervening conditions, action/interaction strategies, and consequences. For example, our analysis showed that type of resident-staff relationship was influenced by task configuration and that the co-occurrence of these two categories related to other factors, such as length of employment and training. As part of axial coding we compared data across participants and homes, using analytic diagrams and charts to facilitate analysis. In the final stage of coding—*selective coding*—major categories are organized around central explanatory concept or *core category* (Strauss & Corbin, 1998). Specific analyses and core categories are explained further in chapters 4, 5, 6, 7, 10, and 11.

In the memoing process, we recorded three types of notes: observational, methodological, and theoretical (Muller, 1995). Methodological notes helped track problems, changes in research procedures, and issues regarding relationships with participants. Theoretical notes, which contain insights, observations, interpretations, and questions about the data, facilitated linkage between data collection and analysis and helped identify recurring patterns and themes in the data (Strauss & Corbin, 1998). At the end of study of each

facility, researchers prepared a summary memo that listed tentative conclusions and insights about the site. The research team met regularly throughout
the project to discuss ongoing analysis, which facilitated the identification of
missing themes to be pursued in subsequent interviews.

Because of the large volume of data, we used a software package for qualitative data management (Ethnograph 5.0). Ethnograph is designed to analyze
narrative text by producing counts and frequencies of textual occurrences that
assist the researcher in coding and by further identifying interrelated occurrences of coded categories (Walker, 1993).

Characteristics of Study Participants

Here we present selected characteristics of study participants: facilities and
direct care and administrative staff. The following chapters present more detailed and in-depth descriptions.

Sample Characteristics

Selected characteristics of sample ALFs according to size (small, medium,
and large) are shown in Table 3.1. More than half (67%) are corporately owned,
and the large majority (87%) are for profit and (82%) are freestanding. In the
majority of them (76%), all or most resident rooms or apartments are private
(rather than shared). Two are affiliated with a nursing home, and six have
independent living apartments on the same campus. As a group, large homes
have been in business less time than either the small or medium homes. The
two longest-tenure homes (25 years) are in the metropolitan Atlanta area. One
is African American–owned, is for-profit, and has 24 residents; the other is
nonprofit, has a Jewish affiliation, and has 33 residents. Sixty-six percent are
located in urban areas, including all the large homes. Just under half of small
homes (44%) are in rural locales, with four (9%) in completely rural areas or
with populations less than 2,500.

The mean minimum and maximum facility fees are $1,763 and $2,859,
respectively; as shown in Table 3.1, fees tend to increase with facility size.
Only nine (50%) of the small homes participate in one or more of the Medicaid-waiver programs that subsidize fees for low-income residents. The mean
minimum and maximum hourly pay rates for DCWs are $7.13 and $9.83,
respectively; like fees, rates also increase with facility size. Opportunities for

Table 3.1   Facility Characteristics, by Facility Size

Characteristic	Small (N=18)	Medium (N=13)	Large (N=14)	Total (N=45)
Corporate (%)	50	92	79	67
For-profit (%)	78	77	93	87
Median tenure (in years)	7.2	9.2	6	104
Urban (%)	56	77	100	66
Mean fee (min/max)	$1,498–1,983	$1,772–2,803	$2,097–4,037	$1,763–2,859
Mean salary (min/max)	$6.63–8.39	$6.94–9.65	$7.91–11.74	$7.13–9.83
Medical insurance (%)	22	77	100	62
DCU (%)	0	31	77	31
LPN/RN on staff (%)	39	23	100	53
Mean turnover rate	117	55	63	82

health care benefits varied similarly. Only 22 percent of small homes offered medical insurance to employees, compared with 77 percent of medium homes and 100 percent of large homes.

Almost a third (31%) of the medium and a little over three-fourths (77%) of the large ALFs have special dementia care units (DCUs). Two of the large homes are dementia-specific. A little over half (53%) of sample ALFs have either an LPN or RN on staff, including all the large homes. Facility turnover rates range from a low of 0 to a high of 333 percent, with a mean of 82 percent and a median of 63 percent. Turnover rates were calculated based on the number of staff who had left during the 12 months before the study period in each home.

Table 3.2 shows selected characteristics of the all residents and DCWs in the sample ALFs. These data were derived from reports of facility directors. With the exception of two small homes and one medium home, the majority of the resident population of sample ALFs is female. Most residents are white. In only two small homes was the majority of the population nonwhite. Resident care needs varied widely across individual ALFs, from a low of no residents needing assistance with three or more activities of daily living (ADLs) to a high of 100 percent. Overall, 42 percent required this level of care. Only a minority of residents needed assistance in the form of one- or two-person transfers. The proportion of residents diagnosed with dementia varied similarly across homes, with a range from 0 to 100 percent. The proportion with dementia

Table 3.2 Facility Sample: Resident and Staff Characteristics, by Size (in percentages)

Characteristic	Small (N=18)	Medium (N=13)	Large (N=14)	Total (N=45)
Resident Census	346	427	919	1,692
Female	84	74	80	76
White	93	94	97	95
Need assistance with 3+ ADLs	38	37	46	42
Have dementia	38	39	50	47
Need 1-person transfer	8	11	15	13
Need 2-person transfer	4	3	4	4
65+	85	93	99	94
DCW Census	143	177	397	717
White	70	46	25	39
CNA	31	31	49	42

for the sample as a whole is 47 percent. As expected, the large majority of the residents in the sample are over the age of 65.

Unlike the residents, a minority of DCWs in the sample homes are white (39%), although the proportion of white staff decreased with size (70% in small, 46% in medium, and 25% in large). Differences by facility size were largely a factor of geographic location. Rural locations were found only for small homes, and, although 3 of the 18 small homes have no white staff, the majority of staff are white in 13 homes and all are white in 5 of the 13. Overall, 42 percent of DCWs are certified nursing assistants (CNAs).

Characteristics of Interview Participants

Table 3.3 shows the personal characteristics of the DCWs who participated in either type 1 or type 2 interviews. Almost all (99%) are female, 61 percent are nonwhite, and 82 percent are native-born. The largest foreign-born group comes from Africa (10%). The large majority of the DCWs are between the ages of 25 and 54 (71%), with a mean of 40 years. The majority (61%) are unmarried, and a little over half (53%) have children living at home; 85% provide support to someone else, either living in or out of their home. Most (84%) had at least a high school degree or the equivalency, and 43 percent have current CNA training. Participants have been working on average in the LTC field for 7.8 years and in their current facility for 2.5 years.

Table 3.4 shows the race and nativity of DCW participants according to location and size of the facility where they work. As shown, the majority of

Table 3.3   Personal Characteristics of Direct Care Staff (N=400)

Characteristic	%	Characteristic	%
Gender		Marital Status	
Female	99	Married	39
Race		Never married	31
Black	57	Divorced	19
White	39	Separated	7
Other	4	Widowed	4
Country of Origin		Dependents	
United States	82	Children living at home	53
Caribbean	4	Support others outside home	32
Africa	10	Education	
Other	4	Less than high school	16
Age		HS diploma / GED	47
18–25	17	Trade school	8
26–35	23	Some college / assoc. degree	24
36–45	22	College degree	5
46–55	25	CNA training	43
56–65	11	Employment History (mean	
65+	2	number of years)	
Mean	40	LTC (± SD)	7.8 ± 7.4
		Facility (± SD)	2.5 ± 2.7

nonwhite DCWs work in areas 1 and 2 and in the medium and large facilities. With respect to nativity, the majority of foreign-born DCWs work in area-1 homes and large homes. All except one of the DCW participants in the small homes are native-born.

Table 3.5 shows personal characteristics of the 44 administrative staff who were interviewed. Like DCWs, they are predominantly female (70%), though less so. A higher proportion are white (87%), and they are older, with a mean age of 47 years. As would be expected, administrators are better educated than are DCWs. With respect to LTC training, 14 percent of administrators have CNA certificates, 9 percent are LPNs, 17 percent are RNs, and 16 percent have an AL administrator license. Most have considerable LTC experience. Although one has been in the field for only 8 months, average time in the field was about 13 years. Length of time working in AL is somewhat less, with a mean of 8.7 years. Facility tenure was even lower on average, with a mean of about 6 years. Experience as an administrator or manager ranges from 5 months to 32 years, with a mean of about 11 years.

Table 3.4   Race/Country of Origin of DCWs (%), by Facility Area/Size (N=400)

	Area 1 (N=158)	Area 2 (N=112)	Area 3 (N=130)	Small (N=87)	Medium (N=111)	Large (N=202)
Race						
Black/African American	77	63	27	31	52	70
White/European American	19	34	68	63	44	26
Other	4	3	5	6	4	4
Country of Origin						
United States	60	98	95	99	89	71
Caribbean	9	0	1	0	5	5
Africa	24	0	1	0	5	17
Other	7	2	3	1	1	7

Georgia Assisted Living Facilities in the National Context

Facilities and Residents

As noted, AL is defined broadly in Georgia, and the ALFs represented in this study include a wide range of sizes and types. Based on their characteristics, they may be categorized according to various classificatory schemes described in the literature. Using an empirically derived typology, Zimmerman and colleagues (Zimmerman & Sloane, 2007; Zimmerman et al., 2001) categorize facilities as *small, traditional,* or *new model,* based on various structural characteristics, including size, tenure, and resident profiles. Our sample includes only homes with 16 or more beds, and the majority (76%) can be classified as *new model,* with approximately one-third of the small and medium homes and only one of the large homes falling into the *traditional* type. None fits the criteria for a *small* category, which refers to homes with fewer than 16 beds. The facilities in our sample also fit the broad inclusionary criteria for AL used by Hawes and colleagues in the only existing national AL studies (Hawes et al., 1999, 2003).

With respect to regulation, Georgia ALFs would fall under Mollica's (2007) *umbrella model,* which allows one set of regulations to cover two or more kinds of housing or service arrangements. In Georgia, all sizes and types of facilities are licensed under one category and are called *personal care homes* in statute.

Table 3.5   Personal Characteristics of Administrators
(N=44)

Characteristic	%
Gender	
Female	70
Race	
Black	11
White	87
Other	2
Mean age (± SD)	47 ± 10.86
Education	
Less than high school	5
HS diploma / GED	12
Trade school	5
Some college / assoc. degree	33
College degree	22
Some postgraduate	2
Graduate degree	21
Long-term care training	
CNA training	14
LPN	9
RN	17
AL administrator license	16
Employment history (mean number of years)	
LTC (± SD)	13.2 ± 9.23
AL (± SD)	8.7 ± 6.22
Facility (± SD)	6.3 ± 6.17
Administrative experience (± SD)	11.2 ± 8.46

Most ALFs are paid for privately, with rates varying widely across sizes and types. The National Center for Assisted Living (2001) reports monthly private-pay fees ranging from $1,000 to $3,500, with an average of $1,873. A Metlife Mature Market Institute (2008) national survey found an average monthly base cost of $3,031 for 2008. Fees in our sample of Georgia ALFs are comparable to those reported in the literature. In 2004, 43 states, including Georgia, had some type of Medicaid-reimbursed services in ALFs, but a relatively small number of beneficiaries are served in this setting—about 102,000 (Mollica, Johnson-Lamarche, & O'Keeffe, 2005). Only three states, Colorado, Oregon, and Washington, have shifted public resources from nursing homes to AL. Only a fifth of homes in our study (all small) participated in a Medicaid-waiver program.

Residents in Georgia ALFs are similar to those throughout the United States described in other studies: the majority are white, elderly, and female, and a substantial proportion require assistance with three or more ADLs (Assisted Living Federation of America, 2006; Hawes et al., 1999; Morgan, Gruber-Baldini, & Magaziner, 2001). In our study sample, 47 percent of residents are reported to have dementia. Other studies show that close to 50 percent of AL residents have Alzheimer disease or another type of dementia (Gruber-Baldini, Boustani, Sloane, & Zimmerman, 2004; Sloane, Zimmerman, & Ory, 2001). These residents are cared for in a variety of AL settings that provide dementia-specialized services, including freestanding dementia-specific facilities and secured DCUs that operate within larger ALFs. The number of ALFs with DCUs nationwide is unknown, but one of the largest estimates comes from a survey in Massachusetts (Stocker & Silverman, 1996) showing that 18 percent of ALFs offered specialized dementia care (Sloane et al., 2001). In Georgia, eight ALFs are freestanding, dementia-specific facilities, and 32 percent of ALFs with 16+ beds include a DCU (Georgia Chapter of the Alzheimer's Association, 2005). In our sample, 31 percent of facilities have a DCU, and two are dementia-specific.

Staff

Hawes, Phillips, and Rose (2000) reported the most comprehensive data about AL staff. These data come from a national sample of 569 staff members and represent 41 percent of all ALFs nationwide that meet the researchers' criteria for high-service or high-privacy facilities. Slightly over half (51%) are DCWs. In this sample, 97 percent are female, 68 percent are white, 15 percent had not completed high school, 75 percent had previous LTC experience, and 52 percent had worked in the facility two or more years. No AL national data are available that report characteristics of DCWs separate from other types of workers. Recent national data, however, for nursing homes show that nursing assistants in this setting are predominantly female (92%) and middle-aged, with a median education level of high school graduate or GED; 39 percent are black, and 26 percent have never been married (Squillace, Harris-Kojetin, Rosenoff, & Remsburg, 2006). The workers described in both the AL and nursing national data are similar to the DCWs in our sample, although a higher percentage of Georgia staff are nonwhite (61%), which is not unexpected in a southern state; 18 percent are foreign-born. Other data indicate that DCWs in LTC settings in the United States more and more are women of color, both foreign- and native-born (Redfoot & Houser, 2005).

In Hawes and colleagues' national study of ALFs with more than 10 beds (Hawes et al., 1999), 71 percent of facilities had either an RN or LPN working full- or part-time. In our sample, 53 percent of homes overall and 100 percent of large homes have a licensed nurse. No data are available about AL administrators.

Conclusion

The participants in our study—both facilities and DCWs—represent the range of ALFs and DCWs found throughout the United States. In the chapters that follow, we will provide in-depth information about these workers, their experiences, and the diverse workplaces they inhabit.

REFERENCES

Assisted Living Federation of America. 2006. *Assisted living: What is it? Facts, and definitions.* Retrieved September 20, 2005, from www.alfa.org/public/articles/details.cfm.
Ball, M. M., Perkins, M. M., Whittington, F. J., Hollingsworth, C., King, S. V., & Combs, B. L. 2005. *Communities of care: Assisted living for African American elders.* Baltimore: Johns Hopkins University Press.
Ball, M. M., Whittington, F. J., Perkins, M. M., Patterson, V., Hollingsworth, C., King, S. V., et al. 2000. Quality of life in assisted living facilities: Viewpoints of residents. *Journal of Applied Gerontology* 19, 304–25.
Balzer, W. K., Kihm, J. A., Smith, P. C., Irwin, J. L., Bachiochi, P. D., Robie, C., et al. 1997. In J. Stanton & C. Crossley (Eds.), *Users' manual for the Job Descriptive Index (JDI; 1997 Revision) and the Job in General scales.* Bowling Green, OH: Bowling Green State University.
———. 2000. In J. Stanton & C. Crossley (Eds.), *Users' manual for the Job Descriptive Index (JDI; 1997 Revision) and the Job in General scales.* Bowling Green, OH: Bowling Green State University.
Charmaz, K. 2006. *Constructing grounded theory: A practical guide through qualitative analysis.* Thousand Oaks, CA: Sage Publications.
Cohen, J. 1988. *Statistical power analysis for the behavioral sciences.* Hillsdale, NJ: Lawrence Erlbaum Associates.
Creswell, J. 2003. *Research design: Qualitative, quantitative, and mixed methods approaches.* Thousand Oaks, CA: Sage Publications.
Georgia Chapter of the Alzheimer's Association. 2005. Unpublished data.
Georgia Department of Labor. 2006. Unpublished data.
Georgia Office of Regulatory Services. 2006. Unpublished data.
———. 2007. Unpublished data.
Georgia State Health Planning Agency. 1993. *Personal care homes in Georgia.* Atlanta: State Health Planning Agency.

Groger, L., & Straker, J. 2002. Counting and recounting: Approaches to combining quantitative and qualitative methods. In G. Rowles & N. Schoenberg (Eds.), *Qualitative Gerontology* (pp. 179–200). New York: Springer.

Gruber-Baldini, A. L., Boustani, M., Sloane, P. D., & Zimmerman, S. 2004. Behavioral symptoms in residential care/assisted living facilities: Prevalence, risk factors, and medication management. *Journal of the American Geriatrics Society* 52, 1610–1717.

Hawes, C., Phillips, C. D., & Rose, M. 2000. *High service or high privacy assisted living facilities, their residents and staff: Results from a national survey.* Washington, DC: U.S. Department of Health and Human Services.

Hawes, C., Philips, C. D., Rose, M., Holan, S., & Sherman, M. 2003. A national study of assisted living facilities. *The Gerontologist* 43, 875–82.

Hawes, C., Rose, M., & Phillips, C. 1999. *A national study of assisted living for the frail elderly: Results of a national survey of facilities.* Beachwood, OH: Myers Research Institute.

Johnson, G., & Johnson, W. 2000. Perceived overqualification and dimensions of job satisfaction: A longitudinal analysis. *Journal of Psychology* 134, 537–55.

Kiyak, H. A., Namazi, K. H., & Kahana, E. F. 1997. Job commitment and turnover among women working in facilities serving older persons. *Research on Aging* 19, 223–46.

Kreft, I., & De Leeuw, J. 2006. *Introducing multilevel modeling.* Thousand Oaks, CA: Sage Publications.

Lambert, E., Hogan, N., & Barton, S. 2001. The impact of job satisfaction on turnover intent: A test of a structural measurement model using a national sample of workers. *Social Science Journal* 38, 233–50.

Metlife Mature Market Institute. 2008. *The Metlife market survey of nursing home and assisted living costs.* Westport, CT: Metlife Mature Market Institute. Retrieved June 1, 2009, from www.metlife.com/assets/cao/mmi/publications/studies/mmi-studies-2008-nhal-costs.pdf.

Mollica, R. 2007. *Residential care and assisted living compendium: 2007.* Retrieved February 2, 2009, from http://aspe.hhs.gov/daltcp/reports/2007/07alcom1.htm#box1-1.

Mollica, R., Johnson-Lamarche, H. S., & O'Keeffe, J. 2005. *State residential care and assisted living policy, 2004.* Portland, ME: National Academy for State Health Policy.

Morgan, D. 1998. Practical strategies for combining qualitative and quantitative methods: Applications to health research. *Qualitative Health Research* 8, 362–76.

Morgan, L. A., Gruber-Baldini, A. L., & Magaziner, J. 2001. Resident characteristics. In S. Zimmerman, P. D. Sloane, & J. K. Eckert (Eds.), *Assisted living: Needs, practices, and policies in residential care for the elderly* (pp. 144–72). Baltimore: Johns Hopkins University Press.

Muller, J. 1995. Care of the dying by physicians-in-training: An example of participant observation research. *Research on Aging* 17, 65–87.

National Center for Assisted Living. 2001. *Facts and trends: The assisted living source book, 2001.* Washington, DC: American Health Care Association.

Patton, M. 2002. *Qualitative research and evaluation methods.* Thousand Oaks, CA: Sage Publications.

Redfoot, D., & Houser, A. 2005. "We shall travel on": Quality of care, economic development, and the international migration of long-term care workers. Washington, DC: AARP Public Policy Institute.

Rogers, W. H. 1993. Regression standard errors in clustered samples. *Stata Technical Bulletin* 13, 19–23.

Sankar, A., & Gubrium, J. F. 1994. Introduction. In J. F. Gubrium & A. Sankar (Eds.), *Qualitative methods in aging research* (pp. vii–xvii). Thousand Oaks, CA: Sage Publications.

Sloane, P. D., Zimmerman, S., & Ory, M. G. 2001. Care for persons with dementia. In S. Zimmerman, P. D. Sloane, & J. K. Eckert (Eds.), *Assisted living: Needs, practices, and policies in residential care for the elderly* (pp. 242–70). Baltimore: Johns Hopkins University Press.

Spybrook, J., Raudenbush, S. W., Liu, X., & Congdon, R. 2006. Optimal Design. Retrieved September 14, 2007, from http://sitemaker.umich.edu/group-based.

Squillace, M. R., Harris-Kojetin, L. D., Rosenoff, E., & Remsburg, R. E. 2006. *A profile of certified nursing assistants working in US nursing homes: Results from the 2004 national nursing assistant survey.* Paper presented at the 59th annual meeting of the Gerontological Society of America, Dallas, TX.

StataCorp. 2007. *Stata Statistical Software: Release 10.* College Station, TX: Statacorp LP.

Stocker, K. B., & Silverman, N. M. 1996. Assisted living residences in Massachusetts: How ready and willing are they to serve people with Alzheimer disease or a related disorder? *American Journal of Alzheimer's Disease* 11, 28–38.

Strauss, A. 1987. *Qualitative analysis for social scientists.* New York: Cambridge University Press.

Strauss, A., & Corbin, J. 1998. *The basics of qualitative research: Grounded theory procedures and techniques.* Thousand Oaks, CA: Sage Publications.

U.S. Census Bureau. 2000. *State and county quick facts.* Washington, DC: U.S. Census Bureau.

Walker, B. 1993. Computer analysis of qualitative data: A comparison of three packages. *Qualitative Health Research* 3, 91–111.

Wenger, C. 1999. Advantages gained by combining qualitative and quantitative data in a longitudinal study. *Journal of Aging Studies* 13, 369–76.

Williams, R. L. 2000. A note on robust variance estimation for cluster-correlated data. *Biometrics* 56, 645–46.

Zimmerman, S., & Sloane, P. 2007. Definition and classification of assisted living. *The Gerontologist* 47 (Special Issue 3), 33–39.

Zimmerman, S., Sloane, P., Eckert, J., Buie, V., Walsh, J., Hebel, J., et al. 2001. An overview of the Collaborative Studies of Long-Term Care. In S. Zimmerman, P. Sloane, & J. Eckert (Eds.), *Assisted living: Needs, practices and policies in residential care for the elderly* (pp. 117–43). Baltimore: Johns Hopkins University Press.

CHAPTER FOUR

Pathways to Caregiving

Michael J. Lepore, Ph.D.
Mary M. Ball, Ph.D.
Molly M. Perkins, Ph.D.
Candace L. Kemp, Ph.D.

The entry of workers into caregiving professions is critical to the existence and quality of long-term care (LTC), including assisted living (AL), but few studies address individuals' motivations for care work (Moody & Pesut, 2006). This chapter examines direct care workers' (DCWs) motivations for employment in LTC, and specifically in AL, and depicts the common pathways to these caregiving professions. Understanding motivations for, and pathways to, care work is integral to understanding why workers choose and remain in AL.

Motivations, including motivations for employment, generally have been categorized as intrinsic or extrinsic, that is, as internally or externally driven (Ryan & Deci, 2000). Intrinsic motivation, Ryan and Deci (2000, p. 55) explain, "refers to doing something because it is inherently interesting or enjoyable," whereas extrinsic motivation "refers to doing something because it leads to a separable outcome." The dichotomous intrinsic/extrinsic definition of motivations, however, has been challenged on several fronts, particularly regarding care work. Rather than identifying motivations as either intrinsic or extrinsic, some social theorists have come to define motivation more broadly, including variables such as culture and group social norms (Markus & Kitayama, 1991; Scheuer, 2000). Because workers differ in what they value and values are culturally determined (not universal), motivators are often "fuzzy" and neither clearly intrinsic or extrinsic (Kreps, 1997, p. 361). In this chapter, we examine personal, cultural, institutional, and societal factors that influence motivations for care work. Findings contribute to an understanding of the nature of motivations for employment, especially LTC employment, and provide guidance for policies and practices to support the entry of workers into LTC. Our two key aims are (1) understanding DCWs' pathways to, and motivations for, employment in LTC, AL, and their current AL workplaces and (2) understanding how workers' motivations relate to individual-, facility-, and community-level factors.

Methods

We use a grounded theory approach (described in Chapter 3) to address our research aims. Qualitative data for this chapter are drawn from open-ended questions in standardized surveys, which were performed with 370 care workers, and from qualitative interviews, which were conducted with 41 care workers. Eleven workers participated in both types of interviews; the total number of interview participants is 400. Methods for selecting interview participants are described in Chapter 3.

Surveys asked open-ended questions addressing workers' motivations for employment in LTC, AL, and their specific AL facilities (ALFs); their tenure in LTC and in their current ALFs; their education and LTC training; and their job immediately prior to their current position and reasons for leaving. Qualitative interviews provided similar types of data, but in greater depth, and explored DCWs' life histories, family backgrounds, informal caregiving experiences, educational and career opportunities over the life course, and current and past jobs.

Profile of Direct Care Workers

Overall, the sample of 400 DCWs is socioeconomically disadvantaged, as illustrated by characteristics of their current LTC jobs as well as by their life histories. Across the sample, the median hourly pay is $8, and the median number of hours worked per week is 36, resulting in an average annual net pay of approximately $16,000. Almost half (46%) of the 370 survey participants stated that they wanted to work more hours than offered at their facilities, and 24 percent of the full sample of 400 workers hold one or two additional jobs. Among the DCWs who have additional jobs, over half (53%) have another position caring for older adults. These second LTC jobs are split fairly evenly between AL, nursing home, and in-home care. Workers with a second job outside LTC hold positions in a variety of female-dominated fields, including child care or other health services (15%), secretarial work (6%), retail (3%), domestic labor (3%), and food service (2%).

The sample's low pay is grounded primarily in broad gender inequalities. Almost all (99%) of the 400 DCWs are female, echoing gender roles in family life, wherein women historically have been the primary caregivers. Indeed, our qualitative data show that many workers in our sample also are experienced as caregivers in family life, and many associate care work with family caregiving. Furthermore, the majority (61%) are racial minorities, which reflects the broader concentration of minorities in low-paying jobs.

Most DCWs in our sample also have limited educations. Although the sample includes a few outliers with college degrees, the majority (63%) have a high school education or less. From our qualitative interviews, we know that for many workers their family backgrounds, including their parents' employment and financial resources and sometimes their parents' or grandparents' care needs, limited their educational options. In this chapter, we illustrate how these life course factors, together with broad community trends, influence their LTC pathways.

A substantial majority of the 400 study participants (65%) had previous jobs in other LTC settings. Those without prior LTC experience included individuals who currently were working for their first employer and those employed in other health care settings, child care, retail, food service, manufacturing, and clerical and domestic work. Table 4.1 shows DCWs' jobs immediately prior to their current AL job, their tenures in LTC, and their tenures in their facilities. More than half (53%) came directly to their current positions from another LTC job. Overall, 60 percent of DCWs had been employed in LTC for over four years and 35 percent for more than 10 years, with a median LTC tenure of about five years, demonstrating considerable LTC experience among the group. In contrast, tenure in specific facilities was much shorter: 80 percent of DCWs had been employed in their facilities for four years or less; just 2 percent had tenures of more than 10 years; and the median tenure was only 18 months.

Below we present three case studies to provide a more in-depth view of DCWs' pathways to LTC. The cases exemplify the range of workers and employment histories in our sample, and their stories provide context for the following discussion of how and why these participants came to work in LTC.

Table 4.1   Workers' Prior Employment, LTC Tenure,
and Facility Tenure (N=400)

Characteristic	%
Employment Immediately before Current AL Job	
Elder care	53
AL	19
Nursing home	19
Private home	11
Other (including day care or senior center)	4
Child care or other health services	15
Assembly line or processing work	9
Retail	7
Food service	7
Domestic work	3
LTC Tenure	
Less than 1 year	15
1–4 years	25
4–10 years	25
10–20 years	35
Facility Tenure	
Less than 1 year	40
1–4 years	40
4–10 years	18
10–51 years	2

Vera

Vera is a 50-year-old African American mother, grandmother, and wife. Like 20 percent of the sample, she came to her current ALF with no care work experience. As a child, Vera lived in a small town in Georgia with her parents and six older siblings. For more than 25 years, her mother worked in a poultry plant and her father worked in a mill. Vera attended school up to the 12th grade but did not graduate from high school. Following in her parents' footsteps, Vera went to work in a mill, where she stayed for 29 years. She left the mill because of the social stress: "There were a lot of clashes and you kind of get burnt out on stuff like that. You get tired of the bickering." Not one to job-hop, Vera thought long and hard about leaving this job: "I am not a person to go from job to job. If I am on a job, I like to try and stay on that job. My mom stayed on her job a long time and my dad did too. . . . At first I was kind of like, 'am I doing the right thing?' I said, 'There are other jobs but I will wait until I find the right job and feel like it is the right job for me.' So that is what I did." For Vera, the "right" job was in AL.

Some of Vera's co-workers at the mill had already taken jobs in AL, illustrating a common transition among the DCWs in our sample from industrial labor to care work. Vera, however, first took a job driving people to dialysis appointments, but after a short while she grew dissatisfied with the job and the danger she faced driving. At this point, Vera found a newspaper ad for a care worker position at her current ALF. Though Vera had no formal care experience, she cared for her mother in the past, and the administrator hired her on a trial basis at $6 per hour. Now, four years later and earning $8.10 per hour, Vera has established a history of job stability, which she intends to maintain: "I hope to be here until I retire."

Claudia

Claudia, 57 years old and white, has 35 years of tenure in LTC. She grew up near the southern Georgia town where she currently lives and works. Coming from a modest background, Claudia graduated from high school but pursued no further education. From childhood, she looked forward to a career caring for older adults: "I always wanted to work with elderly people, there was something about it. . . . It is just, I don't know, something about elderly people." Claudia's first job at age 20 was caring for a lady from her church: "She fell and broke a hip and I went to her house every day and stayed like eight hours and took care of her and this went on for pretty much close to a year." With this job, Claudia began her caregiving career. Her LTC experiences include nursing home, private home, and, now for six years, AL settings.

Jonee

Jonee, like 18 percent of the sample, is an immigrant. Born in Nigeria, she first moved to the United States and Georgia when she was 20 years old. Now, five years later, Jonee is in college studying nursing and health care management. Her long-term goal is nursing, and she considers direct care work an important component of her professional training that provides her with a grounded understanding of health care: "It gives you a better view of things. If you are on top, you can see everything, but you can't see what is going on *really*. You can only see so far."

Jonee's first job was in a restaurant nearby her home, but after six months, she took a DCW position in an ALF. There, Jonee completed certified nursing assistant (CNA) training because her employer paid CNAs at a higher rate. During training, Jonee interned in a nursing home, and her dislike for this setting strengthened her appreciation for AL: "When I got my CNA we had to go to a nursing home to do an internship; it was not a good site. I didn't want to work in a nursing home. It was too much for me. . . . I like this [AL] better; it is more calm and more like a home."

After nine months in her first ALF, Jonee left owing to personnel changes that negatively impacted the social environment: "She [manager] fired the wrong people and it was not a happy place to work. I gave them my two-weeks notice." Jonee then found her current AL employer: "They had someone, as I was leaving the job, [who] told me about this place so I applied and they called me." Now, three years later, Jonee earns $9 per hour.

Motivations for Employment in Long-Term Care

Our grounded theory analysis reveals three primary categories of motivation for employment in LTC: *moral, material,* and *professional.* Morally motivated DCWs (67% of our sample of 400) identified altruistic values for helping others, particularly older adults. In contrast, workers who were motivated by material concerns (33% of the sample) commonly identified financial need as their primary concern. DCWs motivated by professional goals (7% of the sample) emphasized higher career aspirations and considered LTC a stepping-stone to achieving these goals. We also found that for 33 percent of workers social network members who served as informants and employment advisers acted as conduits to LTC by channeling workers' moral, material, and professional motivations.

Moral values, material needs, professional goals, and social networks are not independent motivators. Rather, these motivators interact, and all are influenced by multiple community, institutional, and individual factors. Societal gender norms about caregiving route women to care work (often via family care), as illustrated by the almost total dominance of women in our sample. Individuals' job choices also are constrained by the options for employment in each community. At the institutional level, the low criteria for employment (education, training, experience) in LTC, and particularly in AL, also influence motivations. At the individual level, DCWs' religious and family backgrounds guide their moral values and motivations; education and age influence their professional goals and motivations; and family care responsibilities and employment histories affect their material needs and motivations. Additionally,

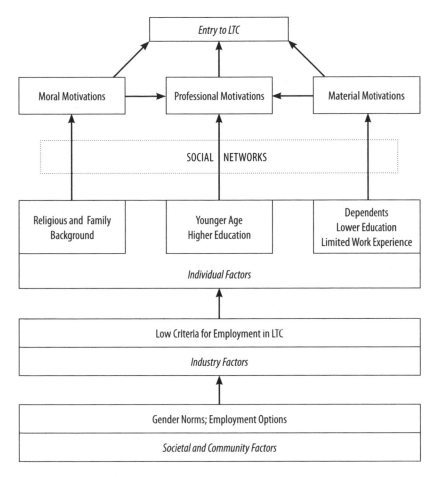

Figure 4.1. Motivations for Employment in Long-Term Care

more than a third (35%) of workers reported multiple motivators. For instance, a worker may be morally *and* professionally motivated to enter LTC and may be encouraged by her social network. In the following pages, we examine each type of motivation and illuminate how it is influenced by various factors. Figure 4.1 depicts the relationship between community-, institutional-, and individual-level factors and workers' motivations.

Moral Motivations

A large majority of DCWs (67%) reported moral motivations for LTC employment; this group included workers of varying age, education, nativity, race, and gender. We identified four subtypes of moral motivations: (1) valuing care for older adults; (2) valuing care in general; (3) attributing familial meanings to care work; and (4) attributing religious meanings to care work.

Most morally motivated workers (59%) reported valuing care for elders, whether or not the older persons are family. For example, Claudia wanted to take care of older adults since she was a child. Other workers who value caring for older adults said things like "I love to take care of old people"; "I think it is a good work to work with elderly. I care about them"; or "I love working with older adults. I love to communicate with elderly and be with them. I like the elderly in general." Expressing a broader moral view, 29 percent of morally motivated DCWs came to LTC because they value care in general, not specifically elder care. Illustrating this moral motivation, one worker simply explained, "I like taking care of people."

Family values for care and caregiving relationships were reported by 16 percent of morally motivated DCWs. Many believe their relationships with LTC residents resemble family ties. One of these workers explained, "I like to work with older adults; the residents are like my family." Vera similarly explained, "I know the residents are not my family, but I still kind of look at them as family. They are older people and they have children and when their children aren't here we have to be children to them . . . like they are your mama or grandmama, in a sense."

Some morally motivated DCWs previously had provided family care. Mandi, a 33-year-old who has been employed in LTC since age 18, chose the field this way: "I used to help my grandmother, which made me feel good since I was helping." In contrast, other workers' motives related to *lack* of opportunity to perform family caregiving. For example, Sheryl, aged 22, is unable to help her own grandmother: "I have a grandmother and I can't really take care of her. I like working with the elderly, help them, the last few years they have, to live peacefully." Further strengthening the likeness between family care and LTC employment, some DCWs actually care for family in a LTC facility. An example is Shelly, a 23-year-old whose grandmother lives in her current ALF: "My grandmother lived here for four years and passed away here—[I came to work here] so I could get closer to her."

Finally, some morally motivated DCWs (7%) reported a religious influence, most often describing care work as a "calling" or a "blessing." Overall, religious beliefs influence workers' care motivations by providing them with an understanding of care work as divinely inspired. One African American woman explained, "I am a Christian and I live for help. This is like a mission for me. I help with my heart." Mary, who is white, said, "This is just something God sent for me to do. I was one of the blessed ones. Not everyone can do this type of job."

Material Motivations

Overall, DCWs have limited educations, few employment options, and scarce economic resources. Many work in LTC simply because they need a job. In fact, 33 percent of workers expressed such material motivations, reflecting the basic need for income, not a specific desire for caregiving. As with moral motivations, material motivations were found among a diverse group of workers, and they were influenced by multiple factors at the individual, industry, and community levels.

Workers' socioeconomic conditions are the primary influence on material motivations for LTC employment. Generally, material motivations originate, or become activated, at a point of increased financial need. For 9 percent of DCWs, the motivation for LTC employment originated from a job loss. For instance, when Dana lost her housekeeping job, her best employment option was LTC, even at $5.75 per hour: "I got laid off. I did cleaning for school. I heard about this job." Glory's situation was similar: "My other job closed down. I looked in the paper and saw this job. I came down and they hired me." Sherry, a 35-year-old African American woman, described a comparable route: "I came to long-term care only because I lost my other job. . . . I did not have plans to do elder care."

DCWs also experienced heightened economic need after a major change in their families, such as divorce, birth, death, a family member's job loss, or entry into college. An example is Terri, a 63-year-old American Indian, who chose LTC 40 years ago: "I got married and was out of a job. Then my husband and I got a divorce and I couldn't find anything in the field I'd been in [doctors' offices]. I saw an ad and came in." Gayle, 58 years old and white, followed a similar path 20 years ago: "I got into it by accident. My husband lost his job and I had to get the first job, which was at a nursing home." Another woman needed to pay for her daughter's college education. Overall, individuals' family responsibilities were a common influence on their decisions to choose a job in LTC.

Our findings show that the low employment criteria for direct care work (see Chapter 10, this volume) support material motivations. Other jobs with minimal requirements, including food service, domestic work, and retail, compete with the LTC field. Denise, with 13 years' LTC tenure, echoes the experience of many materially motivated DCWs: "Just a way to keep getting paid. My job opportunities are limited." Betty, a 52-year-old African immigrant, provides another example: "When I first moved to New York it was very hard for me to get a job—it wasn't like I wanted it [a LTC job]."

Personal socioeconomic factors also interact with community-level factors, especially the local economy and aging demographics, in directing workers to LTC. Four percent of our sample went directly to LTC from a mill or factory. For example, Peggy, a 43-year-old with a high school education, said, "I was laid off at the mill and there was a job available at a nursing home; I applied to the nursing home and they hired me." Vera's AL employer relies heavily on these displaced workers. "Just about all of us worked at the mill," Vera explained.

Professional Motivations

Just 7 percent of the DCWs in our study chose the field of LTC because they viewed it as a stepping-stone to more professional health care employment, particularly nursing. Jonee represents such workers. She was 25, a CNA, in a nursing program, and believed her LTC experience would be beneficial to a health care career. Like Jonee, the other DCWs with professional motivations are young women with more education. Their median age of 24 is much younger than that for the total sample (median age of 40), and most (79%) have at least two years' college education, compared with only 29 percent of the overall sample. Professionally motivated DCWs also have fewer months' tenure in their facilities than all workers (median of 7 compared with 28) and in the LTC field (15 compared with 60). Conceptual linkages between direct care work, nursing, and the medical field support professional motivations for LTC employment. That is, professionally motivated workers view direct care jobs as low-level positions on a career continuum that leads upward to nursing jobs and medical positions (e.g., medical assistant) that require substantially more training and entail considerably less hands-on contact than do direct care jobs. Amber, 20 years old, white, employed in AL for only five months, and in college studying nursing, illustrates this perception: "I am going into nursing, and I thought long-term care work would have a medical aspect." Julie, one of Amber's co-workers, expressed similar motives: "I want to be a physician's assistant, so this is what I want to do for the experience."

Social Networks

About a third of workers (33%) take jobs in LTC because of recommendations made by their social networks, including friends, family members, casual acquaintances, and professional colleagues. Social networks are conduits to employment in LTC that channel the three primary (moral, material, and professional) motivations. For example, in addition to being morally motivated, 41-year-old Cora was influenced by her sister: "My sister was in elder care. I fell in love with the elders. I was in nursing homes for 10 years." Similarly, Faye, aged 52, was led by her religiosity and her family: "Mother was in it [LTC] and I got in it and stayed. I like dealing with elderly, helping them—I'm a minister on the side too." In contrast, Vette, a 24-year-old African American, went to work in LTC because her social network supported her material motivations. She explained, "At the time, I had no job. My mama started here and they needed someone else. I really needed a job and Mama put me on to it." Social networks also guide professionally motivated workers. Trina, aged 43, explained, "I always wanted to be a nurse. Most of my family is in the nursing field."

Choosing Assisted Living

Our findings show that the three primary motivations for choosing the field of LTC (moral, material, and professional) also operate in DCWs' decisions to choose work in AL rather than in another LTC setting and that social networks have similar influences. AL, though, occupies a special niche within LTC, and certain characteristics of the AL social and physical environment and the content and design of AL care work jobs (see Chapter 5, this volume) separate this setting from either nursing homes or private homes and influence individuals' employment decisions. We found that these organizational-level factors interact with those at the individual level (e.g., education, employment experience, family history, health, values), as well as with certain factors at the community level (e.g., LTC regulations) to influence decision making. In this section we examine how people chose AL within the overall LTC context.

Assisted Living versus Nursing Homes

Differences in four key setting aspects influence workers' decisions to work in AL rather than in nursing homes: (1) residents' functional status; (2) job content and design; (3) employment criteria; and (4) the environment. Essentially, workers choose AL over nursing homes based on the belief that residents are less impaired, the work is easier and more gratifying, the criteria for employment are lower, and the environment is more like home. Figure 4.2 depicts the influence of these organizational (industry and facility) factors on

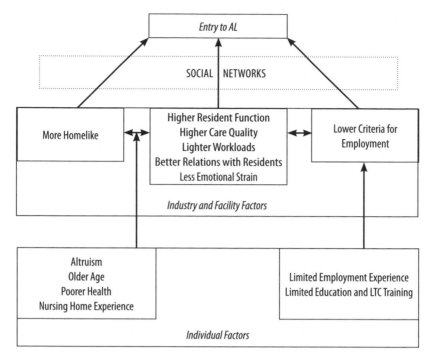

Figure 4.2. Motivations for Employment in Assisted Living versus Nursing Home

the decision-making process. As the figure shows, organizational factors are interactive and are influenced by certain worker characteristics, including age, values, health, employment experience, and education. Below we discuss how these factors act and interact to influence workers' employment decisions.

Residents' Functional Status

A common view expressed by DCWs is that AL residents, compared with residents in nursing homes, are higher functioning, both physically and mentally. We found that these perceptions of residents' functional status underlie workers' motivations for choosing AL. James, one of the six men in our sample, exemplifies this perspective: "I like AL because there is still a lot of stuff that they [the residents] can do, and they still have a lot more freedom than a nursing home. In a nursing home there is more skilled nursing; in AL it is not."

As this quote indicates, a resident's functional status influences *what* care workers do, or the content of their jobs, which, as discussed in Chapter 5 of this volume, primarily involves providing hands-on care, as well as companionship, to residents. Medication management, housekeeping, food service, and other duties revolve around the primary task of resident care. Consequently, differences between residents in AL and in nursing homes, especially differences in functional status, have the potential for fundamentally altering a worker's job experience across these settings. In addition to job content, residents' functional ability impacts job design, including workload, which in turn exerts influence on workers' opportunities for relationship development and the degree of physical and mental stress they experience. Functional status also affects relationship development directly through its effect on communication.

Job Content and Design

About 25 percent of participants chose to work in AL rather than a nursing home because they anticipated the work would be "lighter" or "easier." Such descriptors typically refer to both the type and level of work (see Chapter 5, this volume). That is, because AL residents are less impaired, their care needs are fewer *and* less physically taxing. In many cases, workers' expectations derive from their employment histories. Yolanda, a 35-year-old with eight years of experience in LTC, explained, "It's easier to work in AL. I worked in a nursing home for one year, and it was terrible: hard work, overworked."

Concerns about workload and physical strain also are influenced by health concerns and age. For example, Ebony, a 25-year-old, reported, "In the nursing home, the work is more difficult and easier to get injured." Similarly, Jana, aged 46, explained, "Nursing homes are too much with my bad knees." Health concerns often are compounded by age, as illustrated by Beatrice, who is 61 years old: "With my age, my health wouldn't hold out with heavy lifting." Similarly, Laurette, one of the oldest workers in the sample, states: "I'm not as able to do as much work now as I'm 75."

Additionally, workload issues sometimes join with attitudes toward pay (see Chapter 11, this volume). That is, several workers indicated that low pay was more acceptable when commensurate with the workload. Katrina, aged 50 and with 15 years in LTC, explained, "Nursing homes did not pay much; less work at AL than a nursing home." Likewise, another woman reported leaving the nursing home where she had worked and going to AL because she was "overworked *and* underpaid."

Last, some participants' concerns about workloads were related to their desire to develop relationships with residents (see Chapter 7, this volume). For example, Dena, who had 10 years of nursing home tenure, explained, "There is too much work in a nursing home—no time to give attention to residents." Another worker similarly reported, "Nursing homes are so rigorous, a lot of work, low level of care. At AL; it's just assisting. You have more quality time with the residents." By influencing the amount of "quality time" workers have with residents, workload also influences the quality of their relationships.

Five percent of participants chose employment in AL because they expected their relationships with the residents to be better than in a nursing home. Like their views toward workload, employment histories are informative. Some workers specifically link the residents' communication abilities to the development of relationships. For example, one DCW explained, "I've worked in both AL and nursing homes; it's a challenge in both. Here there are people [residents] you can communicate with, can listen to their stories more efficiently than in nursing homes." More commonly, workers attribute the higher quality of relationships with residents to the lower workloads in AL, which permit more one-on-one time for building relationships. Sally, aged 42 with 17 years in LTC and 3 years in her current ALF, explained, "I got tired of the nursing home—running too short on help. Somebody told me about AL, and you get to do more one-on-one, and it's not as stressful as the nursing home." Reflecting the closeness that sometimes develops with residents, several workers depicted AL as "homelike."

Expectations of residents' functional status also shape workers' notions of the emotional strain that work in either setting would entail. Some workers find the high frailty levels of nursing home residents too depressing. Overall, 9 percent of participants chose AL because they expected the job to be emotionally easier, with less likelihood of depression or mental stress. Again, workers' attitudes are filtered through the lens of past jobs. A woman who had worked in nursing homes, as well as six different ALFs, explained, "I never want to go back to nursing home work. It is too much mentally [stressful]—dealing with a lot of sick people. I had nightmares about the residents. AL is easier." Vera also avoids nursing homes for this reason: "With them [nursing home residents] I feel like I just couldn't help them enough."

Additionally, some DCWs are drawn to AL specifically to avoid dealing with death, an occurrence they expect to be less frequent in AL. One worker explained, "I didn't really want to get into a situation where I knew people were going to die soon."

The combination of influences related to workload, relationships with residents, and emotional strain suggests that workers' choice of AL demonstrates concern about care quality. After all, quality care is difficult to provide if work-loads are too heavy or relationships are nonexistent. Twenty-eight DCWs (7%) chose AL because of their belief that care quality would be better than in nursing homes. For some, previous nursing home work substantiated this belief. Margaret, an Asian immigrant, reported her experience: "The AL care is more for the people. In nursing homes, there are too many residents, you can't help them, you don't have time to really help people, make sure they're clean, they eat, are feeling well. In nursing homes, it's a broken heart." Some workers were influenced by neglect and abuse in nursing homes. Chandra, who recently went to AL after more than four years of nursing work, explained, "I left the nursing home because I did not like the way they treat the elderly. . . . They do not get the care and attention they need." Another DCW reported a similar experience: "I did not like the nursing home; the residents were not treated right. They were being abused and I did not like that." Some workers were influenced by the experience of family members who had received poor care or been abused in nursing homes.

Employment Criteria

The criteria for employment in AL are lower than those for nursing homes, and this difference attracted 7 percent of DCWs to AL. In Georgia, like most other states, pre-employment training and educational requirements are minimal (see Chapter 10, this volume). In contrast, nursing home workers must complete federally specified CNA training. One worker explained how this difference impelled her to choose AL: "Nursing homes require a license, and I do not have a license, and I get on-the-job training here." Another worker similarly reported, "The nursing home, you really had to have a CNA license to work there, unless you worked in housekeeping and I didn't want to do that. Over here we don't have to have a CNA to work."

Workers' caregiving experience also influenced their choice of AL. Specifically, lack of elder care experience contributed to some decisions. One DCW explained, "The nursing home wants you to have experience with the elderly. They tried me here right away."

Physical Environment

The physical environment of ALFs in comparison with nursing homes also attracts workers. Five percent of the sample sought a work environment that was more homelike and cleaner than a nursing home. Workers' attraction to these environmental factors relates to their preferences regarding job content and design. That is, they believe that the homelikeness of ALFs supports the development of a positive social environment, including close relationships with residents, and they equate both homelikeness and cleanliness with the provision of high-quality care. Workers' employment histories, particularly their experiences in nursing homes, contribute to these environmental motivations.

The homelikeness of AL is particularly attractive to some workers. For example, one DCW described going to AL because it is "more homey—the setting, the people." Another worker similarly described AL as "more homey, home-atmosphere." Some workers believe homelikeness benefits the residents, which in turn increases their job satisfaction. For example, a previous nursing home worker said, "Most of the people here consider this as home, and working for them makes me happy."

Additionally, some workers are attracted to the cleanliness of AL; several particularly reported wanting to avoid the "smell" or "odor" of nursing homes. Such environmental concerns are sometimes interwoven with concerns about care quality. One DCW explained, "The smell of nursing homes is too much. I can't handle it. Many residents are left up in the dirty facility in diapers and it smells bad."

Assisted Living versus Home Care

Whereas the majority of workers compared AL with nursing home employment, fewer (less than 10% of our sample) made comparisons with in-home care. Only 11 percent of DCWs went to AL from in-home care, compared with 19 percent from nursing homes. Additionally, most DCWs with home care experience had worked as private employees of the care recipient rather than for an agency.

Ultimately, three key differences between AL and in-home care motivated participants' selection of AL: job and scheduling stability, the availability of health care benefits, and the social environment. Motivations for employment in AL rather than in-home care are depicted in Figure 4.3. Overall, these choices are guided by an expectation that AL jobs would have greater stability, better pay and benefits, and a livelier social environment. These organizational factors and their interactions with individual-level factors, including workers' employment histories and health, are discussed below.

Reflecting their in-home care experiences, several workers chose AL jobs because they are steadier and more predictable. One AL worker described her

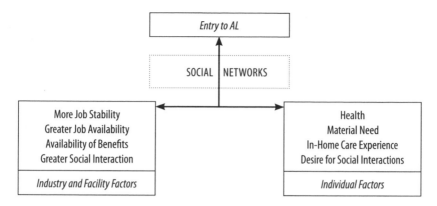

Figure 4.3. Motivations for Employment in Assisted Living versus In-Home Care

reasons: "The private duty is like you have a patient, or person you are taking care of. Okay, maybe they have a terminal illness. Then in a few months they are gone. If they have something broken, it heals back and they don't need you. You pretty much go from one job to another job. So it is not permanent. AL is. You're there; you know you have your job."

In addition to stability, more consistent scheduling is a factor. A woman who had been a private sitter for 11 years and in AL for 4 provides an example: "I needed a break from the responsibility of home health, private duty. I'm now on an actual schedule with time off." A few DCWs moved to AL for health care benefits. One explained, "Private home doesn't have benefits and Clayton [current ALF] is a good place to work."

Compared with the solitude and physical boundaries of a private home, AL offers greater opportunities for social interaction in a comparatively large venue, pluses for some DCWs. One who had provided in-home care for eight years describes her switch to AL: "I really don't care to privately sit; it is more confining. I like to be up and about and be around people." Some DCWs achieve in Al the best of both alternatives. One explained, "Nursing home work is too depressing; private home work is unstable. This is the best of both."

Social Networks

Eleven percent of DCWs chose AL because of their social networks. Some had family members who were AL residents, including mothers and grand-mothers. Participants who previously were home care aides or personal sitters often were led to AL by their care recipients. Others were steered by friends who were employed in AL.

Some workers indicated they assumed a passive role in the AL choice. For instance, one reported, "It [AL] chose me, just by accident, from private duty led to AL. I came to take care of one resident and it led to this." Likewise, a DCW who had provided child care in her home went to AL because her sister-in-law, a nurse, told her about CNA training, which she pursued. She described a subsequent visit to her current ALF, during which she was "forced" to accept her job, as "the point of no return." She has remained in the job for more than five years.

Some DCWs guided to AL by networks were new to the field. One whose textile mill closed reported, "I had a friend who was working here—she told me about this job." DCWs who had worked in other LTC settings also were steered by networks. Frankie, aged 59, had 20 years of LTC experience before beginning her five-year AL tenure: "There was a position available in an AL facility that my friend told me about. I applied and got the job."

Choosing a Facility

DCWs' choices of particular ALFs relate primarily to a facility's location and hiring and recruitment practices, reflecting workers' environmental and material motivations. Similar to their role in previous choices, social networks act as conduits to specific facilities.

Approximately 15 percent of DCWs chose their current ALFs primarily because of its location, in most cases proximity to their homes. About 45 percent were influenced by hiring and recruitment practices, including employment criteria, methods of advertising, and speed of contacting applicants (see Chapter 10, this volume). In some cases it was the fit between an applicant's limited education and experience and a facility's own minimal hiring criteria that influenced facility choices. Anita, a 56-year-old African American with a 10th-grade education, provides an example: "Marlene [the administrator] is the main reason I chose to work here. She took a big chance on me because I didn't have caregiving experience."

Although few facilities advertised for workers, our findings indicate that advertisements can influence facility choice. Advertisement methods included postings in newspapers and online. Terri, a 63-year-old with four years' tenure in her ALF, answered a newspaper ad: "They had an ad in the paper, and I had to go to work fast." Only large corporately owned ALFs attracted workers through online advertising. Online postings attracted workers both with descriptions of jobs available and with additional details about employment benefits. One DCW explained: "I found it online. [The corporation] has a Website and offers tuition reimbursement." Online advertisements were particularly influential for workers who were relocating: "I knew I was moving; I looked online, faxed my résumé, and I got a call the next day. It is the only place I applied to." Corporations also sometimes are able to retain workers by allowing transfers to other AL properties, the experience of one worker: "The company treated me well, and the corporate office people asked me to come here when I moved. They helped me get a job here and keep my benefits."

Employer practices of contacting applicants promptly also influence facility choices. Coco, a 24-year-old with two years in her current ALF, explained: "I was filling out applications and this facility was my first call back." Prompt contact is particularly effective because of workers' urgent need for income.

About 40 percent of DCWs chose their ALFs primarily because of their social networks, which in general guided workers to available jobs. Quanda, a 53-year-old with six years in her ALF, provides an example: "This is the one that needed help. My ex-daughter-in-law worked here and let me know." In addition, social networks sometimes informed workers about an ALF's reputation regarding quality of care or employment practices, the experience of Siena, who has been in her current ALF for three years: "Co-workers. I knew them before. They told me about this place. They like working here. I came and I liked it." The decision of Nicola, aged 27, was similar: "I knew two people who worked here; I heard good things." ALFs that permit family members to work together sometimes benefit from DCWs recruiting family members. Beverly, aged 63 with four years in her facility, illustrates this route: "My sister was a nurse here and she talked me into coming here and I knew the people already."

Discussion

As a society, we care *about* the well-being of older adults, but owing to the shortage of workers across LTC, we are increasingly less able to care *for* them. By examining DCWs' pathways to, and motivations for, employment in LTC, AL, and particular ALFs, this study reveals opportunities for the implementation of policies and practices that could help alleviate the national care crisis. Findings also include theoretical implications regarding the nature of motivations for employment and provide guidance for future research.

Our study was limited to the state of Georgia, but our findings reflect the dominant characteristics of care workers that have been identified nationally, internationally, and historically: almost all care workers are women. Care is gendered, as unpaid labor in family homes and in LTC, where mostly women perform care for little pay. Dilworth-Anderson and colleagues (2005, p. S261) explain how gender shapes pathways to care: "Caregiving is a 'gendered' experience whereby American cultural values, as well as those in specific cultural groups, socialize male and female children into defined roles that prevail today and are evident in who cares for elders in this society." In short, women and men are socialized to perform different roles, the role of care is largely reserved for women, and as a result mostly women follow pathways to care.

The employment histories of DCWs in our sample illustrate the influence of gender on employment pathways: most of their employment histories were limited to caregiving and other forms of "women's work"—jobs dominated by women, including housekeeping, cooking, and domestic work. Additionally, all these jobs include tasks performed by women at home, such as providing hands-on care, maintaining the physical environment, and serving meals (see Chapter 5, this volume). Similarities between women's work in the home and in LTC are also highlighted by DCWs' descriptions of LTC in familial terms and by their descriptions of ALFs as homelike. Overall, normative gender roles are central to many care workers' employment histories, and they thereby depict *gendered pathways to care.*

In contrast, other pathways to care are market-based; *market-based pathways to care* originate in socioeconomic changes, not in normative gender roles. Market-based pathways are depicted by workers who enter LTC after being displaced from a job in a factory or mill. Such transitions entail crossing paradigmatic market and job content divides, from the mechanized and efficient production of goods to the personalized provision of care (Held, 2002). For this reason, market-based and gendered pathways to care differ in terms of smoothness and fluidity.

Additionally, some pathways to care are neither gendered nor market-based but spurred by various turning points (Crosnoe & Elder, 2002) in employment or family life. Common turning points leading to employment in LTC include job losses (one's own or a spouse's), divorce, a child's entry into college, and the death of a family member, especially one for whom the care worker provided care.

Though DCWs' pathways to LTC vary, most had relatively low educational levels and limited employment histories and job options. As a result, the motivations for LTC employment identified in this chapter represent workers' selection of LTC from among a few limited options, including housekeeping, retail, and food service. Within this general context, the majority of participants indicated that they were morally or materially motivated to take employment in LTC, to select a job in AL over another LTC setting, and to choose a specific ALF. Professional motivations were less common but still influential. Additionally, social networks were significant sources of guidance for DCWs reporting each type of motivation and at each level of analysis (LTC, AL, ALF).

The moral value of care work—its association with altruism and benevolence—attracted the majority of DCWs in our sample to LTC, and within LTC these values greatly contributed to workers' selection of AL. Findings indicate that altruistic values for care are grounded in familial and religious beliefs: workers' experiences with their families and teachings from their religions support the view that altruism and benevolence are *good*, thereby making care work morally meaningful and an attractive employment option. The environmental factors that attract workers to AL, particularly homelikeness, also reflect the influence of familial beliefs on workers' motivations. Pillemer's (1996) findings similarly suggest that the most important reasons for choosing LTC work are to help others, to feel meaningful, and to serve society. The choice of AL over nursing homes because of care and relationship quality also affirms the influence of moral values on DCWs' employment trajectories. Likewise, multiple studies have shown that relationships with residents are a central component of job satisfaction and retention among DCWs (Ball et al., 2009; Berdes & Eckert, 2001; Foner, 1994; Chapter 7, this volume). Overall, the strong influence of moral motivations on DCWs' entry into LTC, selection of AL, and satisfaction and retention provides empirical support for Moody and Pesut's (2006, p. 16) motivational theory, which asserts, "Goals emerge from values."

Though moral values and other cultural artifacts have been construed as justifications or rationalizations for individual choices, rather than as motivations (Boltanski & Thevenot, 1999; Swidler, 2001), the prevalence with which care workers rely on moral reasoning to make employment decisions supports the position that moral values and cultural beliefs have motivational force and shape behaviors (Lakoff, 2002). Studies on motivations for employment conducted in China, where moral values are subject to government sanctioning, also show that cultural beliefs, whether or not sanctioned by the government, influence workers' job choices (Bai, 1998). Among DCWs, however, moral values *also* appear to play a justificatory, or rationalizing, role. Few would take employment without need for income, but only one-third reported entering LTC for material reasons (two-thirds reported moral motivations). Given our sample's relatively low levels of education and limited employment histories, we expect that material, extrinsic motivations had an even greater influence on participants' entry into LTC but may have been underreported owing to impression management, to which interviews are particularly susceptible, especially among marginalized persons (Goffman, 1963, 1967). In the context of this relatively poor and untrained workforce, the imbalance between reported moral and material, or intrinsic and extrinsic, motivations suggests that moral values are used to rationalize and justify decisions that are likely, first and foremost, materially motivated. Ultimately, these findings support theories of moral values as justificatory and motivational, and theories of motivations as neither exclusively intrinsic nor extrinsic but blended or "fuzzy" (Kreps, 1997) and influenced by culture and social norms (Markus & Kitayama, 1991; Scheuer, 2000).

Professional motivations were reported by only a small percentage of DCWs, all of whom were younger and more educated and had been working in LTC for a shorter period of time than the overall sample. In general, these workers consider LTC employment a stepping-stone to a more professional—better paying, more highly respected—career in nursing. In this context, nursing represents the fulfillment of both care workers' moral and material motivations. That is, like the direct care jobs examined in this study, nursing would validate workers' moral value of caring for others, but nursing would satisfy workers' material needs to a greater extent than direct care work. Because few, but more highly trained, workers are professionally motivated for LTC employment, attracting more of them would help ease the care crisis; strategies for achieving this aim are a core component of the policy implications discussed below.

Like our participants' professional motivations for LTC employment, their motivations for employment in AL, rather than another LTC setting, are dual: moral and material. They went to work in AL rather than a nursing home or in-home care because they expected AL to reflect their moral values more fully, with higher care quality, and better satisfy their material needs, with more job stability and better pay and benefits. However, the DCWs in this study who previously provided in-home care were employed privately, rather than through a home health agency, which likely influenced their experiences of, and perspectives toward, in-home care. Depending on the type of in-home care employer (see Howes [2008] and Stacey [2005]), pay, benefits, and job security may differ.

Environmental factors, especially the "homelikeness" of AL, are also attractive. Overall, workers consider the physical and social environment of AL superior to that of nursing homes or in-home settings. Though conceptually distinct from moral concerns, workers' environmental predilection for homelikeness reaffirms the *home* source of moral values and motives.

Finally, workers' facility choices are primarily motivated by material concerns. They seek specific jobs in the context of LTC and AL—that is, in a field and in a setting that are consistent with their moral values—to meet their material needs. Many identify available jobs at specific ALFs through their social networks, and some are attracted to particular ALFs by the proximity of facilities to their homes. Employers' hiring strategies, especially the speed of making hiring decisions, also strongly contribute to facility choice, reflecting the urgency of workers' material needs.

Whether DCWs' employment motivations are moral, material, professional, or environmental, their social networks guide them to LTC, AL, and specific ALFs. Family members, friends, past and present co-workers, and passing acquaintances all support workers' employment motivations. Some social networks support moral motivations by reinforcing the importance and enjoyment of developing relationships with LTC residents; some support material motivations by alerting workers to available jobs; environmental motivations are supported by social networks that inform workers about the quality of social relations in AL; and professional motivations are supported by social networks that encourage workers to take LTC employment while training for a career in nursing.

The fluidity of gender-based pathways to LTC and the dearth of men in care work signify direction for increasing the supply of LTC workers, making pathways to LTC smoother for men. Societal gender roles steer women to care work but deter male workers, for whom transitioning to LTC employment would entail transgressing gender roles. Making the transition to LTC smoother and more fluid for men will entail altering gender roles so that care work is not just for women. Policies that support increased caregiving among men in family life, such as the implementation of paternity leave or family leave for men with dependent parents, would likely contribute to this effort.

At the industry level, the primary factor to attract workers to LTC, and an influential factor attracting workers specifically to AL and particular ALFs, is the low level of criteria for LTC employment, particularly in AL. To continue to attract workers, it is important for LTC to retain positions with minimal requirements. However, to attract and retain more professionally motivated workers, who are the smallest percentage of workers in our study, LTC providers must develop more opportunities for professional development, especially opportunities for training in nursing and LTC management, the career aims of most professionally motivated workers. Career ladders that are incorporated with training and education and lead from entry-level direct care positions to jobs with additional responsibilities, including medication management, care planning, and supervision of co-workers, would likely increase professionally motivated workers' entry into, and retention in, LTC. Additionally, LTC providers with both AL and nursing home facilities may benefit from providing DCWs with opportunities for CNA training and linking this training to a transition from AL to nursing home work. Various professional development pathways for care workers have been identified. (For details, see Bishop et al., 2008; Parsons, Simmons, Penn, & Furlough, 2003; Richardson & Graf, 2002.)

In addition to the low level of training required for AL employment, several features of AL attract workers away from nursing homes, including the higher functional status of residents, the lower workloads, the higher care quality, and the more comfortable environment. Additionally, workers chose AL over in-home care for its livelier social environment and greater job stability and access to benefits. LTC providers who design care work jobs and environments to match workers' preferences may ultimately attract more workers, but several barriers to such design exist. First and foremost, resident functioning inevitably declines over time, forcing providers to choose between allowing residents to age in place or discharging residents as they decline (Ball et al., 2004; Chapin & Dobbs-Kepper, 2001). Employers may allow residents to age in place *and* keep workloads relatively manageable and care quality relatively high by altering staff-to-resident ratios in accordance with residents' needs. Additionally, AL attracts materially motivated workers from nursing homes by offering pay that workers consider more equivalent with their workloads and from in-home care by offering better benefits and more stable employment. Though LTC providers are limited in their ability to increase pay or benefits without concomitantly increasing residents' fees, they can offer workers consistent and stable employment.

Finally, at the individual level, care workers' family and religious backgrounds most strongly influence their moral motivations: family lives, especially major financial changes, strongly influence workers' material motivations, and workers' social networks steer them to LTC, AL, and specific ALFs. Informed by these findings, LTC providers may implement recruitment strategies that use workers' social networks more fully, perhaps particularly workers' religious organizations and families. In addition to simply recruiting in churches, providers may actively recruit through current workers' social networks by offering workers bonuses for recruiting friends or family members who come to, and stay in, their facilities.

Owing to market and industry dynamism, policies must also be flexible enough to respond to ever changing demands for workers. Currently, deindustrialization is forcing workers out of factories and mills, where many have been employed for decades. Routing these workers from industrial labor to LTC, rather than to another entry-level but less essential field, like food service or retail, may be critical to meeting the increasing demand for care workers. Typically, individuals' social networks provide this service informally by alerting workers to available LTC positions. However, organized community practices—for instance, authorizing market LTC providers to recruit workers from within factories that are closing or downsizing—may more successfully guide greater numbers of workers to LTC.

Conclusion

Although this study provides guidance for policies and practices that can attract more individuals to care work, it also reveals a danger facing LTC: cultural values motivate workers to enter LTC but are not permanent or universal, and as they change, care work may become even less attractive. Acknowledging the potential for moral values to lose motivational force, Virginia Held (2002, p. 26) warns, "Many people are not yet indifferent to values other than market ones, but it is unclear how long this will last." Ultimately, as the population continues to age and demands for LTC continue to grow, both the material value and professional stature of care work will need to be enhanced.

REFERENCES

Bai, L. 1998. Monetary reward versus the national ideological agenda: Career choice among Chinese university students. *Journal of Moral Education* 4, 525–40.
Ball, M. M., Lepore, M. L., Perkins, M. M., Hollingsworth, C., & Sweatman, M. 2009. They are the reason I come to work: The meaning of resident-staff relationships in assisted living. *Journal of Aging Studies* 1, 37–47.
Ball, M. M., Perkins, M. M., Whittington, F. J., Connell, B. R., Hollingsworth, C., King, S. V., et al. 2004. Managing decline in assisted living: The key to aging in place. *Journals of Gerontology: Social Sciences* 59, S202–12.

Berdes, C., & Eckert, J. 2001. Race relations and caregiving relationships: A qualitative examination of perspectives from residents and nurse's aides in three nursing homes. *Research on Aging* 1, 109–26.

Bishop, C. E., Weinberg, D. B., Dodson, L., Gittell, J. H., Leutz, W., Dossa, A., et al. 2008. Nursing assistants' job commitment: Effect of nursing home organizational factors and impact on resident well-being. *The Gerontologist* 48 (Special Issue 1), 36–45.

Boltanski, L., & Thevenot, L. 1999. The sociology of critical capacity. *European Journal of Social Theory* 3, 359–77.

Chapin, R., & Dobbs-Kepper, D. 2001. Aging in place in assisted living: Philosophy versus policy. *The Gerontologist* 1, 43–50.

Crosnoe, R., & Elder, G. H., Jr. 2002. Successful adaptation in the later years: A life course approach to aging. *Social Psychology Quarterly* 4, 309–28.

Dilworth-Anderson, P., Brummett, B. H., Goodwin, P., Williams, S. W., Williams, R. B., & Siegler, I. C. 2005. Effect of race on cultural justifications for caregiving. *Journals of Gerontology: Social Sciences* 60, S257–62.

Foner, N. 1994. *The caregiving dilemma: Work in an American nursing home.* Berkeley: University of California Press.

Goffman, E. 1963. *Stigma: Notes on the management of spoiled identity.* Englewood Cliffs, NJ: Prentice-Hall.

———. 1967. *Interaction ritual: Essays on face-to-face behavior.* Garden City, NY: Anchor Books.

Held, V. 2002. Care and the extension of markets. *Hypatia* 2, 19–33.

Howes, C. 2008. Love, money, or flexibility: What motivates people to work in consumer-directed home care? *The Gerontologist* 48 (Special Issue 1), 46–60.

Kreps, D. M. 1997. The interaction between norms and economic incentives: Intrinsic motivation and extrinsic incentives. *AEA Papers and Proceedings* 2, 359–64.

Lakoff, G. 2002. *Moral politics.* Chicago: University of Chicago Press.

Markus, H. R., & Kitayama, S. 1991. Culture and the self: Implications for cognition, emotion, and motivation. *Psychological Review* 2, 224–53.

Moody, R. C., & Pesut, D. J. 2006. The motivation to care: Application and extension of motivation theory to professional nursing work. *Journal of Health Organization and Management* 1, 15–48.

Parsons, S. K., Simmons, W. P., Penn, K., & Furlough, M. 2003. Determinants of satisfaction and turnover among nursing assistants. *Journal of Gerontological Nursing* 3 (3), 51–58.

Pillemer, K. 1996. *Solving the frontline crisis in long-term care.* Albany, NY: Delmar/Thompson Learning.

Richardson, B., & Graf, N. M. 2002. *Iowa caregivers association evaluation of the certified nurse assistant (CNA) mentor program: Surveys of long term care facility administrators, CNA mentors and mentees. Program evaluation summary.* Iowa City: National Resource Center for Family Centered Practice, University of Iowa School of Social Work.

Ryan, R. M., & Deci, E. L. 2000. Self-determination theory and the facilitation of intrinsic motivation, social development, and well-being. *American Psychologist* 1, 68–78.

Scheuer, S. 2000. *Social and economic motivation at work: Theories of motivation reassessed.* Copenhagen: Copenhagen Business School Press.

Stacey, C. L. 2005. Finding dignity in dirty work: The constraints and rewards of low-wage home care labor. *Sociology of Health and Illness* 6, 831–54.

Swidler, A. 2001. *Talk of love: How culture matters.* Berkeley: University of California Press.

CHAPTER FIVE

"We Do It All"

Universal Workers in Assisted Living

Mary M. Ball, Ph.D.
Carole Hollingsworth, M.A.
Michael J. Lepore, Ph.D.

Assisted living (AL) is a burgeoning industry, but like the broader long-term care sector, it is strained by an endemic shortage of direct care workers (DCWs). Little has been written about these hands-on workers, neither about their personal characteristics nor about their job experiences in AL, but understanding who DCWs are and what they do in each long-term care (LTC) setting is critical for developing well-informed policies and practices that support recruitment and retention.

Despite lack of information about direct care jobs in AL, numerous accounts exist of nursing home work (see, for example, Gubrium, 1975; Savishinsky, 1991; Shield, 1988). In his classic treatise *Living and Dying at Murray Manor*, Gubrium (1975) portrays the job of a nursing home aide as primarily "bed and body work." Other research also characterizes nursing home work as consisting chiefly of the provision of activities of daily living (ADL) tasks, such as bathing, dressing, toileting, and feeding (U.S. General Accounting Office [GAO], 2001). AL care, in contrast, has been described as more *universal*, meaning that, in addition to personal care, DCWs carry out a variety of other duties, including assisting with activities, medications, and meal service and performing multiple housekeeping tasks (Ball et al., 2000; Hawes, Phillips, & Rose, 2000).

In addition to differences in job content, studies indicate that nursing home aides experience higher levels of physical and emotional stress compared with DCWs in AL, primarily because of the increased frailty and cognitive impairment of nursing home residents (Gruber-Baldini, Boustani, Sloane, & Zimmerman, 2004; Sloane, Zimmerman, & Ory, 2001; Spillman, Liu, & McGuillard, 2002). Differences in job content and workload have implications for DCW job satisfaction and retention. For example, nursing home studies cite the physical demands of the work, heavy workloads, and lower staffing levels as leading to dissatisfaction (Cohen-Mansfield & Noelker, 2000; Ramirez, Teresi, Holmes, & Fairchild, 1998) and turnover (GAO, 2001; Smyer, Brannon, & Cohn, 1992). These stress factors also have been found to indirectly influence satisfaction and retention in AL through limiting DCWs' ability to develop relationships with residents (Ball et al., 2009; Chapter 7, this volume). Bonds with care recipients have been identified as a primary component of DCW job satisfaction and a deterrent to turnover in nursing homes (Berdes & Eckert, 2007; Bowers, Esmond, & Jacobson, 2000; Foner, 1994; Grieshaber, Allen, & Deering, 1995; Monahan & Carthy, 1992), AL (Ball et al., 2009; Chapter 7, this volume), and home care settings (Feldman, Sapienza, & Kane, 1990; Karner, 1998).

Much remains to be learned about how job design factors affect satisfaction and retention in AL. Although DCWs may consider AL employment more appealing than nursing home work, owing to the promise of lighter workloads and less emotional strain (Chapter 4, this volume), we do not know how they view the universal configuration of their jobs or how the array of duties influence the development of relationships with residents.

Moreover, certain characteristics of AL make understanding DCWs' experiences particularly challenging in this setting. Each state regulates AL differently (see Chapter 2, this volume), resulting in substantial differences across states in how AL is configured and defined (Mollica, Sims-Kastelein, & O'Keeffe, 2007). Within states, facilities embody further differences, including size, fees, admission policies, and staffing practices (Zimmerman et al., 2003). The work of Zimmerman and colleagues has led to the development of initial facility typologies, which differentiate three types of assisted living facilities (ALFs) based on facility-level characteristics, including size, tenure, and staffing. These typologies have been developed further by relating structural characteristics to process and resident case-mix domains (Park et al., 2006).

Such variation across ALFs, paired with the problems of DCW turnover and shortages, highlights the need to examine links between ALF types and DCW job experiences and outcomes. Although the work cited above contributes significantly to the ongoing effort to define the world of AL, no studies have examined how DCWs experience their jobs in these variable work settings. The facilities in the study reported on here capture the diversity found in ALFs throughout the United States (see Chapter 3, this volume). They range in size, physical design, location, ownership, organizational structure, funding, fees, and resident and staff profiles. Thus they promise to reflect the experiences of DCWs across the United States. In this chapter we focus on the everyday jobs of the DCWs in these ALFs. We explore what they do in a typical day, how their jobs vary across facilities and workers, and the multiple factors that influence their work experience. We also consider how DCWs' job expectations (see Chapter 4, this volume) compare with their job reality and how their experiences influence their attitudes toward their jobs.

Methods

The data for this chapter derive from surveys of 370 DCWs and from in-depth, qualitative interviews with 42 DCWs and 44 administrators. In the survey, we asked DCWs to identify their specific job role and to specify the tasks that they complete in a typical day. We also asked them what aspects of their jobs they find most satisfying and most frustrating and their perceptions of workload. Qualitative questioning explored in more depth what a typical workday entails and DCWs' attitudes toward various job components. We asked administrators to describe a variety of facility policies and procedures, including those relating to staffing and resident admission and discharge, and to tell us about their own job responsibilities and the duties of DCWs and other staff in their facilities. We also asked about their perceptions of how DCWs experience their work. In analyzing these different types of data, we followed the principles of grounded theory (Strauss & Corbin, 1998; see Chapter 3, this volume, for details of sampling and data collection and analysis).

Case Studies

We begin with four case studies that offer DCWs' own representations of a typical day at work. Although the cases illustrate a range of experiences in diverse environments, many similarities exist. The four cases highlight the concept of "universal worker." Each DCW carries out a variety of tasks in her or his daily job. Yet no two jobs sound just alike. A variety of factors influence each DCW's experience. Some relate to the workers themselves, some to their specific work settings, and others to the communities where facilities are located.

Misty

Misty is a 26-year-old single mother of four who has worked off and on over the past six years in one of two small rural sites (Holly Forest and Oak Hill) owned by her great aunt and uncle. The two homes, each with 24 residents, share a parking lot and a kitchen, and both receive Medicaid reimbursement. Oak Hill serves residents with mental illness and thus has a higher proportion of male (32%) and younger (55%) residents than is typical of the sample as a whole. Misty, who works the first shift (7 a.m.–4 p.m.) at Oak Hill, describes her typical day:

> OK, I come in, I clock in, I tell my residents over at Holly Forest good morning, and I go in the kitchen and talk to the cook, and then I go next door and go to each room and tell everyone of my residents good morning. If Wayne [male DCW] works nights (he don't give the ladies a bath), I start my baths before breakfast, and there is two of us over there. I, or whoever is working with me, we get the baths, and while one is getting the bath, one is either changing beds, taking linens off or making up the beds. We get in about 7 a.m., and probably we do all of that and we are finished by 7:30. We pour our juice and we come over here [Holly Forest] and get the breakfast, take it next door. We serve and then we call them [the residents] out [of their rooms] and while they are up we give their medicines and we get the ones that goes off to work and training center (residents with mental health problems), we get them ready, get their lunches and get them out. . . . After we got those out, we go check to see who goes to the doctor, get them and get all of their medical stuff ready and, if they can't go alone, we normally get Margaret to ride with them. And after that, then we start vacuuming and mopping and cleaning the kitchen after breakfast. Then we start doing laundry. . . . Well, in the meantime we set the table, empty the dishwasher and everything and have it ready for the next meal . . . and so in between that time, I clean the bathrooms, make the bed, dealing with residents' needs and giving baths and stuff, because you have more baths in the mornings, and you have got a couple of more baths in between cleaning the bath-

room and lunch time. Then we give our 12 o'clock medicines. Well, we get lunch about 12 o'clock, we take it over, we serve it. . . . After we get the kitchen cleaned, I would say it is probably about 1:30, and we just go back and re-vacuum our hall, go through, check our bathrooms, check our trash, and do laundry in between all of this. Mainly our laundry time is after lunch, because that is really when we ain't, you know, got any work. . . . So and then we put up laundry and we chart our medications, we make sure our med book is done, and then we get some blood sugars and we got some blood pressures that has to be checked daily and every other day.

Ethel

Ethel, aged 50, began working at Hill Haven, a 48-bed rural facility, about four years ago, after 29 years at the local hosiery mill. Ethel describes a typical morning shift at Hill Haven:

Normally I come on in and start waking up the residents who are not up. I just knock on the door and tell them good morning and it is time to get up. Once they get up, I go around and make the beds. If they don't want to make their own beds, I do it. If someone needs assistance in getting dressed, we help them get dressed. If they don't, you just make sure they come to breakfast on time. Then someone might need assistance to get to breakfast, so you take them. We have to help bring the trays out to the table to them. Once we do that, we kind of sit around until they get finished and get the plates up, take it back so the cook can wash the dishes. I eat breakfast at home. I don't eat here. That is when I go do the house cleaning. You do housekeeping; you do the bathrooms. Once you do that, we have towels we have to wash. Then it gets close to lunch time and you have to basically do the same thing. You have to let them know it is lunch time if they don't know. Then you have to help feed them, get finished, then we eat, and then help to clean the kitchen. Basically if you haven't finished with your house cleaning, you finish that up and then you get ready to go on. That is about a day.

Sabrina

Sabrina, aged 24, has worked for seven months at Pine Manor, a 116-bed, corporately owned facility in a large urban area. She describes a typical morning shift as a med tech:

Come to work, clock in, come upstairs, go into my little office area where I have a medication cart. I go in there and see what notes and what has changed during the night. The med tech in the evening would have left me a note saying what happened during the evening. I go in and start pulling my meds to pass them out. I get them all together and I come downstairs and start passing them out. As soon as I come in at 6:30 I am busy and working. It is more busy in the morning. Everybody in the morning gets meds but not everybody in the afternoon does. . . . I have to do paperwork, like ordering new meds, faxing things. I may talk to doctor's office, that type of thing. Taking blood pressure, taking blood sugars. . . . I help out all the time with hands-on care. . . . If someone asks me to do the laundry, I can do the laundry. It is not like since I am a med tech that is the only thing I am obligated to do. I am helping out all over the place. I was helping in the kitchen today, in the dining room. I am all over the building.

Miranda

Miranda, aged 36, is from South Africa. Before immigrating to the United States, she worked as a flight attendant. She describes her morning shift in the dementia care unit (DCU) at her 65-bed facility, where she has worked for a little over a year:

You first clock in and the team that is leaving will tell you how the residents are doing. They write it down, but the most important things they will tell you up front. You look at your assignments. If there are two people [working], you will have like ten people to get up. If you have showers to do, you go in the rooms and start getting the people up and ready and out to the dining room. . . . Mostly you have two or three showers. You do that, get them up and ready for breakfast. By 8:30, they should be in the dining room. They have their breakfast. . . . When we come in, we bring them to the dining room and get them water or orange juice or milk. Some people have cereal before the hot plate. Those that need to be fed, we sit down with them. After that, about 9:30, we clear the tables and put the residents in kind of a circle as we clear. Then you take your stuff [dishes] upstairs. You are kind of running around. We take it on a cart. I might grab a cup of coffee between. You watch the residents as you do all that running around. About 10:30 we wash the tables down and sweep the floor. Then you might get a 10-minute coffee break. You might nibble on something while you do something at the same time. Then it is 11:00 and you set up activities for the residents. They always want to go back to sleep for some reason. We do a sing-along or something. Since there are two of us working, we take turns, so the other one will have gone back to change the sheets or make the beds, whatever needs to be done. We do activities. If the other person comes back, you can go do your beds because there has to be someone there with the residents the whole time. Around 11:30, we bring them back to the tables and set up the dining room, set silverware, napkins. Lunch is at 12:00, so we go upstairs and get the ice and the drinks and bring the food down. We feed them again and that takes like an hour. By 1:00, we take the plates back upstairs. About 1:10 or 1:15, we don't set it up again, we just clean up the floors and tables. By 1:30 you go back to the rooms to change them. Some of them take naps after lunch. You have to change their diapers and make sure they are not wet. Some of them might need a sponge bath if they smell. Some of them will go back to the TV room. By 2:10, we haven't had a lunch break. We are supposed to get 30 minutes. We take the trash from the bathrooms and by the time we are done it is 2:20. Then the next staff is coming in and you have to write in the book or whatever comments you have. Some days they just don't like the food and we will just make a comment about their eating. We might write down bowel movements and how many times you change their diapers so they [management] can see how many times you changed them.

The Universal Worker

The four case studies illustrate the *universal worker* concept. Below we discuss two components of the universal worker experience—task configuration (types of tasks performed) and workload (level of demand)—paying attention to the variation found among workers and facilities and the multiple factors that influence these differences.

Task Configuration

In interviewing DCWs, we asked them whether specific tasks typical of AL care were a part of their usual job. We then asked them to name any other jobs they did regularly that we had not mentioned. Table 5.1 shows the percentage of DCWs who carry out particular tasks on a regular basis, as well as the mean and median number of tasks for all DCWs interviewed and for workers in each size facility.

The high overall number of tasks (mean: 8.49; median: 8) demonstrates that these jobs are consistent with the universal worker concept. Moreover, comparison of mean task numbers by size of home shows that the concept is embodied more fully in small homes compared with medium and large (mean

Table 5.1   DCWs Who Perform Tasks on a Regular Basis, by Facility Size (as percentage)

Task	Small (N=85)	Medium (N=111)	Large (N=204)	Total (N=400)
ADL care	98	98	99	99
Medications	94	68	51	65
Food preparation	62	24	19	30
Meal set-up	94	71	79	80
Meal service	87	70	80	80
Dish washing	66	30	50	47
Light cleaning	96	92	97	95
Heavy cleaning	85	54	46	57
Laundry	90	85	85	86
Activities	71	48	57	58
Documentation	89	84	90	88
Supervision	30	30	21	26
Transportation	38	20	9	19
Other	27	20	10	17
Mean/Median	10.28/11	7.99/8	7.88/8	8.49/8

of 10.28 vs. 7.99 and 7.88). Yet variation by facility size is not evident for all tasks. Almost all DCWs in all home sizes perform regular ADL care, and most also do light cleaning, laundry, meal set-up and service, and record keeping. The percentage of DCWs performing most other types of tasks, though, *decreases* as home size *increases*, with the difference being greater between small homes and the other two size categories. For example, 94 percent of DCWs in small homes assist with medications, compared with 68 percent in medium homes and 51 percent in large homes. Similar differences are seen with heavy cleaning, food preparation, activities, and transportation. Additional tasks named by DCWs included answering the telephone (the most common); facility shopping and maintenance; caring for a resident's dog or cat; and a variety of health care tasks. These "other" tasks are reported more frequently in small facilities (27%) compared with medium (20%), and large (10%).

Interview and observation data reveal that the daily work experience of DCWs also includes activities that were not mentioned as a "job task" by workers: responding to residents' multiple and varied needs (e.g., answering call lights and pagers); monitoring residents' conditions, whereabouts, and behaviors; and handling a variety of problem behaviors, as well as interacting socially with residents.

Factors affecting a DCW's task configuration are related principally to the facility. Key is a facility's organizational structure, which depends largely on size and resource level. Task configuration varies also by shift (morning, evening, or night), a facility's resident profile, and, if a facility has multiple units or areas that vary according to resident care needs, a DCW's particular work assignment.

Organizational Structure of the Facility

The organizational structure of an ALF influences the work experience of the DCWs in multiple ways. For the most part, the organization of study homes increases in complexity as homes grow in size. Below we describe the administrative structure and types of ancillary workers and DCW positions found in the sample homes.

The 18 small homes, with few exceptions, have only one individual in a management position, the director. In a third of these homes, the director also is the owner. Only one, a higher-fee, corporately owned small home, also has an activity director. In two cases where more than one facility shares a common property, individual homes have on-site managers who work under the director. Ancillary personnel (other than DCWs) also are limited in small homes. Only eight have a cook, and just four have a dedicated housekeeper. Several small home owners use family members as staff. In one, the owner's husband handles maintenance and yard work and most of the cooking. Another owner relies on her son and a brother for a variety of duties. At Oak Hill, where Misty works, Misty's aunt, the owner's niece, manages the homes. The only other non-DCW employee is the cook.

In contrast, all but 1 of the 13 medium-sized homes have management positions in addition to the director. The one exception is a rural, low-income home with 30 residents that operates with only the owner/director, a cook, and DCWs. The majority of medium homes have an activity director and dedicated housekeepers; three have dietary aides who handle meal set-up and service. All the large homes have multiple management positions in addition to the executive director, typically including directors of activity, food service, marketing, maintenance, and business. Most also have a manager of DCWs and, if the home has a DCU, a separate person who coordinates staff in this unit. All have housekeeping staff, but only one has dietary aides and one a dedicated laundry person.

The number and type of DCW positions also tend to vary with home size.

Overall, three DCW positions are found. All homes in all size categories have some variation of the universal care worker, under a variety of labels, including care aide, resident assistant, personal care technician, care manager, and caregiver. Also common are a lead caregiver or shift supervisor position and a medication manager or "med tech." Sometimes the lead caregiver and med tech position are combined.

Of the 18 small homes, 13 have only one type of DCW. Four also have a lead caregiver position; 1 has the combined lead caregiver/med tech. Of the 13 medium homes, 6 have only one category of DCW; 5 have a lead caregiver or shift supervisor; and 3 have a med tech. All of the 14 large homes have at least two DCW levels; 4 have three levels. Six have med techs. Slightly over half (53%) of sample homes have an RN or LPN on staff. Table 5.2 summarizes the DCW roles and the various ancillary personnel found in each facility size category.

Misty illustrates the essence of a universal worker, and her role is typical of DCWs who work in small homes with only one type of DCW and few or no ancillary staff. On an average day, Misty helps residents to bathe and dress, assists them with medications, changes beds, does laundry, cleans bathrooms, sets up for and serves two meals, vacuums and mops the kitchen, helps residents get ready to go to day programs, charts medications, and performs blood pressure and blood sugar checks. In between these tasks, Misty tries to squeeze in time to talk to and hug her residents. The director of another small home describes the DCW role as including "everything a person would do to manage their own home." Yet in all small homes, DCWs also assist with ADL care and medications. In the words of another small-home director, "We cook, care, and clean."

Hill Haven, the 48-bed home where Ethel works, has a caregiver supervisor, a full-time activity director, receptionist, lead caregiver position, and kitchen staff, but no dedicated housekeepers. Ethel, like Misty, is a care aide, but she is not responsible for medication assistance or laundry.

Although Sabrina usually performs multiple tasks, her primary role is medication assistance. Sabrina works in one of the six large homes with a DCW position dedicated to medication assistance, commonly called a med tech. The director at this large, corporately owned facility describes the med tech role: "This group of staff members are charged with making sure the residents are receiving the right medication with the right dose at the right time. That is their primary job. They don't generally provide resident care beyond that. However, as part of the team that works with the care managers, they do pitch in."

Table 5.2   Number of Homes with Each Type of Worker, by Home Size

Type of Worker	Small (N=18)	Medium (N=13)	Large (N=14)	Total (N=45)
DCW Roles				
DCW only	13	6	0	19
Lead DCW	4	5	5	14
Combined lead DCW/med tech	1	0	4	5
Med tech	0	3	6	9
Other Workers				
Housekeeper	4	9	14	27
Dietary aide	0	3	1	4
Laundry worker	0	0	1	1
Cook	9	13	14	36
Activity director	1	10	14	25
RN or LPN	7	3	14	24

Sabrina is responsible for mediation assistance for all residents in her 116-bed facility. She also communicates with physicians, orders medicines, and, in her words, is "all over the place" helping out as needed. That is, as a specially trained med tech, she remains a universal worker.

As the case studies indicate, the particular position a DCW holds can influence daily tasks. Table 5.3 shows the variation in task configuration for the typical DCW positions: care aide, shift supervisor, and med tech. These data show that DCWs in all three positions essentially are "universalists."

More than half (58%) of care aides assist with medications, compared with 88 percent of shift supervisors and all med techs. As noted, in most small homes all care aides regularly perform this task. In larger homes, with more than one DCW position, medication assistance usually is performed by the shift supervisor or the med tech. Slightly more than half (53%) of the 45 sample homes have an RN or LPN on staff. In four of these homes, nurses are the primary or only persons who assist with medications.

As Table 5.3 shows, med techs are less likely to perform meal set-up and service and heavy cleaning than the other two positions, but they still engage in multiple tasks. Shift supervisors have the highest mean (9.43) and median (9) number of tasks; 95 percent have supervisory roles compared with 13 percent of care aides and 43 percent of med techs. Typically they have jobs similar to those of care aides, with the addition of supervision and oftentimes medications. A director described the shift supervisor role at her medium-sized facil-

Table 5.3   DCWs Who Perform Tasks, by Position Type
(as percentage)

Task	Care Aide (N=316)	Shift Supervisor (N=42)	Med Tech (N=29)
ADL care	99	100	97
Medications	58	88	100
Food preparation	32	79	14
Meal set-up	84	74	45
Meal service	82	71	64
Dish washing	49	38	35
Light cleaning	97	93	89
Heavy cleaning	62	52	18
Laundry	88	86	68
Activities	60	48	52
Documentation	86	100	97
Supervision	13	95	43
Transportation	18	33	7
Other	16	38	14
Mean / Median	8.41 / 8	9.43 / 9	7.46 / 8

ity: "The supervisor, they all work the floor just like the regular care giver but they are responsible to do the report for the shift. I look to them as the person I would question if I found out something went on during the night or if I had a problem, they are the ones who call me at home."

Shift, Residents' Impairment Level, and Work Assignment

A DCW's shift also affects task configuration. As a rule, the morning shift performs the bulk of ADL care, which leaves the later shifts with more house-keeping. The director of a large home with no dedicated housekeepers and relatively independent residents uses this pattern: "Our folks are not high need. Plus we divide up the duties. The seven to three shift is responsible for bathing and dressing and making beds and fresh towels, and the three to eleven shift is responsible for housekeeping because they are not doing the bathing. When they come in at three, they have set schedules for cleaning the different units and doing the residents' laundry. Then the eleven to seven shift, if we have ironing or pressing, they do it at night, and they dust and [do] quiet tasks in the mall area at nighttime. The majority of the folks [residents] are going to sleep at night."

In some cases, an administrator will alter the typical pattern in order to equalize the care burden or cater to residents. A common practice is for the night shift to do laundry. The director of Ethel's home explained her strategy: "The day shift does all of the cleaning and housekeeping. When they go in the room, they change out the towels and put out the soaps and all that. Then they bring them [the residents] to breakfast and to lunch, but evening shift gives the baths. The only kind of housekeeping they will do is if there is a spill or spot cleaning. Then the night shift will do all the clothes." In a few homes third-shift workers get residents up and ready before breakfast.

In homes where the residents' needs are greater, two-hour checks and incontinence care are regular night duties. Where dementia levels are high, more residents may be awake at night, and tasks thus will include resident monitoring. A DCW in a large, dementia-specific facility explained: "They do not sleep, you would think, they walk all day long, bless their hearts. They got some sun-downers. They stay awake at night too. They might take a little cat-nap, but they do not sleep."

The type of ADL care DCWs perform, regardless of shift, depends also on the overall impairment level of a facility's residents. For example, although Ethel's ADL care only includes assisting a few residents with bathing and dressing, in other facilities ADL care includes a much wider range of tasks. One DCW described the resident in her facility who requires the most care: "I call her Miss Jane. She needs, out of all the residents, she needs the most care. . . . We pretty much have to do everything for her and that is the resident that takes me the thirty minutes."

As noted in Chapter 3, almost a third (14) of the study homes have a DCU. Others have multiple buildings or floors with varying levels of care; two are dementia-specific. A DCW's assignment has bearing on task configuration. For example, Miranda's day in the DCU, which includes heavy ADL care, contrasts with her work experience in the AL section: "Up here [AL] it is different. There are only four that need help getting out of bed. [For] most of them, you just knock on the door." Most DCWs assigned to DCUs, like Miranda, also conduct resident activities, even when facilities have an activity director.

Workload

In addition to task configuration, the DCW job experience is defined also by the amount of work DCWs must perform during a shift and the degree of physical and mental stress they feel, that is, "workload." We asked two questions related to workload in our survey of 370 DCWs: (1) How pressed do you feel to complete all of your work during your shift? (responses on a 10-point Likert scale collapsed into two categories); and (2) Do you have enough time for breaks? (yes or no response). Overall a substantial percentage (42%) of DCWs feel pressed to complete daily tasks, and almost a quarter (24%) feel they lack sufficient break time. When comparing attitudes by facility size, no significant differences are evident regarding feeling pressed: 43 percent in small homes, compared with 36 percent in medium homes and 45 percent in large homes. Regarding break time, however, DCWs in large homes are significantly more likely ($p = .000$) to report not having enough time for breaks (34%) compared with workers in medium (15%) and small (11%) homes.

Both quantitative and qualitative data reveal that DCWs in all size homes experience both low and high levels of workload stress. Misty feels her job is "pretty laid back," despite her portrayal of a nonstop day. Misty's perception, though, contrasts with that of another small-home worker: "There are some times it is hard to take a break. If it is not a family member, it is a resident. Here comes Ms. Ethel: 'I didn't eat today'; 'Yes, you did, dear'; 'What did I eat?' If it is not something like that, it is a family member coming up in here chatting with you. We don't get a break. When you do sit down to eat, they interrupt you. 'I hate to interrupt you, but I need a pill.' Something." Administrators expressed similarly contrasting attitudes. In the eyes of one small-home owner, DCWs have a "very stressful job" because "they are the ones on the front line." Yet, in the view of an administrator of a medium home, "No one here has a stress load. No one does."

Although some DCWs described work that is more constant than physically demanding, others said that they experience elevated levels of physical stress. A DCW in a large home explained: "Just trying to get them up out of a chair or a wheel chair, standing them up and changing their clothes, getting them up, it takes sometimes three of us to do that with some of the heavy ones."

Our analysis revealed numerous individual- and facility-level factors that affect DCWs' workload. Typically more than one factor is operative, and often factors are interactive and dynamic. We found also that task configuration and workload have common influences and, in turn, influence each other.

Individual-Level Factors

Individual-level factors that affect workload and its perception include a DCW's job tenure, experience, and training; work style; age; and health.

Misty's view of her job as "pretty laid back" is colored by her long tenure at Oak Hill. Over time her job has become easier: "At first, you know, when I started working, like six years ago, I thought it was like overwhelming, how am I going to get this done, but after I have worked for so long it is just a breeze really." A med tech in a large home expressed a similar view: "When you first start giving medications it is a slow process because you are learning."

How an individual prefers to arrange her or his job tasks, or "work style," also influences workload perception. When asked whether she ever had difficulty finishing her work, Ethel replied: "I don't have any trouble. I try to keep a routine. Once you get a routine you can basically go on and get through what you do." Some workers prefer to "stay busy." Others require more breaks. One DCW in a large home clarified: "Some people have breaks and some don't, you know. I guess, like I say, you work at your own pace and you try to work it in, but I don't. But some people, 'Hey, you are entitled to thirty minutes.' They will take the thirty minutes and the work is still left undone." Another said: "If you get down to it and do it like you are supposed to, yeah, you can do your work. You sure can." Additionally, a DCW's sense of responsibility regarding her or his job can affect workload. One DCW explained: "Sometimes I do [feel pressed]. I am like this: If I start something, I like to finish it. I don't like to leave stuff undone."

Other DCWs described how health issues affect whether or not they feel stress. One explained: "Like I say, if I am having a bad day or if I have a headache or didn't get any sleep the night before, I will ask a co-worker, the other med tech that works with me, 'Do you mind doing meds today?' I just don't feel up to it or I didn't get any sleep and I don't want to put the residents at risk. I might make a mistake and give someone the wrong medicine because I am tired and haven't had any sleep."

Facility-Level Factors

The facility-level factors we identified as affecting workload include shift, work unit, resident impairment level, emergencies, staff shortages and staffing strategies (including the use of sitters), DCW teamwork, and presence of a break room.

Although not a universal experience, first shift tends to be harder, in the eyes of both DCWs and administrators. One first-shift worker in a large home said: "It is a lot to do sometimes, but you can't do it all. But one main thing, you get thirty minutes deducted out of your check but you never get a break. I mean, you should be able to, you know, go get something to eat, or come back in thirty minutes, or just sit down for a second, but you can't really do that. Three to eleven is the easier shift." The director of Miranda's home expressed a similar viewpoint: "A lot of them will say they don't have time for breaks. I can see how days often don't have time for breaks, but I know evenings do have time for breaks." In this home five of the six first-shift workers stated that they felt pressed to complete their work, compared with one of six on the second shift. The heavier first-shift workload largely results from higher levels of ADL care. Some administrators attempt to balance care burden by reallocating tasks (e.g., transferring laundry to third shift). One explained her strategy: "We looked at every duty and looked where it could be done and where you could have an equitable situation with the distribution of duties. That way it makes it fair. The eleven to seven shift sets up for breakfast, so when the seven to three shift comes in everything is ready to go. The last thing they do is pour juice and make a pot of coffee. They iron the table clothes at nighttime so we have fresh tablecloths. I think we have done a great job with dividing up duties so you do not overload one shift." Still, burdens tend to be higher during residents' waking hours. As one night-shift worker said, "I think it is easier because you don't have too much interacting with the residents. So there is nothing stopping you. You just go straight to your work."

Sometimes workload "depends on the day." As one DCW in a small home said, "Some days and some days not [feels pressed]. It depends on what kind of day the residents are having, a lot of it." Almost all DCWs and administrators reported that when emergencies occur, such as a resident's health crisis or even death, all bets are off. One director of a medium home said, "We are like any other facility, I don't care how much staff you have, sometimes when you have an emergency situation, you deal with it and those situations take more staff time." A DCW concurred: "Sometimes you get rushed if emergencies happen or something. You get a little off schedule and you get a little rushed to catch up and get out of here on time." Crises also can cause significant emotional stress. The owner of a small home described an acute health crisis in her home: "I had another woman, she had a brain hemorrhage. Well, when they [staff] walked in there, she was fine in the morning, joking, laughing, said 'I'm going to go in and take a nap, call me before lunch,' and when they went in there, the blood was, you know. That is stress. That is stress. They immediately go into overload."

Fluctuations in routine workload also occur when DCWs do not show up for scheduled shifts and administrators are unable to replace them. In responding to the query about adequate break time, one worker in a large home responded, "It depends basically. Some days, especially if they pulled your help, you may not get a break because the work has got to get done. I can't say I have gotten a break every day the 12 years I have been here for that reason." "Call-outs" and "no-shows" are a recurring problem in most facilities.

As with task configuration, a DCW's workload is affected by a facility's resident profile regarding the level and type of disability. A facility's resident profile largely depends on its admission and retention policies, which are influenced by multiple factors, including its philosophy regarding residents aging in place. The director of a large home where the majority of residents (67%) need help with three or more ADLs and 13 percent require a two-person transfer explained, "With Excel [corporation name] we do believe in caring for the frailest of the frail, and our residents age in place, so they could be at any end of that spectrum." Such variations in resident frailty have an obvious effect on DCW workload. A DCW who works for Excel described care of one long-term resident: "It takes about two people to help him up. He has a lift to get him from his chair to his bed, and it is too small for his weight. He is so big that once you get him in the lift you need people to move it to the bed. He has been here for a while and you ask, 'Why is he here?' because you feel like when they get to this stage they should be at another home."

The relative influence of residents' impairment levels on workload must be considered along with the way in which facilities staff to meet residents' varying levels of need. With few exceptions, directors report adhering to staffing levels that meet Georgia regulations, which specify one staff person for every 15 residents during waking hours and one for every 25 residents at night. Administrators also commonly report that they adjust staffing levels to meet residents' care needs. The director of the large facility with the philosophy of "caring for the frailest of the frail" explained his strategy: "It [staffing level] varies depending on the acuity of the residents, because we have different levels of care. With the different levels of care we can determine quite easily how many staffing hours per day we will need. If we have a high acuity or we have residents who need a lot of assistance, then we could almost double the amount of staff we have if the acuity was much lower." In this facility, only 4 out of the 14 DCWs indicated they do not have enough time for breaks.

The director of a small home where no DCWs felt pressed to complete their work reported a similar strategy: "I think our staff doesn't feel worked to death. That is done on experience. For a while we had five here in the mornings, because we had four people who had been in the hospital or had a fracture and needed a lot of extra time in the mornings to get up and get going. We were running hard with four people, me, the cook, and the two DCWs. So at that point we brought on a part-time person for the day [shift]. Once breakfast has been served and everyone is up and bathed and dressed, it is not as hard to keep up. We do it based on what works. Right now it works." A common strategy in all size homes is to employ a DCW for a short shift during peak care times, usually the first shift.

One director of a medium home communicates regularly with her staff to gauge the need for more workers: "I continually talk to the caregivers and the lead caregiver about, 'Are ya'll overloaded? Can you handle the people you got? Do you need extra people? Do you need people to take swing shift type things?' We just did this on Friday. If they tell me they are overloaded, it is time to get someone else." In this home all the workers felt they had time for breaks, and none felt pressed to complete their work.

In facilities with DCUs, typically these units are staffed at higher levels than are AL sections. The director of one large home explained, "In the assisted living neighborhood during those daytime hours they [DCWs] will have any-where from 12 to 15 [residents]. In the DCU, they will have anywhere from 6 to 7 residents." In the medium home referenced above, the director staffs the DCU with more experienced workers in addition to having a higher staff-to-resident ratio: "We have the most experienced staff in extra care, the ones who have received the most training. As I said before, we have about one caregiver for every five residents. They have to be good; they have to know what they are doing. Even with just five people, it is a heavier load than regular AL, and we make sure they are good enough to handle it." Higher staffing levels, though, are not the case in all homes. For example, Sabrina reported her DCU being frequently "short-staffed" and operating with only two DCWs for 26 residents.

A common practice to minimize DCW workload and allow aging in place is to require residents to hire a sitter when their care needs increase beyond what the facility is prepared to provide. The director of a medium home explained how she staffs the DCU: "If they are a higher level of care and the family doesn't want them to go to a nursing home, then we explain to the family that we need them to get a sitter because we can't have a staff member sit there and hand-feed."

A DCW's work assignment or specific care role also can affect workload. Working in DCUs, where typically the stress of heavier physical care needs is compounded by a variety of problem behaviors, often is more demanding compared with AL assignments. Miranda, for example, had this experience: "You can work five days up here [AL] and no problem and then two days downstairs [DCU] and you are worn out already." Yet, owing to the interplay of multiple factors, not all DCWs had Miranda's experience. Another DCU worker had this to say: "It [DCU] is a different set up; it is not rushed; it is not hurried. You do what you can do in a day. . . . You have things you do with them like make up and shaving the men, and that is in activity time. They [residents] take their time and they are not rushed eating. They can sit there all day if they want to. You are never rushed. When they finish eating, you take them to be toileted. There are always two people over there. It would be hectic if you didn't work together. I don't feel overwhelmed or frustrated." Staffing levels in this DCU, compared with Miranda's, are consistently higher, with a ratio of one DCW to seven residents.

The universality of the DCW role also can lead to workload stress. The DCU worker quoted above contrasted her experience with that of an AL worker in her home: "They get the work done, but they rush. Sometimes you see them and they are running, 'I got to do this and that.' You don't really have enough time to do everything that needs to be done, so you do it hurriedly, the best way you can. They come in and they get the residents up. Some of them are less independent, and you need to be there to help them. They do that, and they serve breakfast. In between serving breakfast, you may have [call] lights going off because somebody needs something. Then you have to run and do this. And there are people that don't come down to breakfast, so they have to get those trays ready to take up to breakfast. They are constantly going, and the call lights go off over here. You don't have that in the DCU, except maybe one person. It gets really hectic."

Some med techs experience significant mental stress because of the critical nature of their job. One explained: "It is a responsibility because if you think about it you have these people's life in your hands. If you give the wrong medication, it can be devastating. You always have to be conscientious and aware that you have the right person and the right medication. You check and you double-check and you triple-check. When I get to the resident I also check the name to make sure I have the right resident. This is Mrs. Jones and I am giving Mrs. Jones her pills. You have to really be on it."

Often workload can be minimized when DCWs are able to share the load with their co-workers (i.e., when there is teamwork). For Miranda, working as a team is dependent on being staffed fully and is critical: "Sometimes you walk in at 6:30 and they have had a bowel movement and you have to wash them. When you don't have the help, it is really frustrating. . . . It is better [with extra person] because you pool everything and it is a team. When it is only you and someone, it is really, there are days when I have tears in my eyes and it is just too much. Emotionally it is too much and I break down."

Whether or not a facility has a room dedicated for staff to take breaks also can influence workload. A DCW in a medium home explained how lack of such a space spoiled her break time: "So, we have to sit out there [dining room] and eat. Whereas there might be one time a week that you sit down to eat your dinner and there is not a resident in there demanding you come and do something for them while you are eating, or either they are up talking and your plate is here and they are talking all over your food." Overall, 80 percent of DCWs reported that having a dedicated break room is important.

Outcomes for Workers

In our survey, we asked DCWs an open-ended question related to their overall job satisfaction: "Considering your job as a whole, what do you find most satisfying?" A large majority of workers (67%) named some aspect of the physical and emotional care of residents. Qualitative interviews yielded similar attitudes toward resident care. In Misty's words, "Caring for my residents. Like the vacuum cleaning, I don't mind doing it. I will do it, but my perspective is caring for the residents." Ethel, Sabrina, and Miranda all had comparable answers: "Come in and work with the group, laughing and talking," "interacting with and influencing residents," and "when I have time to sit down and talk to them."

We also asked workers to tell us what they found most frustrating about their work. Although 14 percent found nothing frustrating, 20 percent named workload stress, either physical or mental. These attitudes represent a variety of stress components: heavy-care residents, meeting multiple resident demands, being short staffed, lack of social time with residents, and simply not having adequate time to do the job.

Our findings also reveal that stress can have significant negative impact on workers and, ultimately, on resident care. The following quote captures one DCW's stressful day: "Days like that, everybody gets frustrated. All the caregivers do because, you know, you feel like, 'well how am I going to get it done?' I don't have time, and you're stressed trying to get it all done. That is not good. It is pressure, and people don't like pressure. I don't like pressure. I don't do well under pressure."

In some cases, frustration relates to a specific task, usually housekeeping. In response to the question, "What do you like least about your job?" one DCW replied, "Probably the least I would say has got to be laundry. I can't stand laundry. That is one of my things I don't even like to do." Qualitative findings suggest that although most DCWs consider housekeeping a given in their jobs, they do not view these tasks as *care*. One said, "But really the housekeeping [is most frustrating] because I feel like I didn't hire on as a housekeeper. I hired on as a caregiver." DCWs also indicate that such chores impede their ability to provide care: "When residents call for help, I want to do more and don't have the time. I'm doing laundry instead of caring for patients." Another worker expressed her frustration with management regarding the universality of her role and the lack of time to provide quality care: "They [management] were talking about things we have to do, and I raised my hand and said, 'We have these things to do as a care manager, and we need to make sure that work is done to perfection before you talk about other things.' The response we got was, 'You are a jack of all trades, not a master of one.' 'You are telling us we don't have to do it right, we just have to do it? You are saying we don't have to go an extra length, we just have to do it?' That is not good. They might think you are spending time doing little things or wasting time and not doing your work but, really, that is what it is all about. We will do everything, but you will not have it done the way you want it done. It makes you not have enough time to do the really important things." By "really important things" this DCW meant having the time to talk to residents—for example, to comfort one who was nervous about an upcoming blood transfusion. She described how "happy" this resident was when she stayed past her evening shift to spend time with her the night before this event.

Just as emotional care improves residents' quality of life, interacting with residents can benefit workers. One explained how residents relieve her stress: "Sometimes I come in here and I am like, ugh, and then they'll say something and start smiling and I forget about why I was feeling that way."

In a few cases, specific tasks related to resident care created frustration. Two DCWs named tasks related to ADL care as most frustrating, and both concerned "cleaning up poop." Several find medication assistance most frustrating. For Sabrina, "just coming in in the morning and unpacking the medication, because it is very time consuming. That's it." As noted above, some DCWs who assist with medications find this job especially anxiety-producing. For another DCW, having to perform a health care task without adequate training was stressful.

Discussion

In this chapter we elucidate the daily work of DCWs in AL. In so doing, we focus on two components of job design: task configuration and workload. Our analysis reveals that numerous multilevel factors affect these two components, and they, in turn, influence each other. Both task configuration and workload are central to how DCWs experience their work.

First, regarding task configuration, our findings show that although "bed and body work" (Gubrium, 1975) is central to the work of most DCWs in AL, across all facilities and job positions DCWs remain by and large universal workers. The concept is embraced more fully in the small homes in our sample, but DCWs in even the largest homes still perform on average about 8 different tasks (compared with an average of about 10 in small homes).

A facility's organizational structure, which typically increases in complexity as facilities get larger, exerts primary influence on the number and specific array of tasks DCWs perform. The least complex structures are found in small facilities with an owner/director and one type of DCW; the upper end of organizational complexity is represented by large facilities with multiple management and DCW positions and a variety of ancillary personnel, such as housekeepers and dietary and maintenance workers. Almost all DCWs perform ADL care, and most also do light cleaning, laundry, meal set-up and service, and record keeping, but other tasks, particularly food preparation and heavy cleaning, are less likely to be part of the DCW job in larger facilities.

In facilities with multiple DCW positions, the particular role a DCW assumes also shapes task configuration. Care aides and shift supervisors tend to have responsibility for a larger array of tasks than med techs, but even med techs are expected to help out in other areas when needed and remain "universalists" to some degree. When facilities have special medication personnel (only one-third of sample homes), care aides as a rule are relieved of this duty. Overall, over half of care aides in all homes assist with medications, and almost all (94%) of those in small homes perform this task. These findings help elucidate the ways in which medications are managed in AL, an area of research that is just beginning to develop and a component of care that can have serious consequences for residents' well-being (Young et al., 2008).

The type and level of functional impairment found in a facility's resident population, determined largely by admission and retention policies, affect both task configuration and workload. ADL care ranges from minimal help with bathing and dressing in facilities where residents are relatively independent to assistance with eating and transferring in facilities with more heavily dependent residents. Generally, workload levels increase along with resident disability levels. The proportion of residents with specific conditions (e.g., dementia, mental illness, and diabetes) also can affect these two job design components. Such resident case-mix differences do not relate necessarily to facility size, although the large facilities in our sample have somewhat higher proportions of residents needing help with three or more ADLs (46%) and diagnosed with dementia (50%), compared with small facilities, where 38 percent of residents have both these characteristics (see Chapter 3, this volume). Great variation in these facility characteristics, however, also is present *within* facility size categories.

How facilities organize work according to shifts also affects both task configuration and workload. Our findings show that DCWs on the morning shift typically perform the bulk of ADL care and DCWs on other shifts do more housekeeping. Although administrators often attempt to equalize care burden by redistributing noncare tasks across other shifts, first-shift workers also tend to have heavier workloads. Moreover, we found that case-mix factors can influence the effect of shift on job design. For example, in facilities with large numbers of heavy-care residents and/or residents with dementia, night-shift work includes more ADL care *and* is more taxing. Work assignment also is relevant. DCU workers typically engage in a wider range of ADL and other tasks (usually including activity provision) compared with DCWs assigned to AL sections, and they tend to experience greater physical and mental stress. The experience of most DCU workers illustrates the interactive effect of task configuration and workload. These findings regarding job position, assignment, and shift indicate the importance of matching workers and positions and thus have implications for both job applicants and administrators during the hiring process and also when considering job advancements and other changes during tenure.

With regard to the relevance of existing ALF typologies (Park et al., 2006; Zimmerman et al., 2003) for understanding task configuration and workload, our findings indicate that the categorization of Park and colleagues (2006), which includes process and case-mix domains and additional structural indicators (e.g., aide and RN staffing levels), is most instructive. These are the type of facility-level characteristics, rather than size or tenure, that most influence the job experience of DCWs. Although additional work is needed, such typologies could be used to inform facility hiring and staffing policies and practices.

Our findings are clear that the facility factor with the greatest influence on workload is how well a facility staffs to meet residents' care needs, which inevitably change over time as a result of acute health crises and gradual decline associated with chronic illness. Although most administrators in our sample claim to adjust staffing levels as needed, in general staffing patterns are based on Georgia requirements. This practice means that DCWs who work in the facilities with the most impaired residents tend to experience the greatest workload stress. The principal strategies facilities employ to meet residents' ongoing and changing needs are to add staff during peak care times, to staff higher in DCUs, and to require residents to hire sitters when their needs increase beyond the capacity of regular staff.

Another facility factor that has bearing on workload is the presence or absence of a dedicated staff break room. Our findings show that being completely away from residents for even short periods relieves stress and adds value to break time. The large majority of DCWs in our sample stated that having such a space is important to them.

Our data also show the importance of teamwork in the overall work experience. Working together in completing particularly challenging tasks (e.g., dealing with heavy-care or resistant residents), as well as multiple tasks, eases job stress and increases satisfaction. These findings suggest that paying attention to co-worker relationships in scheduling and assigning DCWs would be a productive strategy (see Chapter 6, this volume). They also further illustrate the importance of high staff retention because relationships among co-workers, like relationships between DCWs and residents, also require time to develop.

We found that DCWs' knowledge and skills gained through training and experience serve to expedite task completion and lessen stress, whereas lack of training for specific tasks (e.g., transferring) exacerbates stress. This finding reinforces the importance of pre- and posthire training and indicates that pairing experienced and inexperienced workers may be a fruitful strategy for educating new hires as well as increasing work efficiency. Such mentoring arrangements within LTC facilities also are encouraged by others (e.g., Stolee et al., 2005).

In addition to illuminating the DCW work experience and the factors that influence it, our findings regarding task configuration and workload have implications for job satisfaction and retention. Regarding the universality of the work, of principal importance is the influence of multiple task performance on DCWs' relationships with residents—the most satisfying aspect of their job and a contributor to retention (Ball et al., 2009; Chapter 7, this volume). One issue involves the competition of noncare tasks with tasks that allow direct contact with residents and thus the development of relationships (see Ball et al., 2009; Chapter 7, this volume).

Another issue relates to a worker's professional caregiver identity. Some DCWs resent performing housekeeping and other noncare tasks because they consider such duties as distinct from what they perceive to be their bona fide job—giving care. It is through the hands-on care of residents that DCWs receive *professional* as well as *moral* affirmation (see Ball et al., 2009; Chapter 7, this volume).

Some initiatives to change the culture of nursing homes, such as the Green House model (Rabig et al., 2006) and the Eden Alternative (Thomas, 1996), promote the universal worker concept. Such initiatives are intended to change the culture of LTC from large, impersonal, atomized care settings to smaller, personalized, holistic care settings. Our findings suggest that the trend toward universal design in these culture change initiatives may not be wholly beneficial for DCWs or residents, who also value relationships with their paid caregivers (Ball et al., 2000, 2005; Eckert, Zimmerman, & Morgan, 2001).

In terms of the effect of workload on job outcomes, one-fifth of our sample identified workload stress as the most *dissatisfying* aspect of their job. Stress is both physical and mental and pertains to providing heavy physical care, responding to residents' multiple demands, short staffing, lacking social time with residents, and simply not having enough time to do the job. Qualitative research focusing on DCWs' relationships with residents also identifies workload stress as a key factor impeding relationship development (Ball et al., 2009; Chapter 7, this volume), thus indirectly impacting job satisfaction and retention.

In addition, survey data show that 42 percent of DCWs feel pressed to complete their daily work. Although little variation was found in this variable according to facility size, slightly more than one-third (34%) of DCWs in large homes reported not having enough time for breaks, compared with 15 percent and 11 percent in medium and small homes, respectively, representing a significant difference. Moreover, regression analysis revealed a significant relationship between feeling pressed and job dissatisfaction (see Chapter 8, this volume) and intent to leave (see Chapter 9, this volume). Nursing home studies also cite the physical demands of the work, heavy workloads, and lower staffing levels as leading to dissatisfaction (Cohen-Mansfield & Noelker, 2000; Ramirez et al., 1998) and turnover (GAO, 2001; Smyer et al., 1992).

Conclusion

All these findings point to the importance of maintaining staffing levels in AL that afford DCWs manageable workloads. This job design factor is far reaching in its potential effect on DCW job satisfaction and retention. It also has implications for recruitment of workers to AL in light of the fact that DCWs choose AL over nursing homes in large part because of an expectation of a less stressful work environment, which supports their *moral* motives for care work (see Chapter 4, this volume). Although the universal nature of the job has some bearing on job satisfaction, our findings indicate that dissatisfaction relates more to the increased workload associated with multiple task performance—particularly its negative impact on time with residents—than to the content of the tasks.

These findings also are highly relevant to the ongoing discussion of how to define and regulate AL. The impairment level of AL residents is increasing (Golant, 2008; Spillman et al., 2002), as is the proportion of residents with dementia (Gruber-Baldini et al., 2004; Sloane et al., 2001), both trends with potential impact on the type and level of care DCWs provide. To maximize DCW job satisfaction and retention—as well as residents' quality of care and life—facilities that serve these frailer residents must employ staff in sufficient numbers and with the requisite skills (or be willing to train them) to meet residents' changing care needs. Because most facilities staff in accordance with state regulations rather than resident case mix, such hiring and training criteria may require governmental regulation. Additionally, our findings support a type of AL regulation that would allow for multiple types of DCW positions, ranging, for instance, along a universalist-specialist scale, with each DCW type being matched with relevant training requirements. Akin to the complexity of

DCW jobs is the complexity of AL. Given the central role of DCWs to the operation of AL, and, ultimately, to residents' quality of life, an optimal strategy for defining and regulating AL may be to ground both definition and regulation in the perspectives and experiences of DCWs, which, as this chapter shows, are quite variable. A multilevel typology of AL ordered by resident case mix, therefore, may best reflect the central complexities of this increasingly important LTC setting.

The findings presented in this chapter have relevance for a wide variety of AL settings as well as for nursing homes. With respect to task configuration, data from the only national AL study (Hawes, Phillips, & Rose, 2000) indicate that the experiences of Georgia workers are similar to those in ALFs nationwide, where being a universal worker is the norm. In addition, variation in job configuration based on factors such as facility size and organization structure and DCW shift, position, and training likely would be found for other workers in comparable ALFs. Our findings related to workload level and its effect on job experience and worker satisfaction should be universally applicable to DCWs in both ALFs and nursing homes.

REFERENCES

Ball, M. M., Lepore, M. L., Perkins, M. M., Hollingsworth, C., & Sweatman, M. 2009. "They are the reason I come to work": The meaning of resident-staff relationships in assisted living. *Journal of Aging Studies* 23, 37–47.
Ball, M. M., Perkins, M. M., Whittington, F. J., Hollingsworth, C., King, S. V., & Combs, B. L. 2005. *Communities of care: Assisted living for African American elders*. Baltimore: Johns Hopkins University Press.
Ball, M. M., Whittington, F. J., Perkins, M. M., Patterson, V. L., Hollingsworth, C., King, S. V., et al. 2000. Quality of life in assisted living facilities: Viewpoints of residents. *Journal of Applied Gerontology* 19, 304–25.
Berdes, C., & Eckert, J. M. 2007. The language of caring: Nurse's aides' use of family metaphors conveys affective care. *The Gerontologist* 47, 340–49.
Bowers, B. J., Esmond, S., & Jacobson, N. 2000. The relationship between staffing and quality in long term care facilities: Exploring the views of nurse aides. *Journal of Nursing Care Quality* 14, 55–64.
Cohen-Mansfield, J., & Noelker, L. S. 2000. Nursing staff satisfaction in long-term care: An overview. In J. Cohen-Mansfield, F. K. Ejaz, & P. Werner (Eds.), *Satisfaction surveys in long-term care* (pp. 52–75). New York: Springer.
Eckert, J. K., Zimmerman, S., & Morgan, L. 2001. Connectedness in residential care: A qualitative perspective. In S. Zimmerman, P. Sloane, & J. K. Eckert (Eds.), *Assisted living: Needs, practices, and policies in residential care for the elderly* (pp. 292–313). Baltimore: Johns Hopkins University Press.

Feldman, P., Sapienza, A., & Kane, N. 1990. *Who cares for them? Workers in the home care industry.* New York: Greenwood Press.

Foner, N. 1994. *The caregiving dilemma: Work in an American nursing home.* Berkeley: University of California Press.

Golant, S. 2008. The future of assisted living residences: A response to uncertainty. In S. Golant & J. Hyde (Eds.), *The assisted living residence: A vision for the future* (pp. 3–46). Baltimore: Johns Hopkins University Press.

Grieshaber, L., Parker, P., & Deering, J. 1995. Job satisfaction of nursing assistants in long-term care. *Health Care Supervisor* 13 (4), 18–28.

Gruber-Baldini, A. L., Boustani, M., Sloane, P. D., & Zimmerman, S. 2004. Behavioral symptoms in residential care/assisted living facilities: Prevalence, risk factors, and medication management. *Journal of the American Geriatrics Society* 52, 1610–17.

Gubrium, J. F. 1975. *Living and dying at Murray Manor.* Charlottesville: University Press of Virginia.

Hawes, C., Phillips, C. D., & Rose, M. 2000. *High service or high privacy assisted living facilities, their residents and staff: Results from a national survey.* Washington, DC: U.S. Department of Health and Human Services.

Karner, T. 1998. Professional caring: Homecare workers as fictive kin. *Journal of Aging Studies* 12, 69–82.

Mollica, R., Sims-Kastelein, K., & O'Keeffe, J. 2007. *Residential care and assisted living compendium, 2007.* Prepared for the U.S. Department of Health and Human Services. Washington, DC: National Academy of State Health Policy.

Monahan, R., & Carthy, S. 1992. Nursing home employment: The nurse's aide perspective. *Journal of Gerontological Nursing* 18 (2), 13–16.

Park, N. S., Zimmerman, S., Sloane, P. D., Gruber-Baldini, A. L., & Eckert, J. K. 2006. An empirical typology of residential care/assisted living based on a four-state study. *The Gerontologist* 46, 238–48.

Rabig, J., Thomas, W., Kane, R. A., Cutler, L. J., & McAlilly, S. 2006. Radical redesign of nursing homes: Applying the green house concept in Tupelo, Mississippi. *The Gerontologist* 46, 533–39.

Ramirez, M., Teresi, J., Holmes, D., & Fairchild, S. 1998. Ethnic and racial conflict in relation to staff burnout, demoralization, and job satisfaction in SCUs and non-SCUs. *Journal of Mental Health and Aging* 4, 459–79.

Savishinsky, J. S. 1991. *The ends of time: Life and work in a nursing home.* Westport, CT: Bergin & Garvey.

Shield, R. R. 1988. *Uneasy endings: Daily life in an American nursing home.* Ithaca, NY: Cornell University Press.

Sloane, P. D., Zimmerman, S., & Ory, M. 2001. Care for persons with dementia. In S. Zimmerman, P. D. Sloane, & J. K. Eckert (Eds.), *Assisted living: Needs, practices, and policies in residential care for the elderly* (pp. 242–70). Baltimore: Johns Hopkins University Press.

Smyer, M., Brannon, D., & Cohn, M. 1992. Improving nursing home care through training and job redesign. *The Gerontologist* 32, 327–33.

Spillman, B. C., Liu, K., & McGuilliard, C. 2002. *Trends in residential long-term care: Use of nursing homes and assisted living and characteristics of facilities and residents* (#HHS-100-97-0010). Washington, DC: Urban Institute.

Stolee, P., Esbaugh, J., Aylward, S., Cathers, T., Harvey, D., Hillier, L., et al. 2005. Factors associated with the effectiveness of continuing education in long-term care. *The Gerontologist* 45, 399–405.

Strauss, A., & Corbin, J. 1998. *Basics of qualitative research: Techniques and procedures for developing grounded theory* (2nd ed.). Thousand Oaks, CA: Sage Publications.

Thomas, W. H. 1996. *Life worth living: How someone you love can still enjoy life in a nursing home.* Acton, MA: VanderWyk & Burnham.

U.S. General Accounting Office. 2001. *Nursing workforce: Recruitment and retention of nurses and nurse aides is a growing concern* (Report No. GAO-1-750T). Washington, DC: GAO.

Young, H. M., Gray, S. L., McCormick, W. C., Sikma, S. K., Reinhard, S., Trippett, L., et al. 2008. Types, prevalence, and potential clinical significance of medication administration errors in assisted living. *Journal of the American Geriatrics Society* 56, 1199–1205.

Zimmerman, S., Gruber-Baldini, A. L., Sloane, P. D., Eckert, J. K., Hebel, J. R., Morgan, L. A., et al. 2003. Assisted living and nursing homes: Apples and oranges? *The Gerontologist* 43 (Special Issue 2), 107–17.

CHAPTER SIX

Co-worker Relationships in Assisted Living

The Influence of Social Network Ties

Molly M. Perkins, Ph.D.

W. Mark Sweatman, M.B.A.

Carole Hollingsworth, M.A.

Considerable research exists on the quality of workplace relationships in long-term care settings. Most centers on relationships in nursing homes (see, for example, Berdes & Eckert, 2001; Bowers & Becker, 1992; Chen et al., 2007; Foner, 1994; Powers, 1992; Tellis-Nayak & Tellis-Nayak, 1989). Recently, some research has investigated relationships in assisted living (AL). These studies focus on staff members' relationships with residents (Ball et al., 2009; Gaugler, 2005) and with family members (Ball et al., 2005; Kemp et al., 2009). To date, no published research has explicitly investigated co-worker relationships in AL.

From 2003 to 2004 we conducted a small pilot study investigating the quality of workplace relationships among staff (N=61) in two high-retention AL facilities (ALFs) located in metropolitan Atlanta: a 36-bed nonprofit facility and a 90-bed for-profit facility with a special care dementia unit. Grounded theory analysis of these data show that staff use a process we label "getting by" to meet basic needs, manage day-to-day problems (e.g., combative residents), and accomplish personal and job-related goals (Perkins, Sweatman, et al., 2004; Perkins et al., 2005). Strategies staff use to "get by" shape the unique social environment of each home. An important strategy is finding a "good" job. We found that communication through social networks serves as an informal ranking system that guides staff to the good jobs. Close bonds between staff who had previous ties result in the development of a cooperative support system that promotes job satisfaction and commitment but makes it difficult for new staff to fit in. Based on its fit with the literature (see, for example, Benson, 1986; Foner, 1994), we label this cooperative support system "work culture." This analysis provides a starting point for the current larger study focusing on staff relationships in 45 ALFs located throughout the state of Georgia, which vary in size, geographic location, resident and staff profile, and organizational structure (see Chapter 3, this volume, for detailed information regarding sample selection and study procedures, including adherence to university institutional review board [IRB] protocols and operationalization of variables, such as facility size and geographic location).

Conceptual Framework

Given the demographic profile of AL workers, work relationships in AL generally involve relationships among women. Based on our preliminary research and a recognition of the gendered aspect of staff relations in AL, we draw on a body of feminist literature that focuses on women's workplace relationships, the meanings that women attach to these relationships, and women's individual and group-level strategies for coping with unpleasant and often oppressive work conditions (see for example, Benson, 1986; Foner, 1994; Kanter & Stein, 1979; Lamphere, 1985; Zavella, 1985). This literature grows out of ethnographic studies of women laboring in a variety of low-wage occupations, including factory work, clerical work, and service occupations, such as retail and care work. Inspired in part by the publication of Harry Braverman's (1974) seminal text *Labor and Monopoly Capital,* common themes running through this literature include female workers' strategies of adaptation and resistance to managements' authority and development of a worker consciousness or a collective identity (Foner, 1994; Lamphere, 1985). These constructs typically are discussed in terms of coping strategies (e.g., collective action that includes rituals, games, unofficial rules, and group norms), which form in response to repetitive and often tedious low-skilled labor and result in the development of an informal work culture.

More than a decade ago, Foner (1994) found evidence of such an informal work culture operating in a New York City nursing home. Her findings show that the solidarity it creates among co-workers fosters closer relationships among workers and helps make life "at the bottom" more tolerable, but it also creates a situation in which group norms and expectations (peer pressure) sometimes lead otherwise well-intentioned workers astray and even, in some cases, compromises residents' care. Another negative aspect includes the formation of exclusionary cliques. Our preliminary research, which we describe above, supports many of Foner's findings.

Consistent with a grounded theory approach, we use this body of research as a sensitizing framework to inform our research questions and to position our research within relevant theoretical contexts. These concepts do not limit the direction of our analyses, and by acknowledging them we provide an additional safeguard against forcing preconceived ideas and theories onto our data (Charmez, 2006; Clarke, 2005).

The specific research aims are (1) to explore the nature of workplace relationships across a range of AL settings; (2) to identify what conditions shape the construction of these relationships; and (3) to understand how these relationships influence satisfaction and retention in different types of AL settings.

Methods

For this analysis, we use qualitative data from semistructured interviews with 41 direct care workers (DCWs) and 44 administrators. Interviews with both sets of informants include questions regarding the quality of co-worker relations, including those with shift supervisors and administrators; what factors influence these relationships; and how these relationships influence DCWs' overall work experience. We also analyze data from observations and informal interviews, as well as theoretical memos completed by researchers at the conclusion of data collection in each of the 45 homes, which include researchers' insights and data on emerging themes. Descriptive information we present to describe the study population and provide context for the qualitative data is based on data from interviews with 400 DCWs who completed either a qualitative interview or a survey. Consonant with a grounded theory approach, our goal is discovering processes linking phenomena to one another and generating theory (Charmaz, 2006; Strauss & Corbin, 1998). The core category that emerges in this study is a process we label "maintenance of just-close-enough ties." We describe this process and associated constructs below.

The Gendered Nature of Staff Relationships

Consistent with our preliminary findings, results from the current study show that gender provides an important context in which relationships within AL are shaped. A recurring theme is that a workplace composed mainly of women poses unique challenges. A DCW in a large (116 beds) urban facility related the quality of co-worker relations to hormonal levels, which tend to fluctuate: "There are a bunch of women [working here] and we all have menstrual problems. Everybody has their times when they buzz and bicker and then everybody has times when they are fine." Similarly, a female administrator in a small (24 beds) urban home stated, "It's women working together. When problems come, it is usually female-oriented." A male administrator in another small (16 beds) urban home, who acknowledges that his perceptions about female staff may be sexist, described what he has observed: "Most of what I am seeing, this is a chauvinist thing, what I have seen here, most of the staff are female and they build relationships and most of them become friends. If they don't become friends, they are the opposite and, believe me, that can be problematic. I have seen some fights that I could never see [develop among] men. Little bitty things, wow." Several participants described common problems, such as gossip and clique formation, in terms of female dispositions.

Another recurring theme is the tendency to refer to DCWs as "girls." We observed this tendency among female and male administrators, as well as among DCWs themselves. In several cases, participants' use of the term "girls" conveys DCWs' lower status position within the facility hierarchy. An administrator in a medium-sized (34 beds) urban home described her chain of command: "Starting from the top, [there is] myself as the administrator, I have one assistant, I have a shift leader for each shift, [and] the girls report to her."

Factors Leading to Solidarity, Autonomy, or Alienation in Staff Relations

Several factors—turnover; the facility's reputation; race and culture; shift assignment, work location, and teamwork; and the ability to fit in—influence staff relations. In the current study, we do not find evidence across homes of a cohesive work culture or a worker consciousness, as defined by the literature. Based on results from this study, then, we define staff relations in terms of solidarity, autonomy, or alienation.

Turnover

Our findings show that DCW and administrator turnover has a major influence on how relations in each home are characterized. In contrast to facilities represented in our preliminary study, several homes in this study have high turnover rates, with one-fourth (25%) of facilities reporting turnover rates of 100 percent and higher. We find high turnover rates in facilities of all sizes, as well as in both urban and rural locations. Our findings also show considerable turnover among facility administrators.[1]

Several DCWs reported negative consequences resulting from administrator turnover. A DCW in a large (65 beds) urban home described how the departure of an administrator can negatively impact staff satisfaction and alter the culture of a home: "The new director came in and she fired my supervisors and [some of my co-workers whom] she heard about. She fired the wrong people and it was not a happy place to work." A common practice of new administrators is to bring supervisors and staff with them from their former facilities, which often contributes to dissention and feelings of alienation among staff. A DCW in a large (74 beds) urban home stated: "He [the administrator] started this unequal treatment, because he brought his own staff from [the other facility]." In two large homes, this problem was exacerbated by resultant differences in the racial profile of staff and administrators.

The Facility's Reputation

Consistent with our preliminary findings, results from this study show that the reputation of a facility, which frequently is communicated by word of mouth through informal social networks, is a key factor motivating DCWs to seek employment in a particular home (see Chapter 4, this volume). A sudden change in the reputation of a facility can have a notable impact on DCWs' connection to a facility and other workers. A DCW in a medium-sized (38 beds) urban facility described how the change in an administrator adversely affected the reputation of her facility, contributing to her feelings of detachment: "This [facility] has a bad reputation. When I first came here, it didn't have that reputation, because the administrative staff was different. . . . I would like to see the place full. I would like to see people knowing when you said, 'The Glenn,' everybody is like, 'Oh, I heard of that place. It is a good place.' Whereas now, you say you work at The Glenn and [DCWs in other ALFs] say, 'Oh, I know Jane [the administrator],' . . . bad, bad [reputation]."

Findings show that, in addition to the qualities of the administrative staff and other employees, the good standing of a facility rests on the reputation that it has in the community for caring for residents. A DCW in a large (120 beds) urban home said, "When a [resident] is coming to a place like this, they ought to be treated with respect, dignity, and honor. The reason I come to this particular [ALF] was because I always heard of Green Gables and I always heard they had a good reputation." Similarly, a DCW in a small (24 beds) rural home described how she chose her facility: "I heard good things about the care [the owner] gave."

Our findings show that working in a facility with a good reputation for resident care fosters a sense of solidarity among staff. A DCW in a small (17 beds) urban home stated: "We are more like on the same page about resident care, their medications. We can sit down and talk about something and if I can't pick a word, [other DCWs] may finish it, because they know [which resident] I am talking about." A DCW in a medium-sized (47 beds) urban facility explained that staff can work toward the same goal and maintain a sense of solidarity without necessarily liking one another: "We don't have to all like each other, but we have to take care of the residents." Another DCW in small (15 beds) urban home, who links her motivation for caregiving with religious values, said that she values the "Christian atmosphere" that characterizes her workplace.

Findings show that a key source of frustration and alienation is DCW turnover and administrators' inability to recruit good employees or discipline staff who call out, which impacts DCWs' workload and ability to provide good care. A DCW in a small (24 beds) facility expressed her frustration: "[The owners] have a hard time getting good help and all of the help that comes in here don't pitch in and that is frustrating." Another source of frustration is staff absenteeism, a problem that, according to a DCW in a large (56 beds) urban facility, is compounded when administrators do not address it: "[DCWs who call out] know that [the administrators] don't get rid of anyone. I don't think it is fair for the people who are here when you have someone who is constantly calling out. Sometimes, I think [the administrators] take it for granted that I am not going to call out."

Race and Culture

Other factors influencing staff relations are racism and cultural differences, which occur primarily in larger facilities located in urban locations.[2] These two factors are major sources of dissention and alienation. Interestingly, we also find that racial bias and racial and ethnic group affiliation promote solidarity and a collective identity among certain factions of workers in these homes. In the current study, we observed considerable conflict between African and African American DCWs, which promotes social cohesion between staff members within the two groups. Many African workers expressed the attitude that they as a group are better educated and have a superior work ethic compared with African American staff. In one large (74 beds) urban home characterized by considerable racial conflict between African DCWs, the white executive director, and African American DCWs (several of whom the executive director brought with him from another corporate location), many African DCWs expressed the view that African American staff are lazy and get by on the job through sycophancy toward the white administrators: "We [the African staff] come to this country to work ten times harder to make a better life for our families. We don't have time to kiss butt like the [African American] staff." Similarly, African American DCWs often complained that communicating with "foreign" staff is difficult. An African American DCW in the same large urban home stated, "You can't understand them and there is a lot of times that you just can't get through to them." Of note, we observed similar perceptions of racial favoritism among white, Asian, and Hispanic staff working in another large (66 beds) urban facility, where the administrators are African American. A Hispanic DCW complained: "She [the African American executive director] took my hours and gave them to this woman because she is black and I am Hispanic." The same DCW also conveyed her own racial prejudice: "I like working with Asian and Hispanic co-workers. They are disciplined. If the supervisors are not here, we can do the job. Black girls, if the supervisor is not here, they do nothing."

We also found that some racial discord relates to cultural beliefs surrounding caregiving practices. An African American DCW in a medium-sized (31 beds) urban home described her view: When we [blacks] give baths, most of us, because of the skin, we are going to put moisturizer on everybody. Some of the Caucasian people, when they are giving baths, I guess they are just used to getting them [the residents] out and drying them off and putting their clothes on."

In some regions of the state, long-standing racial prejudice limits employment opportunities for nonwhite DCWs and negatively affects their job experiences. An administrator in a small (19 beds) home located in a predominantly white small-town community in the north Georgia mountains described her experiences: "The Ku Klux Klan is still on the mountain. They [residents of the community] are so prejudiced and make no bones about it." One DCW employed in this home is an American Indian, and she reported that she has experienced racial discrimination from other staff, who are all white, as well as some residents who have mistaken her for black.

In many cases, administrators' racist attitudes or lack of cultural competence contributes to racial conflict. In one large (60 beds) urban home, a white administrator openly refers to her African American staff as "the street group." In another large (120 beds) urban home, a white administrator's use of the word *them* when describing her problems related to managing African staff is instructive: "One of the things I have come to learn managing people from Africa is that they would never make eye contact and the way they would interrelate is different from managing someone from America. There are certain things you need to learn about their culture to know how to manage them." A DCW in a large (65 beds) facility who indicated that she was thinking about leaving her job described her frustration after a white administrator directed racial slurs toward her and the executive director failed to address the issue: "Susan cussed me out and called me the 'n' word. I reported the incident but of course nothing was done and Susan still works here. I see that I am not needed here because anybody can treat you anyhow and get away with it."

Shift Assignment, Work Location, and Teamwork

Shift assignment, work location, and teamwork are additional factors influencing staff relations. Conflict between shifts is common and in many cases helps build solidarity among DCWs working on the same shift. Much of this conflict is related to a lack of communication between shifts, resentment over work left undone, and the perception that the workload on other shifts, such as the night shift, may be lighter. An administrator in a large (69 beds) urban home described a common scenario: "A lot of people get possessive about their shift and they work so well together that they think they are the best shift in the world and no one came take care of the residents like we can on our shift." A DCW in a large (81 beds) urban home explained how animosity develops between shifts, especially toward the night shift: "Every shift thinks the other shift is not working like they should. You feel like the other shift has it easier than you do. Everybody is always looking for a quick thing to blame on the other shift instead of owning up to it. We couldn't get to this or second shift didn't do this or third shift didn't do that or [staff on the third shift] don't do anything all night. So why didn't they do it? Instead of one day they didn't do it, it is every day they didn't do it. No doubt about that. We blame the third shift for everything." When asked about problems related to staff performance, an administrator in a small (24 beds) urban home said that the conflict between shifts is one of the biggest difficulties she confronts: "They are constantly looking for anything that the other shift did not do to complain about." Several administrators recognize that a lack of knowledge regarding the work that is done on other shifts contributes to the problem, and a strategy some use is to schedule staff to work across shifts, which helps alleviate some of the conflict.

Several staff members who work the night shift indicated that they feel somewhat alienated and cut off from administrators and other staff, many of whom suggested that the night shift does not work as hard. Several administrators said that they know a problem exists but indicated taking little action to address it. One administrator in a large (65 beds) urban home admitted that he may even contribute to the problem: "I haven't been as good [at communicating] with third shift because I don't like to get up in the middle of the night and they don't always come for the [staff] meetings [which are held during the day]."

Given the value that many DCWs place on resident care (see Chapter 7, this volume), it is possible that some of this lack of connection between night staff and other DCWs may be due in part to night staff's limited role in resident care. One DCW in a large (69 beds) urban home admitted that her job, which mainly consists of cleaning offices and doing laundry, is somewhat easier because she does not have much contact with residents: "It is easier because you don't have too much interacting with the residents, so there is nothing stopping you. You just go straight to your work." Thus, whereas some night staff suggested that they feel alienated, others working the same shift indicated a sense of autonomy. A DCW in a large (60 beds) urban facility said, "I have control over my shift because there is nobody there but me. I am the only one at night on my floor and I try to do everything possible that I am supposed to do."

Although most staff expressed a value for teamwork, many, regardless of shift, indicated that they prefer to work alone and at their own pace. A DCW in a large (160 beds) urban facility voiced a feeling held by many: "I work until the work is done and I get it over with, right. But when I work with someone who doesn't work like that, I don't hold it against them, but sometimes when it is like that, I would rather be by myself. I get the job done quicker by myself than I would with somebody that is slow or just going to slow me down." A DCW in another large (75 beds) urban home expressed a similar preference: "I like to work with other people, but when I get in my zone, when I am doing what I do, I like to work by myself."

Often DCWs relate their value for teamwork with working toward a common goal of providing good resident care. When asked what teamwork means to her, a DCW in a large (56 beds) urban home expressed a common view: "Everyone coming together for the benefit of the residents." In several cases in which staff conveyed a value of working together to complete tasks, they referred to the requirements associated with meeting the needs of heavier-care residents, a situation we often observed among staff working in dementia care units (DCUs). Although the work conducted in DCUs is generally more labor-intensive compared with work in other areas in a facility, we found that staff often take pride in this distinction, which helps promote group solidarity. A DCW in a large (57 beds) urban facility stated: "There were some of us designated to work in [the DCU] because of the way we can interact with residents."

Another common strategy we observed is for DCWs to forge a close working relationship with at least one other person who has a similar work ethic and work style. A DCW in a medium-sized (54 beds) rural home described the necessity of having such a relationship: "Clara's sister was diagnosed with breast cancer and I worked all of her weekends for a month. To me that is teamwork. If I needed off, she would work for me." In another medium-sized (38 beds) urban facility characterized by some racial conflict among staff, one Latino worker indicated that she thinks about leaving her job all the time but stays primarily because of her close working relationship with one other person assigned to her shift. In several cases, we found that DCWs develop their closest relationship with a shift supervisor and that many supervisors may act as intermediaries in the communication (e.g., regarding scheduling, workplace conflicts that develop) between staff and upper level management.

In some cases, these close working relationships cut across racial and ethnic lines. A white DCW in a medium-sized (27 beds) urban home, who admitted she does not typically get close to anyone at work, said that she has developed a close working relationship with an African American DCW whom she shares similar values with and describes as a "Christian lady." Similarly, a white DCW working in a medium-sized (44 beds) rural home acknowledged that "race is an issue" for some employees but said that her religious values include acceptance of racial differences. She described the bond she shares with an African American DCW, who works with her on the same shift: "I know all of her people and she knows all of mine." In these examples, religious and cultural (i.e., connection to family and place) values are important factors in the development of these relationships.

In some cases, the physical design of a facility, similar to shift assignment, influences the creation of solidarity among subgroups. We observed this situation in several large homes where staff are segregated on different floors, in facilities with DCUs, and in a few places where residents are housed in different buildings located on the same campus. A DCW in a large (81 beds) home described the quality of relations among staff in a DCU: "Most of us who worked in the Alzheimer unit was like a close knit family and everybody worked together. We didn't have much of a relationship with [staff on] the other [AL] side." In several facilities where separate work spaces exist, including those found in two small homes where residents are housed in more than one building on the same property, this environmental separation also provides staff with some freedom from direct supervision by administrators and supervisors, which also is valued by many.

Fitting In

Across facilities in this sample, we found that newly recruited staff often have difficulty transitioning into a new job. Our findings indicate that some of the difficulty they encounter is related to the effect that their need for orientation and training has on other DCWs' workflow. Sometimes, this problem is compounded when a new person has no previous connection with current staff. In several cases, we found that this inability to fit in can result in turnover of new staff. An administrator in a large (59 beds) urban home acknowledged the challenges that new staff face: "I don't think it is easy for new staff. [My staff] are not the most welcoming unless it is someone that they know. If it is a total stranger, I don't think they are real receptive to that." An administrator in another large (57 beds) urban home described a similar situation: "It can be difficult for new people. If they are brand new and nobody knows them, then it can be difficult." A DCW in a medium-sized (35 beds) urban home described how she and other staff in her facility view new hires: "We get along pretty much the same, except for the new people, because they just don't know anything." With regard to the perceived ability of new hires, an administrator in a small (19 beds) urban home said that her staff will often say things like "She can't remember anything" and "She is not going to be any good." Another administrator in a small (20 beds) rural home indicated that once her staff set their mind against a new hire, she does not try to retain the person, regardless of that individual's qualifications: "They will say, 'I know that girl's reputation.' Even if it is not founded and just rumor, [I know] it is not going to work, if she is not well liked for whatever reason, even if she is well qualified."

In situations in which administrators' economic constraints or local economic conditions limit the pool of potential staff, the employment of DCWs with a dubious background or a poor work ethic, including a lack of commitment to caregiving, contribute to relationship problems. In some cases, administrators reported staffing problems, such as theft, including theft of drugs, and substance use. Key values of DCWs with strong job commitment include working with like-minded staff, including those in administrative roles, and affiliation with a facility with a good reputation. We found that, when these values are not supported, DCWs are likely to become alienated and less committed to their jobs. An administrator in a large (59 beds) urban facility with an 88 percent turnover rate estimated that 75 percent of the staff who leave her facility leave because of problems related to co-workers. Similar perceptions are reported by staff and administrators across homes.

Negotiating Risks

Like low-wage workers employed in other sectors of the service industry, these staff represent an economically marginal group. More than half (59%) earn $8.50 or less an hour. Many, particularly those who lack income from another job or support from another wage earner, are at risk of falling below the established federal poverty level, which for a family of four is currently $21,200 (U.S. Department of Health and Human Services, 2008). A large percentage (61%) are unmarried, and more than half (53%) report that they are supporting children under the age of 18. Close to one-third (32%) are supporting people living outside their homes. Many (26%) of these are immigrant workers who support family members back in their native countries. As we note in Chapters 4 and 9 in this volume, other factors linked to DCWs' economic vulnerability include gender, race, education, geographic location, and work status. Owing to low wages and, in many cases, limitations on available work hours, including unpredictable drops in hours, many (24%) of DCWs report that they work one or more additional jobs to survive economically.

When compared with the national profile of low-wage workers, these workers are older on average, with a mean age of 40. Twenty-five percent are aged 50 years or older. The combination of low socioeconomic status and increasing age contributes to the likelihood of health problems, and, as we note in Chapter 11 in this volume, 41 percent of DCWs in this study lack medical insurance. The percentage of DCWs without medical coverage is higher (54%) in facilities located in rural areas, which tend to employ a larger percentage of older workers.

In some cases, the profile of administrators mirrors that of staff. Seven out of 42 administrators we interviewed have a high school diploma or less. Two, both operators of small, low-income facilities, have what some staff might view as dubious backgrounds. One, who operates a home in an urban area and recruits most of his staff from homeless shelters, reported a history of homelessness and drug use. The other, who operates a home in a rural area, currently moonlights as a bail bondsman and nightclub operator. Although other administrators have more traditional backgrounds, including training in long-term care, all struggle to balance the needs of residents and staff while trying to protect their bottom line. As we note in Chapter 11 of this volume, some small business owners, especially those in rural areas, who cannot take advantage of economies of scale and face disadvantages related to the local labor market must struggle harder to meet these demands.

Participants' economic vulnerability and, in many cases, marginal social position dictate what strategies they use to survive economically. Ironically, we find that the survival strategies participants use often result in risks to their economic security, a process we label "negotiating risks." This process, which we have identified previously among similar groups (see Ball et al., 2005; Perkins, Ball, Whittington, & Combs, 2004), in some cases poses risks to residents' quality of care.

A common strategy DCWs employ is "job hopping" in search of that elusive "better" low-wage job. An administrator in a medium-sized (27 beds) home referred to this strategy as "the grass is greener" phenomenon and described how it often backfires: "The reason they were leaving was that they wanted to find a better job. It always looks better on the other side. I would say that one-third of them want to come back after they leave. They say they realize it is much worse out there than they thought, but I have a policy that if someone leaves, if they don't give a two-week notice or work out their two week notice, they can't come back."

Often, information conveyed through DCWs' social networks leads them to seek better job options, frequently involving a search for better pay and more hours. Having ties with other staff employed in a new location can ease a job transition. However, as we indicate above, as new employees DCWs often face significant challenges related to their stigmatized position as a "new" person who "can't remember anything" and is "not going to be any good." In addition, as new employees, these DCWs often have less job security than staff with more tenure if the resident census drops. Scheduling of work hours and whether or not an administrator is sensitive to a DCW's individual needs often hinge on relationships that develop over time.

As we note in Chapter 11 in this volume, administrators use a variety of strategies to save money on staffing, including cutting hours to accommodate drops in the resident census, keeping wages low, and limiting health benefits. We found that, ironically, these strategies promote staff dissatisfaction and turnover. As indicated in previous chapters, turnover is financially costly. Recent estimates suggest that the total cost per employee is at least $2,500 (Seavey, 2004).

As we illustrate above, we also find that staff turnover has a substantial negative impact on the social environment of a facility, including the quality of staff relations, which also influences turnover. In addition, turnover disrupts continuity of care, which in turn has a negative influence on resident care. These findings show that the inability to provide good quality care to residents is another important factor that leads to dissatisfaction among staff and reduces their organizational commitment (see Chapter 7, this volume).

Administrators faced with high turnover and a limited labor pool often must lower their standards for hiring. In some facilities, we found that the presence of staff members with dubious backgrounds also negatively impacts the social environment within a facility and, in many cases, tarnishes a facility's reputation. These findings show that a facility's reputation, which is communicated through DCWs' social networks, can place further constraints on an administrator's ability to recruit quality staff.

A value of staff, many of whom are struggling financially and face significant problems balancing family and work, is empathy and support from administrators, which we find foster organizational commitment. A DCW in large (62 beds) urban home described her relationship with her administrator:

"She is like a big umbrella. She makes sure you are protected. She will only let you go, if you let yourself go." However, in some cases, administrators' attempts to help staff have a negative outcome, especially in the case of staff with greater personal problems. An administrator in a small (24 beds) rural home described her experience attempting to help a recovering drug addict: "One [DCW] was an excellent worker and I have to defend her. She had problems with drugs, but she beat it and was doing good. I think it [her illness] was her gallbladder, and they rushed her to the hospital. Her husband begged them not to put morphine in her. When she was finally over the surgery, she was hooked again. It took us all but a day and a half and we found that the meds were missing."

Administrators in three homes with high turnover rates reported that theft is a significant problem. Because of difficulties monitoring night staff, DCWs who work these shifts often are suspect, which adds to their stigmatized position. A common strategy these three providers use is making unannounced nighttime visits. A DCW in one of these facilities described her administrator's behavior: "One night, she came out here to try and slip through the window." This staff person reported that on another night she and other employees were "caught" with Walmart bags, which the administrator subsequently discovered were filled with toiletry items staff had purchased for residents. No doubt such negative interactions with administrators have a damaging impact on DCWs' job attitudes.

Maintenance of Just-Close-Enough Ties

Consistent with our preliminary finding, we found that social networks (relationships staff have with family, friends, and former co-workers and employers) are a key factor leading DCWs into these ALFs. In the current study, 33 out of 41 staff who completed qualitative interviews reported that they chose their facility based on what they heard about the facility from others. Six of the 41 said that they were actively recruited by an administrator or manager at the facility. In addition, many of these staff reported that they had previously worked with another DCW or one of the supervisors at another facility. An administrator in a medium-sized (35 beds) home described this recruiting pattern: "A lot of staff members have joined me from my previous community." However, as we note previously, this strategy sometimes has a negative impact on staff already present in the home.

In contrast to previous findings, findings from the current study show that network ties are not necessarily close ties. In addition, we found that this pattern of job referral does not always lead to a cohesive social environment. DCW and administrator turnover, and strategies participants use to negotiate risks, are important intervening factors that influence the culture of these homes. Racial, ethnic, and cultural differences, lack of communication, and physical and social distance also have an important impact.

In this study, we found that an important strategy DCWs use to get by on the job is to maintain some distance from co-workers. Staff value teamwork as means for providing good resident care, but many, when given the opportunity, like to work alone and at their own pace. As noted, staff turnover and the presence of new employees often disrupt DCWs' workflow, which leads to frustration. Conversations we had with DCWs indicate that conflict between shifts and gossip are to be expected and one way to cope is to maintain just-close-enough ties to provide good care to residents and get by on the job but also to maintain a degree of separation.

A recurring theme is establishing boundaries. Although we found some close ties in a few small homes, especially those that include staff who are biological family members, we found that most DCWs do not cultivate close relationships with co-workers. As we illustrate previously, a common strategy is to forge a close relationship with just one or two people who have a similar work ethic and work style. Sometimes this relationship is with a supervisor or an administrator. By establishing boundaries, staff find that they can avoid conflicts, including becoming the subject of gossip. Many DCWs work more than one job and are struggling to balance work and family life and, because of limited time and resources, do not want to incur the emotional costs or social obligations associated with close work ties. In relation to her workplace relationships, a DCW in a small (15 beds) urban home stated: "Unless you are going to a funeral, everything stays there [at work]. I don't care too much for mixing business with pleasure." Another DCW in a medium-sized (44 beds) rural home, where most staff had been recruited from a local mill that had closed and had work relationships that spanned over 20 years, expressed a similar view: "It's not that I don't care for them, but once you leave here, you don't take your work home with you."

Administrators seem keenly aware of this need to establish boundaries, and many promote the practice themselves. An administrator in a small (15 beds) urban home stated his philosophy: "I constantly mention boundaries to staff. What makes good neighbors is good fences. With co-workers, let's not cross the line. [The relationship] should be pretty professional and of an adult nature. When it is time to work, it is time to work." Another administrator in a large (56 beds) urban home expressed a similar viewpoint: "I have mixed feelings about the relationship building for staff, because sometimes I find that the closer they are, the more difficult it is for those who are not [part of] the group. It can [result in] cliques."

Discussion

Over the past several decades, numerous studies have focused on the plight of poor people. Since the publication in 1974 of Carol Stack's groundbreaking ethnography, *All Our Kin*, much literature has been written aimed at dispelling negative stereotypes and confronting societal and institutional forces that contribute to these individuals' economic marginality and stigmatized image, including factors contributing to joblessness (see, for example, Anderson, 1990; Dodson, 1998; Wilson, 1996). Recently, researchers and policy makers have begun to focus on the struggles of low-wage workers, our nation's invisible working poor, individuals who work hard but teeter precariously on the brink of poverty (Munger, 2007; Newman, 1999; Shipler, 2005; Shulman, 2005). For many of these workers, a crisis, such as a family emergency, illness, or an unexpected bill, could be the catalyst leading to impoverishment. We found that some strategies workers use to survive economically place them at increased financial risk (Ball et al., 2005; Perkins, Ball, et al., 2004).

Our previous study of five small African American–owned and –operated ALFs in Georgia (Ball et al., 2005; Perkins, Ball, et al., 2004) reveals some of the personal struggles and financial hardships faced by operators and staff in these low-wage workplaces, but, to date, little of the growing literature that addresses low-wage workers in the United States (for example, see Munger, 2007; Newman, 1999; Shipler, 2005; Shulman, 2005) provides much information regarding the experiences of care workers. Thus the unique challenges faced by this segment of the low-wage workforce remain relatively unknown. In this chapter and throughout this book, we highlight the important contributions of DCWs, including their commitment to caregiving; describe the creative strategies they use to get by on the job and survive economically; and bring to light the distinct challenges they face.

For the most part, AL staff fit the national profile of low-wage workers (Schochet & Rangarajan, 2004). They are predominantly female, most lack a college education, and many are minorities and immigrants. A distinction of low-wage workers represented in this study is that many are older on average, compared with the national profile, who as a group tend to be young adults under the age of 35 (Schochet & Rangarajan, 2004). In defining these workers as low-wage, we use a common benchmark, which is an hourly wage that results in annual earnings that fall below the established federal poverty level for a family of four. We find that certain factions of DCWs, such as those living in rural areas, are particularly disadvantaged. Given the current economic downturn and rises in unemployment in both rural and urban areas, these workers as a group represent an especially vulnerable population.

Similar to staff in nursing homes, AL staff are culturally diverse. Although the findings show that bonds formed among racial and ethnic lines can promote group solidarity, consistent with previous research in nursing homes (Berdes & Eckert, 2001; Foner, 1994), findings also show that cultural differences, including differences in language, customs and beliefs, as well as country of origin, often lead to conflict, which is damaging to the AL social and work environment.

In addition to cultural conflict, findings from this study highlight several other important factors that affect co-worker relationships and influence DCW turnover in AL, an outcome that has a negative effect on administrators, residents, and DCWs themselves, including potential serious economic implications. A key strategy DCWs use to maintain viable employment is use of social networks. In contrast to our previous studies of AL staff (Perkins, Sweatman, et al., 2004; Perkins et al., 2005) and small AL operators (Ball et al., 2005), we found that these network connections do not necessarily represent close ties. Based on the literature, we characterize these ties as "social leverage networks," a form of social capital related to the concept of "weak ties" (Granovetter, 1973, 1983, 1995), which research shows can be critical for economic survival among low-income groups (Briggs, 1998; Dominguez & Watkins, 2003). Like Dominguez and Watkins (2003), we found that DCWs' ability to benefit from their social connections requires a delicate balance between friendship and family-based ties, which require an emotional investment and can result in time-consuming social obligations, and informal support or so-called social leverage ties, a type of social support that provides access to information, as well as opportunities for material or professional advancement. These findings are consistent across geographic locations, including rural areas and small towns often characterized by dense social ties. Findings indicate that, in these small, close-knit communities, where DCWs may experience a lack of anonymity, for many, setting boundaries with co-workers may also be a way of preserving some privacy.

We found that the meanings DCWs attach to the relationships they develop in their workplace have an important influence on their commitment to a given facility and the likelihood of their remaining in a given job. In this study, we define commitment as the "cost" associated with giving up a social connection or an identity (Burke & Reitzes, 1991; Stryker, 1968). In the context of workplace relationships, previous research shows that, compared with men, women tend to develop more intense and intimate ties (Wiley, 1991). These findings are supported by research we present earlier in this chapter on women's workplace relationships. In the current study, we found that gender, in contrast to race, does not necessarily promote a group identity or help build solidarity among DCWs. Rather, in this study, we found that a key source of group solidarity and job commitment is DCWs' occupational identity as care workers.

According to Stryker (1968), the various identities that constitute the self are organized hierarchically according to salience. Following this perspective, the salience of a particular identity, such as that of care worker, is confirmed in a particular social setting through an individual's social connection to others in that setting. In this context, commitment is reinforced through others' affirmation of a valued identity or role. For most people in the workforce, a major factor in self-definition is occupational identity. In the case of marginalized work, such as low-wage care work, workers often use a variety of defense tactics to help enhance this identity (Ashforth & Kreiner, 1999). In previous research, we found that DCWs strive to elevate their status as caregivers through affirmation from residents (Ball et al., 2009) and affirmation from residents' family members (Kemp et al., 2009). The current study, which builds on these findings, shows that the lack of affirmation from administrators and co-workers, as well as negative perceptions DCWs have regarding the reputation of their workplace or other staff, especially with regard to the quality of resident care, can jeopardize DCWs' valued identity as caregivers and reduce their organizational commitment.

Conclusion

These findings have important implications for interventions to promote organizational commitment and reduce turnover, which can improve resident care and reduce threats to DCWs' and facility operators' economic security. Findings show that the reputation of a facility, including hiring and retaining employees who have similar values regarding resident care, is a key factor in staff satisfaction and commitment. An important goal should be to educate administrators about the importance of a facility's reputation and the factors that influence it. We found that lowered standards for hiring and many of the cost-cutting strategies administrators use to get ahead financially, such as cutting staff hours when the resident census drops, may result in staff turnover and adversely affect the reputation of a facility, potentially placing providers at economic risk. In turn, we found that DCWs intent on improving their own financial situations and work environments often hop from job to job and find themselves more economically vulnerable after changing jobs (i.e., as new employees at the bottom of a facility hierarchy). Steps should be taken to break these vicious cycles.

Findings presented in this chapter and throughout this volume also show that cultural conflict is a significant problem. The increasing racial and ethnic diversity of the AL workforce, which includes a growing number of immigrants, heightens the need for strategies to promote cultural competence. Other potential sources of relational conflict that administrators need to recognize and address include competition between shifts, new staff until they are acculturated into the setting and other staff members who disrupt workflow, staff who are perceived as receiving special privileges or favoritism from supervisors, and a perceived lack of trust and respect from employers. Findings show that night staff face unique challenges, and steps should to be taken to see that these workers are better integrated into the facility culture. Results indicate that other workers' perceptions regarding the night shift's lack of interaction with residents contributes to their lower-status position, providing further evidence of the importance that DCWs place on their role as caregivers. As noted in several chapters throughout this volume, affirmation of this value is an important first step toward hiring and maintaining a good-quality workforce.

NOTES

1. Data we present here on staff turnover were collected from administrators at the time of their interview. Turnover is calculated as the number of employees who left during the previous year divided by the total number of DCWs employed in the previous

year multiplied by 100 to obtain a percentage. Data we report on administrator turnover were obtained when we called facilities one year after completion of staff interviews. These data show that almost one-third (30%) of administrators left their job. Although this information does not reflect conditions at the time that qualitative data were collected, it is presented here as context for the qualitative findings.

2. As we note in Chapter 3 in this volume, 18% of staff are foreign-born, and all these DCWs work in homes located in urban areas. For the most part, the racial, ethnic, and immigrant compositions of staff present in the study homes reflect geographic (urban versus rural) and regional differences in concentrations of minority populations found throughout the state. Although Georgia has a relatively sizable black population, including a large percentage of blacks who live in rural counties (i.e., part of an area known as the southern Black Belt), several rural counties located in the northern mountain region of the state are predominantly white and historically have been home to few blacks.

REFERENCES

Anderson, E. 1990. *Streetwise: Race, class, and change in an urban community.* Chicago: University of Chicago Press.

Ashforth, B. E., & Kreiner, G. E. 1999. "How can you do it?": Dirty work and the challenge of constructing a positive identity. *Academy of Management Review* 24, 413–34.

Ball, M. M., Lepore, M. L., Perkins, M. M., Hollingsworth, C., & Sweatman, M. 2009. "They are the reason I come to work": The meaning of resident-staff relationships in assisted living. *Journal of Aging Studies* 23, 37–47.

Ball, M. M., Perkins, M. M., Whittington, F. J., Hollingsworth, C. King, S. V., & Combs, B. L. 2005. *Communities of care: Assisted living for African American elders.* Baltimore: Johns Hopkins University Press.

Benson, S. P. 1986. *Counter culture: Saleswomen, managers, and customers in American department stores, 1890–1940.* Urbana: University of Illinois Press.

Berdes, C., & Eckert, J. M. 2001. Race relations and caregiving relationships. *Research on Aging* 23, 109–26.

Bowers, B., & Becker, M. 1992. Nurse's aides in nursing homes: The relationship between organization and quality. *The Gerontologist* 32, 360–66.

Braverman, H. 1974. *Labor and monopoly capital: The degradation or work in the twentieth century.* New York: Monthly Review Press.

Briggs, X. 1998. Brown kids in white suburbs: Housing mobility and the many faces of social capital. *Housing Policy Debate* 9, 177–221.

Burke, P. J., & Reitzes, D. C. 1991. An identity approach to commitment. *Social Psychology Quarterly* 54, 239–51.

Charmez, K. 2006. *Constructing grounded theory: A practical guide through qualitative analysis.* Thousand Oaks, CA: Sage Publications.

Chen, C. K., Sabir, M., Zimmerman, S., Suitor, J. J., & Pillemer, K. 2007. The importance of family relationships with nursing facility staff for family caregiver burden and depression. *Journals of Gerontology: Social Sciences* 62, P253–60.

Clarke, A. E. 2005. *Situational analysis: Grounded theory after the postmodern turn.* Thousand Oaks, CA: Sage Publications.

Dodson, L. 1998. *Don't call us out of name: The untold lives of women and girls in poor America.* Boston: Beacon Press.

Dominguez, S., & Watkins, C. 2003. Creating networks for survival and mobility: Social capital among African-American and Latin-American low-income mothers. *Social Problems* 50, 111–35.

Foner, N. 1994. *The caregiving dilemma: Work in an American nursing home.* Berkeley: University of California Press.

Gaugler, J. E. 2005. Staff perceptions of residents across the long-term care landscape. *Journal of Advanced Nursing* 49, 377–86.

Granovetter, M. S. 1973. The strength of weak ties. *American Journal of Sociology* 78, 1360–80.

———. 1983. The strength of weak ties revisited. *Sociological Theory* 1, 201–33.

———. 1995. *Getting a Job: A study of contacts and careers.* Chicago: University of Chicago Press.

Kanter, R. M., & Stein, B. (Eds). 1979. *Life in organizations.* New York: Basic Books.

Kemp, C. L., Ball, M. M., Perkins, M. M., Hollingsworth, C., & Lepore, M. L. 2009. "I get along with most of them": Direct care workers' relationships with residents' families in assisted living. *The Gerontologist* 49, 224–35.

Lamphere, L. 1985. Bringing the family to work: Culture on the shop floor. *Feminist Studies* 11, 519–40.

Munger, F. (Ed.). 2002. *Laboring below the line: The new ethnography of poverty, low-wage work, and survival in a global economy.* New York: Russell Sage Foundation.

Newman, K. S. 1999. *No shame in my game.* New York: Random House.

Perkins, M., Ball, M. M., Whittington, F. J., & Combs, B. L. 2004. Managing the needs of low-income board and care home residents: A process of negotiating risks. *Qualitative Health Research* 14, 478–95.

Perkins, M. M., Sweatman, M., Lepore, M., Ball, M. M., Hollingsworth, C., & Sambhara, R. 2005. Workplace relationships in assisted living: How they influence satisfaction and retention. Paper presented at the Joint Conference of the American Society on Aging and the National Council on Aging, Philadelphia, PA.

Perkins, M. M., Sweatman, M., Sambhara, R., Hollingsworth, C., Lepore, M., & Ball, M. M. 2004. *Work culture in assisted living: Key to satisfaction and retention.* Paper presented at the 57th annual meeting of the Gerontological Society of America, Washington, DC.

Powers, B. A. 1992. The roles staff play in the social networks of elderly institutionalized people. *Social Science and Medicine* 34, 1335–43.

Schochet, P., & Rangarajan, P. 2004. *Characteristics of low-wage workers and their labor market experiences: Evidence from the mid-to-late 1990s* (Mathematica Policy Research, Inc. Publication No. 8915-600). Retrieved October 3, 2008, from http://aspe.hhs.gov/hsp/low-wage-workers04/report.pdf.

Seavey, D. 2004. *The cost of frontline turnover in long-term care.* A Better Jobs Better Care practice and policy report. Washington, DC.

Shipler, D. K. 2005. *The working poor: Invisible in America.* New York: Vintage Books.

Shulman, B. 2005. *The betrayal of work: How low-wage jobs fail 30 million Americans.* New York: New Press.

Stack, C. 1974. *All our kin.* New York: Basic Books.

Strauss, A., & Corbin, J. 1998. *Basics of qualitative research: Techniques and procedures for developing grounded theory.* Thousand Oaks, CA: Sage Publications.

Stryker, S. 1968. Identity salience and role performance: The relevance of symbolic interaction theory for family research. *Journal of Marriage and Family* 4, 558–64.

Tellis-Nayak, V., & Tellis-Nayak, M. 1989. Quality of care and the burden of two cultures: When the world of the nurse's aide enters the world of the nursing home. *The Gerontologist* 29, 307–13.

U.S. Department of Health and Human Services. 2008. The 2008 HHS Poverty Guidelines. *Federal Register* 73 (15), 3971–72.

Wiley, M. G. 1991. Gender, work, stress: The potential impact of role-identity salience and commitment. *Sociological Quarterly* 32, 495–510.

Wilson, W. J. 1996. *When work disappears: The world of the new urban poor.* New York: Knopf.

Zavella, P. 1985. "Abnormal intimacy": The varying work networks of Chicana cannery workers. *Feminist Studies* 11, 541–57.

CHAPTER SEVEN

Connections with Residents

"It's All about the Residents for Me"

Candace L. Kemp, Ph.D.
Mary M. Ball, Ph.D.
Carole Hollingsworth, M.A
Michael J. Lepore, Ph.D.

What attracts and keeps direct care workers (DCWs) in jobs that are consistently characterized as physically and emotionally demanding, low wage, and low status? As the collection of work in this book attests, the answer is complex. Nevertheless, existing research suggests that relationships between caregivers and care receivers are potentially important pieces of this puzzle. For example, studies in home care settings (Ball & Whittington, 1995; Chichin, 1992; Karner, 1998; Parks, 2003) and nursing homes (Bowers, Esmond, & Jacobson, 2000) show that care workers and the older adults they care for often develop close, personal connections that not only improve quality of care and life for care recipients but also are meaningful for caregivers and among the most satisfying and rewarding aspects of care work.

Despite their apparent import, almost no research has considered these relationships in assisted living (Ball et al., 2009), which, as suggested in Chapter 5 of this volume, differs in important ways from nursing homes and home care and is the fastest-growing sector in the long-term care (LTC) industry (Mollica, 2002). In one of the few studies examining relationships in these settings, Ball and colleagues (2009) drew on data from two assisted living facilities (ALFs)—a nonprofit with 35 beds and a for-profit with 75 beds—to explore how DCWs experience their relationships with residents. As research in other care settings has shown, they found that relationships are meaningful for DCWs and exert influence on care outcomes. They also identified factors that influence the development, quality, and meaning of relationships, attributing variation to certain facility (e.g., physical environment and workload), staff (e.g., personal characteristics and employment history), and resident (e.g., personal characteristics, history, and functional status) factors. Ultimately, they concluded that relationships with residents are among the most important reasons DCWs go to work and remain in their jobs. As one care worker put it, "They are the reason I come to work."

The analysis presented in this chapter builds on Ball and colleagues' (2009) work in an effort to further understand the meanings of and variations in staff-resident relationships using a larger, more diverse sample of workers (and residents), ALFs, and their surrounding communities. Specifically, we ask (1) How do DCWs perceive and experience their relationships with residents? and (2) What factors affect relationship development, maintenance, and meanings? Throughout we consider the extent to which relationships influence DCWs' caregiving experiences, including their overall job satisfaction and retention.

Methods

Our analysis relies on data from all 45 homes involved in the study, "Job Satisfaction and Retention of Direct Care Staff in Assisted Living." Specifically we draw on semistructured qualitative interviews with administrators (N=44) and DCWs (N=41). We asked both groups about the quality and negotiation of staff-resident relationships, factors influencing these relationships, and the roles these relationships play in DCWs' work experiences and satisfaction. We also consider data from the 370 DCWs' surveys by considering these open-ended questions: What type of relationship do you value most with residents? What do find most (and least) satisfying about working at your ALF? What type of resident do you find most difficult to care for?

Data Analysis

We analyzed our data following the principles of grounded theory methods (Strauss & Corbin, 1998). We began the three-stage method by examining our textual data line by line for emergent categories guided by our research questions and issues raised by participants in a process referred to as *open coding*. Initial codes included relationship type, factors influencing relationships, and relationship outcomes. In this initial phase we analyzed administrator and staff data separately. Next, we conducted *axial coding*. We connected open-coding categories to other categories signifying relationships, intervening factors or conditions, and consequences. For example, we linked relationship type to community-, facility-, and individual-level factors such as community size, location, and degree of staff-resident homogeneity; facility size and relationships-related policies and practices; and residents' and DCW's personal characteristics and relationship goals and strategies. At this point, we interpreted staff and administrator data within the context of one another. In the final stage, we integrated and refined categories to form a larger conceptual scheme through *selective coding* and organized our categories around our core category, "promoting satisfaction and retention through meaningful relationships."

Results

Workers' Perceptions and Experiences

DCWs' relationships with residents are central to understanding their caregiving experiences and attitudes toward work. When asked what they find most satisfying about their jobs, the majority (65%) said "the residents," explaining they "love working with," "taking care of," and "being with" residents. Over half said residents are "the number one" or "only reason" they remain in their job. One succinctly explained, "It's all about the residents for me."

From DCWs' perspectives, rewarding relationships with residents tend to counteract dissatisfying aspects of care work. One explained, "Sometimes I am tired and I think I want to quit, but then I go home and rest and think about these people." Another elaborated, "The [residents] in my building, I am here for them. I won't lie. There have been times I wanted to take my pocketbook and walk out of here, but I couldn't do it. This is my family, my second family. It is not for the benefits and it sure ain't for the money. For 12 years, I might be somewhere else making a lot more money than I make now." Speaking more generally, one DCW noted, "The majority of people stay because they enjoy the residents. It is not for the pay. It is not because everything is so great up in here. It is just for the residents."

Administrators echoed these sentiments, with some conceptualizing staff-resident relationships as DCWs' "second pay check." One remarked: "I think the relationships the staff member builds with the resident is part of the reward. . . . No one is going to get rich doing this kind of work so there has to be something else about it." According to DCWs, relationships with residents and the meanings they attach to them appear to be that "something else."

Not all staff-resident relationships are equally rewarding or meaningful. Our data describe relationships ranging from "close," "personal," and "friend-" and "family-like" to "not that close" and, in some instances, "difficult" or "abusive." One DCW summed up the variation in relationships and outcomes by saying, "I can feel when I get to the door, I am like, 'I don't want to be here,' but then sometimes you go talk to these residents and you'll be like, 'I love this job!' You know, they are such sweethearts. But, I mean, oh my goodness, now don't get me wrong, some of them you want to choke."

Despite the wide range in relationship type, many spoke of residents who are their "heart" or "pets." As one commented, "I have *certain ones* that make me want to come to my job."

Factors Influencing Relationships

Our analysis identifies several multilevel factors that interact and create relational variability. As illustrated in Figure 7.1, factors at the community, facility, and individual (i.e., residents and staff) levels directly and indirectly influence the negotiation of staff-resident relationships and ultimately relationship quality, care outcomes, and the meanings of relationships. In turn, these factors and their relational outcomes influence DCWs' satisfaction and retention.

Community-Level Factors

The size, location, and culture of the community in which an ALF is located can be consequential. In small towns and rural settings "everybody knows everybody" and staff, residents, and their families often have prior connections. DCWs reported seeing residents' family members not only "when they come in" to the facility but also "out in the community, like the grocery store." Some find this familiarity "satisfying," saying it encourages them to get close to residents and "go that extra mile." Speaking of a resident she considers her "heart," one worker explained, "She came here and I knew her. I knew everything about her."

Preexisting familiarity creates a sense of community and closeness that

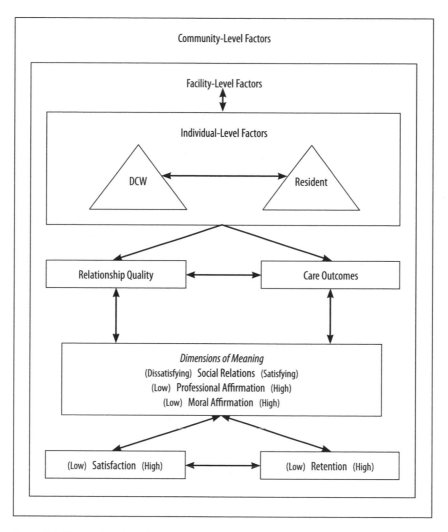

Figure 7.1. Promoting Satisfaction and Retention through Meaningful Relationships: The Relationship Process

is found less frequently in larger, urban settings. Moreover, in small towns, particularly in rural areas, staff and residents are apt to share racial, ethnic, social, economic, and religious backgrounds. For example, when asked about race-related problems, the administrator of an ALF in a predominantly white community where residents and staff are all white responded, "We have never had anything else. That has never been a problem." Although not a necessary condition, homogeneity can facilitate closer relationships. In communities such as larger metropolitan areas where staff and residents come from different backgrounds, differences can create relational barriers. The administrator of an urban facility with a majority black (native- and non-native-born) staff and an all white resident population speculated on the biggest barrier to positive relationships: "Probably race, different generations, race and ethnic background or origin." She commented on certain residents' use of racial language that is "offensive" by today's standards and foreign-born workers' use of their "native tongue," which residents find rude. Ultimately, though, how these behaviors are negotiated depends on facility and individual factors.

Facility-Level Factors

Facility characteristics, including size, ownership, physical layout, and fees, are among the facility-level factors influencing staff-resident relationships. DCWs employed in smaller ALFs generally get to know all residents, which is not always the case in larger settings. Smaller and family-owned ALFs are often described as "homelike," where familiarity promotes "family-like" relationships, suggesting the importance of social and physical environments. Facilities with dementia care units (DCUs) typically design these spaces in ways that promote interaction. One DCU worker noted: "It's a smaller unit and they are all in one place. . . . You are in constant contact so you have a more personal relationship with them." Conversely, some of the larger ALFs are located on campuses with multiple buildings, and workers complained that this layout inhibits interactions with residents. In high-fee facilities, residents are not always able to afford aging in place and leave, which some DCWs find emotionally difficult. Others complained that such facilities attract residents who "have money and are just snotty people" rather than the "down-to-earth" residents found in facilities catering to the less wealthy.

Staff-resident relationships develop within the context of caregiving. For this reason, our analysis indicates that workload, task configuration, and degree of resident frailty—which are interrelated—are consequential to staff-resident interactions. In facilities where the universal worker concept (see Chapter 5, this volume) is more fully embraced and where residents with relatively high levels of cognitive and physical disability are admitted, DCWs often feel frustrated because they lack sufficient time with each resident. One such worker explained, "Everything we do is based on time. . . . You have some that want you to come back to their room and sit down with them but you don't have the time." In another facility with heavy workloads, a care worker complained, "You are rushed for time and you need to go to another room [but] you are in another resident's room." Meanwhile, a DCW in a facility with a high resident-to-staff ratio and increasing resident frailty commented, "I wish I had more time. Now we have more residents and we don't have more staff. We have more residents and half the time." In response to these conditions, some DCWs said they "sneak in some time to talk" or visit when they are "off the clock."

Workers in ALFs with lower levels of resident disability or with less universality in their job descriptions speak of having more quality time to spend with residents. Reducing the number of tasks DCWs perform can create more time for residents. A DCW employed in a small ALF explained, "Sometimes since we have the cleaning lady, I get a chance to talk to [residents]." Likewise, DCWs employed by facilities where social and emotional care is considered essential to residents' well-being reported having more time for resident interaction. One care supervisor explained, "We like for [DCWs] to go up and down the halls, I mean just go in there and visit if they have to, talk to them, just see, because you might have somebody that might be down and sometimes if they are down, we have got a couple of clowns here that really can help out."

Another facility factor affecting relationships pertains to the rotation of staff. Some facilities rotate staff, which ideally reduces the frustration of dealing with the same people. This strategy can positively influence relationships because it distributes the burden of difficult or hard-to-care-for residents. In other ALFs, DCWs routinely care for the same residents. Administrators and workers in these facilities feel this practice leads to knowing "everything about the resident" and promotes familiarity, trust, and bonding. An administrator explained, "If we are switching too much, it will not allow us to be as consistent as we want . . . we have to make sure that the residents for sure are comfortable and to make the staff comfortable." Finally, some DCWs discussed the importance of scheduling and being able to get time off when needed, which helps them to be rested and have positive interactions with residents.

Facilities use various strategies to directly manage relationships. Some attempt to promote interactions through organized activities (e.g., parties, teas, dinners, karaoke nights) involving staff and residents. Certain ALFs communicate resident information to staff through a "communication book" or regular meetings. Some use "bio boards" (often used in DCUs) to display residents' biographical information outside their rooms. Many facilities collect detailed information about residents upon move-in. One administrator explained, "We do have a social and activities book and a form that we fill out on each resident to let the employees know the residents. Does she have any children, whether she was married, these types of things relate to how they are going to know these residents and meet their needs." A few facilities provide one-on-one time with residents as part of new staff training and offer counseling to staff when a resident passes away. Most others do not.

ALFs further govern staff-resident relationships through relational policies. Administrators' preferences for staff-resident relationships vary and tend to supersede formal rules when they are in conflict. For instance, some facilities have policies instructing staff not to get personally attached to residents. Formerly a DCW, one administrator explained why she does not enforce this policy: "I would be telling a total nontruth if I just stood there and said you cannot or you are not supposed to get personally attached, 'cause I do." This type of policy can be frustrating to DCWs, as one indicated by asking, "How do you do that? How do you not get attached to these people when you work with them five days a week, eight hours a day?"

Some facilities encourage DCWs to have close, personal relationships with residents. The administrator of a small, nonprofit ALF explained her approach: "I teach them. It's written policy also. I teach them that at nighttime when they're putting them to bed, rather than just washing their bottoms and putting a diaper on them if they wear diapers and getting them, and just, I say, sling them in the bed but to spend the time, spend that time to talk to them and find out what they're thinking and where their mind is and I said if you're a Christian and you feel comfortable, I said, then when you put them to bed have a short prayer with them. . . . And then, I said, reach over and kiss their forehead and put lotion on their hands and their faces and things. I said treat everyone like it was your grandmother or your grandfather."

Certain administrators instruct DCWs to develop "personal" but not "too close," or "professional" yet "loving," relationships. In one facility an administrator encourages caring relationships but forbids staff from discussing their personal problems with residents because residents care about staff and will worry.

In an effort to discourage "favoritism" and "bribery," most facilities have gift-giving policies either banning or placing restrictions on what, how much, and when residents can give to DCWs. The majority ban residents from giving to staff members, particularly money or valuables. Some facilities allow residents to give gifts, typically "inexpensive gifts," only on "holidays or birthdays" or with a family member's or supervisor's permission. From administrators' perspectives, these practices protect residents and staff. According to one, "We had a resident who was giving out $50 bills and we had some money missing. One shift got forgotten. It was not a pleasant time. Right now they are not supposed to accept gifts from residents. . . . If someone wants to give you a plant or a piece of clothing they don't want anymore, they have to okay it with their supervisor. The reason for that is tomorrow morning they may wake up and say they stole it." Another explained, "One lady told one of the employees to come in and pick a ring out of her ring drawer. . . . It is almost like bribery, I will give you a ring and they will take better care of you. That is not fair to the people who don't have anything to give. I pay them for caring for you. That is what they get." Although there are other ways of expressing appreciation, facility intervention in gift giving affects how residents express thanks to caregivers.

Facility intervention in relationships also occurs when conflict arises. When residents behave in ways perceived by DCWs as inappropriate, such as being abusive or making racist remarks, administrators' degree of support for staff is crucial. With regard to racism, the administrator of an ALF where most residents are white and DCWs are black said, "Sometimes residents use words that aren't appropriate and I let them know. . . . We call each other by name and we don't talk to people in a derogatory manner." DCWs appreciate such support, but it is not universal. For instance, referring to a history of poor race relations in the United States, especially the South, the administrator of a large corporately owned facility in an urban setting claimed: "You are not going to change 80 some years of bigotry," and focuses more "on the staff and helping them deal." Some DCWs accept this response and said that residents do not know any better, but others find it unacceptable. One complained: "One resident curses and yells, talks to staff like they are shit. She's catered to by the administrator and that's not right."

Individual-Level Factors

The resident factors that influence relationships fall into four categories: individual characteristics, health status, attitudes and behaviors, and family involvement. Regarding individual characteristics, DCWs note that residents' race and class (as well as their own) can influence relationships in that differences sometimes lead to residents being more "snooty" and "less appreciative" or in some cases "racist" or "suspicious" toward care staff. Similarities can have the opposite influence. As a black DCW explained, "Since I have been here, I have only known one black person to live here and you know, they [white staff] would give her a shower but then when they washed the hair they didn't know what to do with it. . . . So I would make sure I took care of the hair." As a consequence she spent more time with this resident.

Given that the majority of DCWs and residents are women, gender influences relationships. For example, in some homes, male DCWs do not bathe female residents, which limits contact. However, "good rapport" reportedly develops between male caregivers and recipients. A resident's tenure in the facility influences relationships, as staffed report greater familiarity and closer relationships with long-standing residents. Having a pet can also make a difference by encouraging, or in the case of a dog that bites, discouraging staff from entering a resident's room.

Health plays a pivotal role in establishing the types of relationships staff have with residents, but its effect is not uniform. For example, the effect of a resident's cognitive ability is interpreted in different ways. Some DCWs feel especially close to residents with dementia because they are "needier" and require "more time and care." Even though some DCWs said that residents with dementia are not able to do much, they derive satisfaction from the appreciation they offer and the feeling of being needed. One DCW explained, "You know they don't remember a lot. When you do little things for them, they thank you for it and they will hug you. I mean it is just a real rewarding job working with them." Alternatively, others feel dementia is a barrier to relationships because residents "don't remember stuff" and "forget who you are." Likewise, frailty levels have multiple interpretations. Some DCWs said that they are better able to develop relationships with residents who are less frail because they communicate better. Others suggested that residents who are less frail require less care and consequently fewer interactions: "The ones who can't walk, you have to spend more time with them and other residents get left out." However, a few DCWs said that relationships with residents with greater independence can be stressful because they are "harder to please" and "complain more."

Residents' illness or imminence to death can influence relationships. Some DCWs keep their "distance" or reduce their interactions because they are "scared" or find it "heart-breaking." Others go out of their way to visit. For example, one DCW described her routine after a resident began cancer treatment: "Every night just before I leave, unless she is asleep I always go to her, or she will come out and wait for me by the med station there. And I will sit there and talk with her for at least 30 minutes or an hour. After I finish everything and am off the clock, I just sit and talk with her because, I don't know, for some reason I feel like I may come in here one day and she might not, that could be anybody, I might not come in the next day. So, I want to talk with her before I leave." The death of a resident is an unavoidable yet potentially painful aspect of working in an ALF. As one DCW said, "You take care of them and you love them and it breaks your heart when they die."

Residents' attitudes and behaviors toward staff and other residents influence relationships with care staff. As one worker put it, "Everybody is different." Some residents are open to developing relationships with care staff while others are not. Typically, DCWs have the best relationships with residents they describe as "nice," "caring," "sweet," having a "heart of gold," and who "treat [staff] nice." Some feel closer to and value relationships with residents who take a personal interest in them, whom they can "talk to," and who "listen" and "pray" for or "joke with" them. DCWs also tend to prefer residents who are appreciative, explaining, "It makes my day when you are taking care of them and they say thank you." Another explained feeling rewarded when residents "thank you and you try to think back to what you did and you don't remember and then they come and tell you what you did. It's nice too. I'm not saying they have to acknowledge what you do, but it's nice for them to say they appreciate what you do. And I really like that a lot. They don't have to do that. You know, it's our job to take care of them, but it's nice for them to thank you."

Residents considered "rude," "demanding," or "unappreciative" are especially frustrating. Identifying her biggest frustration, one DCW said, "When residents are very demanding like, 'get me my ice' without even saying, 'thank you.' [It's like] we are their slaves. If they only knew how little we make." Another explained, "We have one resident who is very frustrating and she rings the bell constantly. When you get there you ask what she needs and she says, 'Nothing.'" Residents who "think they are the only ones" and "want all the attention" create stress for workers. DCWs are further frustrated by residents who can, but do not, do things for themselves or who are uncooperative or resist care. Such behaviors negatively influence the quality of staff-resident interactions and ultimately impede the care process.

"Abusive," "hostile," or "combative" residents are associated with some of the most difficult relationships. DCWs find it upsetting to deal with residents who bite, hit, scratch, or kick them or other residents, whom they must, in turn, protect. Some residents are verbally abusive, a behavior that sometimes stems from racism (see Chapters 6 and 8, this volume). Reflecting the legacy of historically poor race relations in the United States, especially in the South, according to DCWs, certain residents think they "are still living in the Jim Crow times." In one facility a white resident routinely makes racial slurs when speaking to nonwhite care staff, saying, for example, "Shut up, you're nothing but a black bitch." Another black care worker described racism in her ALF: "Mr. B is very racist. He would not let you do anything for him. . . . He would call us the 'n' word. He wouldn't let us bring his tray. . . . There is one more lady. . . . She needed a bulb put in her lamp and she said, 'Can you come and put this bulb in for me?' I said, 'Yes, ma'am. I will be right there in a second.' So, Jane, of course, is white and she said, 'Well, that is okay, Jane will do it because I have had so many things taken out of my room.'"

Residents' families who "do their part" in caring for residents often develop good relationships with care staff.[1] In doing so, families often provide staff with information about residents' history and preferences. This practice promotes familiarity and individualized care. DCWs said that seeing a family "who cares" brings them "closer" to residents and "makes" them "feel better" and "want to go an extra length." Alternatively, families who do not provide the perceived necessary support or "neglectful families" are major sources of frustration for DCWs. Neglectful families do not provide care workers with what they need to provide care (e.g., diapers, body wash, clothes). Thus, despite earning low incomes, some DCWs resort to "buying stuff" themselves because "we know they can't get it from their family members . . . they got the money, but they just don't take the time." Neglectful families also offer little social or emotional support to residents. Describing the most frustrating resident to care for, one DCW explained, "She calls and calls and calls for apparently no reason . . . [except] she's lonely. Her family brought her here and since she's been here, I think I've seen them twice." Sometimes DCWs develop closer relationships with neglected residents: "[Residents] that the families don't come to visit or send a card or flowers, or anything, and some of those, it just draws me closer to them. . . . I don't treat any of them different than the other, but it just makes me want to do more. I don't know how to say it, be close to the ones like that because it feels like they have nobody, even though they are out there but they are not here."

The main staff factors affecting the negotiation of resident relationships include their personal characteristics, job-related characteristics, and relationship goals and strategies. As previously discussed, the degree of commonality with residents along gender, class, and racial lines exerts influence. In terms of age, older workers reported that they have more care work experience and that residents relate better to them than to younger DCWs. A staff member's sexual orientation and physical appearance also can influence how he or she relates to and is perceived by residents. A black lesbian DCW explained, "I think some of the residents suspect, but, you know, I don't broadcast it because I am mistaken a lot for a black man. I have several ladies that don't want me to see them with their clothes off. If I walk in the room they will cover up quick because they think a black man is standing there. I give them that respect because I don't have no problem with it whatsoever."

DCWs' personality, attitudes, care experiences, family history, and motivation for care work enter into the negotiation of relationships. Voicing the opinion of many care workers, an administrator explained, "I think it tends to be the staff member's personality. If he or she is warm and giving, then there is a [positive] relationship nine times out of ten. If they are not and they are standoffish and treat it like a job, there is not going to be a relationship." Picking up on this theme, a number of DCWs noted variations in motives for care work, saying, for example, "Some of them are here for the money and the money only. They do their job and go home and that is it . . . but you have to feel it from your heart." Individuals who feel they care from their hearts described themselves as having a "big heart" or being a "people person." These relationships are so central to the lives of certain DCWs that they "worry about" their residents, "go to sleep dreaming about" them, and "look forward to coming in and seeing how" they are doing.

Many DCWs come from caregiving backgrounds. They have provided or observed formal or informal care in their families and view themselves as predisposed to caring (see Chapter 4 in this volume). As one explained, "I have always taken care of people. It is just part of my life. It is what I was raised to do." In a few instances, care workers desire close relationships with residents because it fills "the hole" left by the passing of elders in their families. One worker elaborated: "I came along too late in life to have grandparents. I am taking care of them like I would take care of my family." Some simply "love old people." According to some administrators, DCWs who do not like working with older people often quit.

Care workers' job characteristics, including facility tenure, position, and shift, are relevant to relationships. One DCW explained the influence of her tenure: "I haven't been here long enough to have a specific favorite." DCWs with longer tenure described a different level of familiarity: "Some of the relationships I have had from the beginning, from seven years. Some of them just trust me. They trust I will do the best I can for them." Job position and shift also make a difference in terms of time spent with residents. For instance, med techs and DCWs on the night shift sometimes have less resident contact compared with others. One med tech commented, "A lot of these people, the only contact I have with them is giving them medication. Other than that, I don't really get to develop any kind of one-on-one."

DCWs' relationship goals and strategies are pivotal. Not all workers have the same preferences or approaches to residents. Many prefer close, personal, or "friend- or family-like" relationships, saying, for instance, "We are family and that is the way it is supposed to be. Some of them [caregivers], they don't act like family. That is part of our job, to love and care for them. It is not just to walk in and go, 'hello' and go through the routine. You have to really know people and enjoy them. I love laughing with them. I love to make them laugh." Other DCWs negotiate relationship quality based on the role they adopt. One explained, "I know they are not my family, but I still kind of look at them as family. They are older people and they have children and when their children aren't here we have to be children to them. When you have to see about them, you have to be a caregiver also. I look it as friend and family."

Some DCWs have little interest in developing close relationships with residents, opting for emotional distance. Some prefer to keep it "professional." Others view close relationships as barriers to task completion. In a few instances the preference for emotional distance relates to the pain of having lost a special resident. For example, "The one that I was very, very close to passed away and I have tried not to get close to another one. It has been two of them that has passed away that I was very close to and now I don't know. I just really treat all of them the same without trying to get close to them."

It follows that workers' relationship strategies are based on their preferences and responses to individual resident behaviors. One worker who prefers close relationships explained her strategy: "You get closer to them if you spend more time with them, you learn more about them. They get used to you and then they want to talk to you and they are so outgoing with you." Another worker explained, "I make myself sit down a little bit and talk to them, see what they like and what they dislike, see what the situation is from their point."

Workers who care for "difficult" or "abusive" residents develop a variety of strategies to manage these interactions. Some avoid such residents or attempt to minimize contact by doing their job and "get[ting] out." Others try to ignore the behavior and "don't let it get to" them. Still others view these residents as a challenge to overcome and "kill them with kindness." For example, a black worker from a facility with an all-white resident population explained: "I had this one gentleman, he didn't like black people . . . eventually within six months I had him and he loved me. I gave him baths, I shaved him, I kept him clean and he gave me a compliment in his own way and it didn't make me feel bad. It was kind of funny, he looked at me and he said, 'You know, you're a good ["n" word].' I said, 'Well thank you Ray.' I said, 'I appreciate that.' He gave me a compliment in his own way. That was the best way he could give it to me. From then on we were buddies. You just have to be able to accept stuff like that because back in that time that is what it was. That is the way it was." Not every DCW rationalized or accepted such behavior.

Relationship Quality and Care Outcomes

As discussed, the quality of staff-resident relationships is highly variable. Although not a necessary condition for positive care outcomes, having good relationships with residents positively influences care and vice versa. From administrators' perspectives, residents benefit from their relationships with DCWs. Because relationships develop through the care process, they view staff-resident interactions as meaningful for residents, particularly their satisfaction and quality of life, saying, for example, "I think the staff member is the most important person in whether [residents] enjoy being here or not."

Although DCWs have different strategies with residents, most suggested that familiarity gives way to individualized care, which is thought to have positive care outcomes. One DCW explained, "I like to get to know the people because that way I have an idea you know each day what I'm supposed to do for each individual." Another went further: "The more I like the residents, the better of a job I do. I mean I think that is with everybody. You know with Ann, now she is one where I go in and do what I need to do and get out. . . . But other residents, I try to take time and make them, you know, you always want to make them feel like they are the only person, like they are your favorite person." When residents resist the assistance, care delivery becomes difficult; having a cooperative relationship facilitates the process.

The Meanings of Relationships

The meanings DCWs attribute to their relationships with residents and care work are essential to understanding how they influence work experiences, particularly satisfaction and retention. Our analysis reveals three key intersecting dimensions of meaning. The first pertains to social relations and the extent to which workers find interactions with residents satisfying or dissatisfying. The second and third dimensions—professional and moral affirmation—refer to the degree of professional and moral confirmation DCWs derive from their work with residents. Care workers described a positive relationship between these three dimensions and overall job satisfaction and retention indicating that satisfying social relations and high levels of professional and moral affirmation typically lead to higher overall job satisfaction and retention and vice versa (see Figure 7.1).

Social Relations

Most care workers enjoy interacting and developing relationships with residents. Relationships develop through the care process and are typically personally and professionally meaningful. Some DCWs identify the best part of their work day as the "time when you can sit down and talk with them" and "ask the questions." Many enjoy "kidding around" and "doing things with" residents. One worker's favorite part of caring for residents is "coming in and joking around and loving them, giving them good morning hugs." Others feel rewarded because they "learn something new from each [resident] everyday."

Satisfying interactions with residents make workers "feel good," "happy," and in some cases helps them "cope" with a "bad day" or personal problems. Consequently, many derive satisfaction and meaning from exchanges of support and affection, saying, for example, "I like taking care of these people. I like being around them. They cheer me up and I cheer them up" or "They like hugs and I need them too."

As suggested earlier, however, not all interactions are satisfying or live up to care workers' relational expectations. Some are a tremendous source of frustration, which often is related to an inability to provide what they consider quality care. Relationships thus can simultaneously be the most and least satisfying part of their job. Most DCWs downplayed the overall impact of dissatisfying interactions on their overall job satisfaction.

Professional Affirmation

Professional affirmation is another key dimension of meaning associated with staff-resident relationships and refers to the confirmation that DCWs have done their jobs well. By caring for (the physical act of caring) and in many cases about (the emotional act of caring) residents, care workers view themselves as "making a difference" in residents' lives. They accomplish this goal when they feel their professional efforts have positive physical and emotional outcomes. One worker explained, "I like taking care of people and thinking that I made someone's life a little better." Such an outcome is professionally and, for most, personally rewarding. DCWs find satisfaction in seeing residents feel and look better: "seeing them improve" and "see[ing] people smile and be happy, satisfying their needs." Some DCWs derive satisfaction from having "encouraged someone's life" and motivating residents to live "another day." Such an outcome lets them know they have "touched somebody in a meaningful way."

Resident (as well as family) recognition of and appreciation for caregiver's efforts are essential to the professional affirmation process. In the words of one worker, "It makes me feel good when they say, 'I was wondering when you were coming back to work.' That lets me know I am doing something there that is helping someone. I like being wanted or doing my job good enough for someone to say, 'She is good.' " Workers further explained that when residents express appreciation they feel "rewarded" and "make everything else feel like it's worthwhile."

Feeling valued for their care further reinforces DCWs' job satisfaction. Some feel rewarded because they are "needed" or "wanted" and because residents rely on and trust them to do their jobs well. One worker explained, "It makes you feel so good that they really depend on you." One DCW elaborated: "If I quit, who would take care of my residents? And that would drive me crazy. I'm sitting at home not doing nothing and my residents up here would have to have a new person come in here, learn their medicine, learn them all over again and I am already sitting here knowing everything."

Ultimately, many DCWs feel professionally affirmed because they believe their job is not well suited to all. One caregiver said it "makes his day" when residents and family members tell him they are "so glad" they have "somebody like" him in the facility. Believing they possess specialized knowledge, professional skills, and personal aptitude for care work resonates with DCWs' moral identity (the moral view they hold of themselves and perceive others hold of them).

Moral Affirmation

The moral meanings of care work are key to understanding how DCWs experience their jobs and relationships with residents. Most find care work morally affirming. In other words, caring is an exchange relationship and is viewed as "giving back" to a "generation" who "gave a lot." It makes care workers feel good. One explained, "You know, you are doing something for somebody and it makes me feel good if I know I have done something for somebody and it makes them happy or you said a kind word to make them smile or whatever, then that makes me feel good, you know, because we are all human, we have feelings."

Care work affirms DCWs' moral values for helping and in some cases fulfilling a "calling" (see Chapter 4, this volume). In their words: "It is a job that is giving back. It is helping . . . that is what gets me" and "When I help them, I feel satisfied like it is what I am supposed to do. . . . I think this is God's gift to me." In exchange for caring, DCWs feel morally rewarded, saying, for example, "I can feel the Lord intervene and this is what I do. I will probably do it until I am out of here. I am very proud of it because I have touched a lot of people's lives. Each one I take something and I give something. If I am the last person they see, that is worth it. You can't even imagine that."

Caregivers' perception that they are "making a difference" in the lives of a marginalized and vulnerable segment of the population elevates their moral identities. One worker likes that she makes residents "feel appreciated and not thrown away." Another explained, "I like to talk to the residents about what they used to do, give them some attention. Don't nobody pay them attention."

For many workers, having an elevated moral identity compensates for low material rewards and job status associated with caregiving. Career options are rather limited for this group of workers (see Chapter 4, this volume). Some DCWs have other options for easier work or higher pay but deliberately choose caregiving over other unskilled jobs because of its perceived moral worth. One worker noted, "I feel good working here. I have a medical assistantship so I could work in a doctor's office and get paid more money." Another DCW who left a job at a major retailer explained, "I was making $17 an hour, so, it will be a while before I get up to there . . . my job that I am doing now is rewarding because of the benefits I get from the residents." One administrator summed it up by saying, "If [staff] didn't get a sense of satisfaction doing what they are doing, they wouldn't continue to do it." Ultimately, the relational aspects of care work are meaningful and are central to DCWs' satisfaction and retention in ALFs.

Discussion

In this chapter we explored staff-resident relationships in ALFs from the perspectives of DCWs and administrators in the state of Georgia. Without doubt, these relationships are at the heart of care work and temper caregivers' daily lives. Although DCWs' feelings about and experiences with residents are not universal, the overwhelming majority said that their bonds with residents are the most rewarding part of their jobs and among the reasons they stay. Our analysis identified multilevel factors that shape relationships and the multidimensional meanings staff-resident relationships hold for care workers. Ultimately, our findings confirm and extend previous research and have implications for policy and practice.

To begin, reflecting on our findings and the LTC literature as a whole, little doubt should remain as to the importance of the caregiver–care recipient relationship, regardless of setting. Confirming Ball and colleagues' (2009) findings, our data show that relationships develop within the caregiving process and impact care delivery and quality in ALFs. Good relationships tend to promote effective care delivery and desired care outcomes, which DCWs find satisfying and are undoubtedly good for residents. Thus, as we discuss further below, facilities need to make every effort to promote and maintain positive staff-resident relationships.

We observed DCWs' tendency to focus on positive relationships in their global evaluation of residents and their effect on overall job satisfaction and retention. Although not dismissing them entirely, the majority downplayed negative or frustrating relationships. This strategy allows DCWs to feel good about their work and shapes their view of their jobs and themselves. Put otherwise, there are issues of self-identity at play.

Neysmith and Aronson (1996, p. 12) argue that care work "can be a source of pride and identity." Our findings confirm that DCWs take considerable pride in their work and are happy when they feel they've "made a difference" for residents in terms of their emotional or physical well-being (see also Ball et al., 2009). Their care work and social relations contribute to how they feel about and view themselves personally and professionally. Both identities are intertwined and rely heavily on the perception of "making a difference."

Writing about unpaid care, Finch and Mason (1993) suggest that individuals' moral identities are bound up in the negotiation of informal care within families. This observation is transferable to paid care workers, particularly those who care for and about residents, in many cases viewing them as family or family-like. Culturally, as one is viewed as giving of him- or herself for the sake of others, high moral value is placed on care work. Not only do care workers subscribe to this view, but it is embedded in their perceptions of care work in general and their labors, specifically. Their sense of moral worth is further heightened by caring for what they perceive to be a frail, vulnerable, and overlooked group.

In her feminist commentary on the home health care industry, Parks (2003, pp. 85–86) draws attention to workers' status and treatment in the workplace and emphasizes the relational dimensions of care work. Parks suggests that care recipients' selves are connected to caregivers. In previous analysis (see Kemp et al., 2009) and in our present work, it is apparent that DCWs' selves are also connected to the nature and quality of relationships they have with those for whom they care. In fact, issues of self-identity underlie the connection between staff-resident relationship and satisfaction and retention (see also Ball et al., 2009).

One reason that social relations and professional and moral affirmation are so important to these workers is related to their labor market position. Caring for and about residents helps them realize their professional goals, fulfill their values for helping, and develop socially meaningful connections, but typically this job is not accompanied by significant material rewards or job status (see Chapter 11, this volume). Focusing on the social, professional, and moral rewards allows workers to, as Ball and colleagues (2009) suggest, "renegotiate their low job status" by redefining their identities and the accompanying value of their labor. These authors invoke Goffman's (1963) concept of *impression management* to explain this cognitive process.

In addition to providing an understanding of how and why connections with residents matter, our analysis identifies key community, facility, and resident and staff factors that influence the development, maintenance, quality, meanings of, and experiences with relationships. The use of statewide data and their accompanying community, facility, and individual variations allows us to explore the factors identified by Ball and colleagues (2009) and extend their work. In light of their importance, understanding how and why relationships are variable allows us to make suggestions aimed at strengthening relationships. Factors such as community or facility size and location or commonality of background between staff and residents cannot be changed, but a number of factors are malleable and can be altered in ways that might enhance the development of positive relationships between staff and residents in ALFs.

At the facility level, some administrators were keenly aware that promoting relationships was important and adopted successful strategies such as making time for staff-resident interaction or viewing social and emotional support as an important part of residents' care regimes. In a number of facilities, DCWs expressed frustration with not having enough quality time to spend with residents in their work day. Understanding how a given facility's job configuration, workload, and level of resident frailty affect relationships would go a long way toward making the necessary adjustments to ensure the development and maintenance of positive connections between staff and residents.

As suggested in Chapter 5 in this volume, some administrators attempt to identify DCWs' preferences when they are assigning shifts and tasks. While it is not always feasible to pair DCWs with residents they prefer to care for, identifying and making efforts to do so might reduce the frustration or stress. For example, some DCWs prefer to care for residents with dementia, while others find it difficult and frustrating. Of course, having the right staff person for the job also begins with hiring and attracting the most suitable candidates (see Chapters 4 and 5, this volume).

Our analysis suggests that family members can play a significant role in the development of staff-resident relationships through the quality and quantity of their support (see also Kemp et al., 2009). Facilities can play a role in promoting family member involvement through policies (e.g., open visiting policies) and practices that encourage families' involvement in facility life (e.g., parties, support groups) as well as educating families about their role in the care process. If successful, these efforts will improve the quality of life for residents and contribute to care workers' satisfaction.

Consistent with Ball and colleagues' (2009) research and the quantitative findings presented by Baird and colleagues in Chapter 8 of this volume, we found that racism enters into the negotiation of some staff-resident relationships and is a source of dissatisfaction for DCWs in ALFs. Although these studies were conducted in Georgia, a state with a long history of racial divide,

DCWs' experiences with racism is neither geographically specific nor confined to AL environments, as research in nursing home settings (Diamond, 1992; Dodson & Zincavage, 2007; Foner, 1994) has shown. Dodson and Zincavage (2007, p. 290) found that DCWs in their nursing home study, set in Massachusetts, felt racism was "really unfair" but an almost inevitable "aspect of nursing home work" in the United States. In another nursing home study, set in Illinois, Berdes and Eckert (2001) explored the influence of racial and ethnic differences between nursing home staff and residents. Consistent with our findings, care workers experienced racism from an array of sources including family members, co-workers, and, in some cases, supervisors. Residents were the most common offenders. In Berdes and Eckert's (2001, pp. 113–15) study, DCWs differentiated between "anachronistic racism," in which offenders used unacceptable language that was not meant to be offensive, and "malignant racism." We also found evidence that racist language and actions can be interpreted these ways by some. Yet staff, residents, family members, and administrators did not always agree on what constitutes racism or how racist residents' attitudes and behaviors should be interpreted and subsequently managed. Divergent opinions often lead to staff dissatisfaction.

Berdes and Eckert (2001) found that foreign-born workers were more likely to experience racism in the workplace than African American staff. Our data indicate that there can be additional implications related to ethnic and cultural differences for foreign-born DCWs (e.g., surrounding residents' perceptions of the use of their "native tongue"). Although demographic projections indicate increasing ethnic and cultural diversity in the U.S. population, particularly among older cohorts (Federal Interagency Forum on Aging-Related Statistics, 2008), little indication exists that this diversity will be reflected in the demographic profile of AL resident populations. In these settings, it is typically white residents who are and will be cared for by nonwhite, and increasingly foreign-born, DCWs (Redfoot & Houser, 2005). Creating strategies that promote awareness and address racial, ethnic, and cultural differences will be crucial for staff satisfaction and care quality in all LTC environments, especially in urban areas, where greater staff-resident heterogeneity is apt to be present.

At present, our data show that administrators influence the culture of a home and determine what, if, and how policy and practices are followed. The extent to which facilities tolerate racism on the part of residents (or anyone) is largely dependent on administrators. Workers are angry and frustrated when they feel unsupported by administrators when residents behave in racist or other unacceptable ways. Conversely, feeling supported by administrators in this regard is satisfying for DCWs.

Conclusion

As suggested at the outset, the issue of satisfaction and retention among DCWs in ALFs is not straightforward. Yet our analysis clearly shows the relevance of staff-resident relationships in this regard. These relationships are themselves complex and multidimensional, but they are meaningful to care workers and care recipients. To this end, we should continue exploring ways to enhance these relationships and improve DCWs' work experiences by balancing out the divide between material and moral rewards. As the population continues to age and the demand for LTC increases, doing so is imperative.

NOTE

1. In previous analysis of data from the "Job Satisfaction and Retention of Direct Care Staff in Assisted Living" study, we explored staff-family relationships (see Kemp et al., 2009). We identified a range of relationships as well as the factors influencing them. Insofar as interactions with family members were rewarding or frustrating, they influenced DCWs' work experiences and satisfaction. Yet comparing these findings with research on staff-resident relationships, we found that staff-resident relationships are of greater import for DCWs.

REFERENCES

Ball, M. M., Lepore, M. L., Perkins, M. M., Hollingsworth, C., & Sweatman, M. 2009. "They are the reason I come to work": The meaning of resident-staff relationships in assisted living. *Journal of Aging Studies* 23, 37–47.
Ball, M. M., & Whittington, F. J. 1995. *Surviving dependence: Voices of African American elders.* Amityville, NY: Baywood Publishers.
Berdes, C., & Eckert, J. M. 2001. Race relations and caregiving relationships. *Research on Aging* 23, 109–26.
Bowers, B. J., Esmond, S., & Jacobson, N. 2000. The relationship between staffing and quality in long-term care facilities: Exploring the view of nurse aides. *Journal of Nursing Care Quality* 14, 55–64.
Chichin, E. R. 1992. Home care is where the heart is: The role of interpersonal relationships in paraprofessional home care. *Home Health Care Services Quarterly* 13, 161–77.

Diamond, T. 1992. *Making gray gold: Narratives of nursing home care.* Chicago: University of Chicago Press.

Dodson, L., & Zincavage, R. M. 2007. "It's like a family": Caring, labor exploitation, and race in nursing homes. *Gender and Society* 21, 905–28.

Federal Interagency Forum on Aging-Related Statistics. 2008. *Older Americans, 2008: Key indicators of well-being.* Washington, DC: Government Printing Office.

Finch, J., & Mason, J. 1993. *Negotiating family responsibilities.* New York: Tavistock/Routledge.

Foner, N. 1994. *The caregiving dilemma: Work in an American nursing home.* Berkeley: University of California Press.

Goffman, E. 1963. *Stigma: Notes on management of a spoiled identity.* Englewood Cliffs, NJ: Prentice-Hall.

Karner, T. X. 1998. Professional caring: Homecare workers as fictive kin. *Journal of Aging Studies* 12, 69–82.

Kemp, C. L., Ball, M. M., Perkins, M. M., Hollingsworth, C., & Lepore, M. L. 2009. "I get along with most of them": Direct care workers' relationships with residents' families in assisted living. *The Gerontologist* 49, 224–35.

Mollica, R. 2002. *State assisted living policy 2002.* Princeton, NJ: Robert Wood Johnson Foundation.

Neysmith, S. M., & Aronson, J. 1996. Home care workers discuss their work: The skills required to "use your common sense." *Journal of Aging Studies* 10, 1–14.

Parks, J. A. 2003. *No place like home? Feminist ethics and home health care.* Bloomington: Indiana University Press.

Redfoot, D., & Houser, A. 2005. *We shall travel on: Quality of care, economic development, and the international migration of long-term care workers.* Washington, DC: AARP Public Policy Institute.

Strauss, A., & Corbin, J. 1998. *Basics of qualitative research: Techniques and procedures for developing grounded theory.* Thousand Oaks, CA: Sage Publications.

CHAPTER EIGHT

Job Satisfaction and Racism in the Service Sector

A Study of Work in Assisted Living

Jim Baird, Ph.D.
Robert M. Adelman, Ph.D.
W. Mark Sweatman, M.B.A.
Molly M. Perkins, Ph.D.
Mary M. Ball, Ph.D.
Guangya Liu, M.A.

The proportion of jobs in the low-wage service sector has continued to increase since 1956, when the manufacturing sector dropped below 50 percent of U.S. jobs for the first time (Toffler & Toffler, 2006). Black workers are structurally overrepresented in this growing segment of the labor market, yet often, owing to economic inequality, blacks also are underrepresented among service recipients (Blank, 2001; Blau & Duncan, 1967; Grodsky & Pager, 2001). Thus there is a racial dynamic at play that often raises questions regarding the role of race and racism in the job satisfaction of service workers. Assisted living facilities (ALFs) represent an important setting for this racial dynamic because the racial gap between staff and residents is especially wide. Low-wage occupations in long-term care facilities are disproportionately filled by black workers, and blacks are significantly underrepresented as consumers in these facilities (Gaugler, Keith, & Leach, 2003; Hawes, Rose, & Phillips, 1999; Murtaugh, Kemper, Spillman, & Carson, 1997; Wallace, Levy-Storms, Kington, & Anderson, 1998).

However, black workers in assisted living (AL) have leveraged experience working in health care, gaining mobility into supervisory positions, though these are often low- and entry-level jobs. AL, then, is of particular interest because of multiple contrasts in racial composition: a predominantly white resident population cared for by disproportionately black caregivers and substantial numbers of black supervisors directing both black and white subordinates. We study the predictors of job satisfaction among direct care workers (DCWs), especially focusing on how the race of care workers, their supervisors, residents, and residents' families affect job satisfaction.

AL represents a growing and somewhat unique work environment in long-term health care. Care is provided in a residential setting by DCWs who often earn low wages and perform work that is both physically and emotionally taxing. Staff shortages in AL are predicted as the U.S. population ages and as competition increases for low-wage, service-sector workers (U.S. General Accounting Office [GAO], 2001). Job satisfaction is expected to play a vital role in staff turnover, retention, and continuity of care in AL. However, the role job satisfaction plays in employment experiences in AL has received minimal study; thus we build on previous job satisfaction research but within the context of the AL environment.

Using survey interviews of 319 direct care staff from 45 ALFs in Georgia, we draw from an extensive job satisfaction literature to develop multivariate models that include measures of sociodemographic, human capital, job content, and workplace experiential variables of AL service workers. We use the Job in General (JIG) scale to measure job satisfaction (Balzer et al., 1997). Our objectives are twofold: (1) to identify the factors that affect job satisfaction in AL using existing theory to define applicable predictors in this workplace environment; and (2) to focus on how race and the experience of racism affect job satisfaction. Although considerable research has been conducted on the relationship between job satisfaction and race, only recently have the workplace experiences of DCWs been included in the job satisfaction literature. Consequently, our research fills an additional void in the literature by addressing the effect of racism on job satisfaction in this specific workplace.

Background and Theory
Job Satisfaction

Extensive research has investigated job satisfaction, primarily from the perspective of measuring and predicting how favorably or unfavorably employees view their work situation. Here, we focus on job satisfaction among AL staff, drawing from the sociology of work, organizational behavior, social psychology, and gerontology literatures, with particular emphasis on caregivers. Job satisfaction theory has developed along disparate dimensions at different points in time over the past 50 years. Perhaps the most common thread is that research in this area considers both the importance of intrinsic rewards, those that provide internal benefits, such as a sense of accomplishment, and extrinsic rewards, or external benefits such as "job security and pay" (Herzberg, Mausner, & Snyderman, 1959; Janson & Martin, 1982, p. 1090; Johnson, Mortimer, Lee, & Stern, 2007; Kalleberg, 1974, 1977; Rosenberg, 1957; Spilerman, 1977).

Scholars initially emphasized individual sociodemographic attributes, such as age and race, as key correlates of job satisfaction. Over time, the focus shifted to more economically grounded macro-level structural factors—such as education and training (human capital) or the occupational status of a position—as the main predictors of job satisfaction. These earlier studies minimized the importance of micro-level characteristics of specific jobs, a limitation of the entire body of literature. Recent research has begun to focus on microphenomena, such as workplace relations. Theoretical perspectives guiding this work emphasize the experiential aspects of the job, including workplace attributes such as social interactions and group culture (Wharton, Rotolo, & Bird, 2000).

Scholars studying job satisfaction have spent considerable time examining the influence of race and gender. Because DCWs in AL are predominantly female and disproportionately black, our focus in this review, and subsequently in our analysis, is on the disparate levels of job satisfaction reported between white and black DCWs in a particular (AL) type of workplace environment that may provide broader insights into the health care industry and low-wage service sector. This emphasis is evident in the literature categorized as sociodemographic, where we consider the macro aspects of race, and in the review of experiential factors, where we consider the implications of experiencing racism on job satisfaction.

Sociodemographic Characteristics

The literature relating sociodemographic characteristics to job satisfaction is quite extensive in addressing race and, to a lesser extent, age (Ensher, Grant-Vallone, & Donaldson, 2001; Firebaugh & Harley, 1995; Janson & Martin, 1982; Kalleberg & Loscocco, 1983; Wright & Hamilton, 1978). However, most studies using multivariate analysis also tend to control for marital status and number of dependents. These variables are theoretically relevant based on studies indicating that financial burdens and obligations associated with marriage and dependents increase job and organizational commitment, contributing to higher job satisfaction (Miller, 1980; Phelan et al., 1993; Sikorska-Simmons, 2005).

Older workers tend to be more satisfied with their work than their younger counterparts (Barfield & Morgan, 1969; Kalleberg & Loscocco, 1983; Wright & Hamilton, 1978). Janson and Martin (1982) suggest that this finding reflects differences in generational values. That is, compared with older workers, younger workers tend to place a higher value on job fulfillment; alternately, older workers tend to have lower expectations or, in other words, expectations more compatible with their generational values. A competing hypothesis is that older workers are more satisfied because they typically have progressed in their careers to positions that provide more satisfaction through both intrinsic and extrinsic rewards. According to this theory, increases in job satisfaction with age is the result of life cycle events, such as finding work that better fits the individual (Janson & Martin, 1982; Wright & Hamilton, 1978). Both suppositions suggest that job satisfaction will be positively correlated with age in AL.

The largest body of research addressing sociodemographic characteristics, both theoretically and empirically, focuses on the relationship between job satisfaction and race. The predominant conclusion is that black workers have lower job satisfaction than white workers (e.g., Austin & Dodge, 1992; Firebaugh & Harley, 1995; Martin & Tuch, 1993; Riley, 2000). Findings show that compared with white workers, black workers are more likely to respond to extrinsic rewards, such as higher income and job security, while showing less preference for intrinsic rewards such as a sense of accomplishment (Martin & Tuch, 1993; Shapiro, 1977; Tuch & Martin, 1991). Explanations for these findings focus primarily on the structural constraints that black workers face in the labor market, including the possibility that race affects blacks' disposition toward job satisfaction, regardless of class differences (Tuch & Martin, 1991).

Some scholars emphasize the labor force position of black workers, theorizing that black workers are less satisfied because they are disproportionately engaged in jobs that offer low levels of extrinsic rewards. That is, black workers routinely encounter lower pay and less job security than white workers and report lower job satisfaction as a result (Riley, 2000; Tuch & Martin, 1991). Other structural constraints contribute to this effect as well. For example, black workers' employment opportunities often are spatially restricted to urban areas, where declining manufacturing and lower-wage service jobs predominate (Riley, 2000). Less favorable educational outcomes for blacks due to structural inequalities in the U.S. educational system also limit black workers' opportunities for more satisfying occupations (Martin & Tuch, 1993, p. 885; Shapiro, 1977; Tuch & Martin, 1991).

Within the context of race, Martin and Tuch (1993, p. 885) outline three different models of ways job values originate. One model focuses on different socialization processes between classes. Within this framework, values that are learned from lower-class parents differ from those learned in middle- and upper-class families (Gilbert & Kahl, 1987; Lareau, 2003). A second model emphasizes the socializing effects of the jobs themselves, positing that job values are essentially learned on the job (Mortimer & Lorence, 1979). The third model derives from two theoretical lines both of which consider changes in job values as one elevates, or strives to improve, her or his social class. One line centers on Maslow's (1954) hierarchy of needs in which the need for extrinsic rewards takes initial precedence but, once that need is satisfied, the need for intrinsic rewards becomes more salient. The other line considers increased contact within the educational system as shifting job values away from extrinsic and toward intrinsic rewards (Anderson, 1985).

Other scholars explore aspects of job satisfaction that result from racial differences, as opposed to class differences. For example, Martin and Tuch (1993, p. 897) study racial factors that affect job reward preferences. They conclude, "Given that, historically, workplace relations for blacks have been typified by discrimination and relative disadvantage, it is hardly surprising that black workers would continue to value materially rewarding and secure employment." That is, cognizant of a history of institutional discrimination, a black worker is likely to avoid seeking a new job and, therefore, places a higher value on job security. More recent research confirms this earlier finding that job dissatisfaction among black workers is related to job insecurity (Heaney, Israel, & House, 1994; Lim, 1996; Wilson, Eitle, & Bishin, 2006).

Human Capital

Other theories of job satisfaction emphasize human capital theory and center on education as a predictor of job satisfaction. Intuitively, it seems that higher levels of education would result in more intrinsically rewarding occupations and lead to higher job satisfaction. However, research in this area has consistently failed to establish such a positive relationship. Studies by Quinn and Baldi de Mandilovitch (1975), Wright and Hamilton (1979), and Glenn and Weaver (1982) find that the average net benefit in job satisfaction from education is minimal. This research shows that although education may increase opportunities for intrinsic and extrinsic rewards from work, it also tends to increase job expectations.

Experiential Factors

Investigations of social relations in the workplace are relatively recent and tend to focus on discriminatory experiences. Racism is experienced by black workers along two distinct dimensions: (1) institutional discrimination, involving organizational practices that limit black employees while maintaining the privileges of white employees, and (2) interpersonal discrimination, entailing action or behavior toward black workers premised on biased feelings, attitudes, and beliefs (Hughes & Dodge, 1997).[1]

Discriminatory experiences and the resultant effect on job satisfaction have been shown to result from perceived discrimination, the perception that blacks are unfairly treated based on their race (Mirage, 1994). Ensher and colleagues (2001, p. 66) substantiate the relationship between perceived discrimination and employees' attitudes and behaviors. In particular, they found that "perceived supervisor discrimination was a significant predictor of participants' level of . . . job satisfaction."[2] Hughes and Dodge (1997, p. 593) found that "exposure to racial bias in the workplace is an important feature of [black] women's job experiences . . . highlighting the insidious effects of prejudice and discrimination on job quality." These findings showed that racism was a stronger predictor of job satisfaction than other occupational stress factors, including low task variety and decision autonomy, higher workloads, and ineffective management.

Some evidence indicates that nonwhite DCWs experience racial discrimination in the long-term care workplace (Berdes & Eckert, 2001; Foner, 1994), but research in this area is sparse. Berdes and Eckert (2001) focus on racial differences between residents and caregivers in nursing homes. They suggest that the dominance of white residents and black staff arise from "the under-representation of African Americans in the resident population, the maldistribution of African-American residents among nursing homes, and the overrepresentation of minorities in the ranks of nurse's aides" (2001, p. 110).[3] They identified two types of discrimination occurring in this situation. The first, *anachronistic racism*, consists of behavior that, taken contextually, is not intended to be offensive, while the second, *malignant racism*, is action that is overtly discriminatory. Berdes and Eckert found that nurse aides responded differently to the two types of racism, generally ignoring the anachronistic. Nurse aides often considered the competency of the residents as well as the context in which discriminatory behavior occurred and, to a large extent, reported not being stressed by the racist actions of nursing home residents.

Mercer, Heacock, and Beck (1993), studying Arkansas nursing homes, found that black nurse aides experience frequent discriminatory language and behavior from both supervisors and residents. Other nursing home research has also reported racist behavior of white residents toward black workers (Foner, 1994; Jervis, 2001). Shields and Price's (2002, p. 306) investigation of minority nurses in the British Health Service indicates that "the proportion of ethnic minority nurses who are satisfied with their current job is inversely related to the frequency of racial harassment they experience." In both studies, the number of caregivers reporting experiences with racism directed from patients exceeds 50 percent.

Overall, little research, particularly in the workplace, has been conducted until recently on these less overt forms of discrimination, which Deitch and colleagues (2003) term "everyday discrimination" (see also Schneider, Hitlan, & Radhakrishnan, 2000). Because of this gap regarding covert racism in the literature, combined with the disproportionate number of black workers in health care settings (Gaugler et al., 2003; Murtaugh et al., 1997) and the centrality of race in the job satisfaction literature, we seek to better understand the role of race, in general, and racism, in particular, in job satisfaction among DCWs in AL. Consequently, using this sample of AL workers, we ask a series of questions about race and racism including: Are black care workers more or less satisfied with their job than are white care workers? Are there differences by race and nativity; that is, are there differences in job satisfaction between native- and foreign-born blacks vis-à-vis whites? What role do the experiences of racism play with regard to job satisfaction? Does racism have differential effects on job satisfaction depending on the type of racism experienced (e.g., co-worker racism versus resident racism)?

We also ask research questions about other, theoretically relevant factors, including additional sociodemographic variables, workplace experiences, human capital characteristics, and job content. For instance, are older workers more or less satisfied than younger workers? Are married workers more or less satisfied than unmarried ones? Are workers with higher levels of education, and more specialized training, more or less satisfied with their jobs than those with lower levels of education and less formalized training, respectively? Are there differences in job satisfaction by one's job status, shift, and number of job tasks? Beyond racism, if an employee feels valued, does she or he have more job satisfaction? These are important questions to ask about a workforce caring for a vulnerable population in an occupation that has low levels of remuneration.

Assisted Living Facilities and Direct Care Workers

In spite of poorer overall health and higher rates of chronic disease and disability than whites (Belgrave & Bradsher, 1994; Binstock, 1999; Wallace et al., 1998), elderly blacks use formal long-term care at substantially lower levels than those used by whites (Gaugler et al., 2003; Murtaugh et al., 1997; Wallace et al., 1998). Little demographic data exist that describe residents living in ALFs. However, the limited information we have shows that residents are predominantly white and only a small minority are black (Brooks, 1996; Hawes et al., 1995; Mui & Burnette, 1994).

More than 90 percent of aides in nursing homes and home care are female, and close to one-third are black (Crown, 1994). Recent data show that DCWs in long-term care settings are increasingly women of color, both foreign- and native-born (Redfoot & Houser, 2005). Between 1980 and 2000, the proportion of whites decreased from 75 to 63 percent among native-born DCWs and from 36 to14 percent among foreign-born DCWs. Immigrants from the Caribbean, Mexico, Africa, and the Philippines are increasingly employed as U.S. caregivers (Redfoot & Houser, 2005). The growing overrepresentation of nonwhite workers sharply contrasts with the predominantly white resident population in long-term care.

An analysis of national wage and employment data indicates that nurse aides, on average, receive lower wages and fewer benefits than workers in general (GAO, 2001). The national average hourly wage for nursing home aides in 1999 was $8.29, compared with $9.22 for service workers and $15.29 for all workers. The average hourly wage for home health care aides was $8.67. Only 21 to 25 percent of workers in these settings had employer-provided health insurance and pension coverage. Limited data are available for AL workers. Hawes, Phillips, and Rose (2000) reported that more than three-quarters of DCW respondents earned between $5 and $9 per hour.

A serious shortage of care workers exists in hospitals, nursing homes, ALFs, and home health care settings, and demographic changes over the coming decade are expected to worsen this crisis (Friedland, 2004; Galloro, 2001; GAO, 2001; Redfoot & Houser, 2005; Stone, 2001). The ratio of potential care providers (working-age population aged 18–64) to care recipients (population over age 85) is projected to decline from 39.5 workers for each person 85 or older in 2000 to 22.1 in 2030 and to 14.8 in 2040 (GAO 2001). The availability of workers also is tied to local labor markets, and competition for low-skill, low-wage workers may exacerbate the shortage (Salmon et al., 1999). Our research takes place at the nexus of this shortage, aiming to locate the issue of job satisfaction both within a specific form of care provision and within the broader low-wage service sector, where competition for employees is taking place. Toward this end, we investigate job satisfaction among care workers in AL as an instance of low-wage service work that entails particularly sharp racial contrasts.

Data and Methods

In the interviews with the AL staff, we collected data for the JIG scale (Balzer et al., 1997). The JIG reflects general feelings about the job and permits an overall evaluation of satisfaction regarding the job as a whole. The JIG is easy to administer, relatively short (approximately five minutes), available in several different languages, and requires only an elementary school reading ability (Balzer et al., 2000). The JIG scale, which has been used in hundreds of studies, is well validated, and national norms for the JIG have been developed, allowing researchers to compare participants' responses with those of similar groups of employees (Balzer et al., 2000; Spector, 1997). Internal reliability analyses of the scale have yielded alpha coefficients ranging from .86 to .90 and above (Balzer et al., 2000; Johnson & Johnson, 2000). For our sample, Cronbach's alpha equals .88.

In addition to the descriptive statistics about the respondents, we use these survey data to estimate four regression models predicting job satisfaction. We introduce our independent variables in series of equations, including sociodemographic, human capital, job content, and workplace experiential variables. Because our respondents are nested within AL workplaces, they may not provide independent observations, violating an important assumption about OLS regression. Consequently, we correct for errors in our nested (or clustered) data using Stata's robust and cluster option (StataCorp, 2007). Model 1 considers the effects of sociodemographic variables on job satisfaction. Age, marital status, and number of dependents have each been related to job satisfaction in prior research. Race also has been consistently shown to be a significant predictor of job satisfaction. We include race but also add nativity to account in our analysis for an increasing number of immigrants working in low-wage occupations such as personal caregiving. Model 2 adds variables that indicate human capital factors. These include income, education, tenure in both the current job and in the caregiving profession, and specialized training.[4] Model 3 focuses on characteristics of the respondent's job, particularly those that have been shown to be relevant to workload and job status. We include full- or part-time status, shift, average hours worked per week, number of job tasks typically performed, and a measure of how often the worker is pushed to complete her or his work. Model 4 tests variables, shown to be theoretically relevant in recent work (Wharton, 1993), that have to do with the respondent's workplace experiences. These include experiences with racism and a measure of how valued they feel at work (see the appendix of this chapter for full operationalizations of all variables).

Results

Descriptive Statistics

Table 8.1 provides the descriptive results for the variables used in our analysis. Our final analytic sample is 319 respondents of the larger 370-person sample.[5] The mean score for the JIG is 41.69 on a scale that ranges from 0 to 54, indicating a reasonably high level of job satisfaction. Within our sample, the mean age is approximately 40 years old with about 13 years of education. Almost 40 percent of the respondents are married, and they have an average of about 3 dependents. In terms of race and ethnicity, about 37 percent of the sample identified as a native-born white, nearly 46 percent as a native-born black, and approximately 18 percent as a foreign-born black. The average workweek is about 37 hours per week, with almost 83 percent working full-time. About 39 percent work during the day, and the remainder work afternoon and evening shifts. The mean tenure in the respondents' current job is about 29 months while having accumulated 93.42 months, on average, in caregiving jobs during their careers. Also during their careers, 64 percent of these workers received specialized training in resident care, nursing, or the medical field. Workload stress, measured on a 10-point scale ranging from sel-

Table 8.1 Descriptive Statistics for Variables Used in Analysis (N=319)

Variable	Mean	Standard Deviation
Dependent Variable		
Job in General Scale	41.690	11.388
Independent Variables		
Sociodemographic Variables		
Age (in years)	39.884	13.110
Marital status (married)	.395	.490
Number of dependents	3.248	2.608
Native-born white (reference category)	.370	.484
Native-born black	.455	.499
Foreign-born black	.176	.381
Human Capital Variables		
Current salary	$8.381	$1.679
Education (in years)	12.672	1.721
Tenure in current job (in months)	28.837	31.609
Tenure in caregiving (in months)	93.422	97.973
Specialized training	.643	.480
Job Content Variables		
Job status (full-time)	.825	.381
Hours worked per week	37.068	7.541
Shift (day shift)	.386	.488
Workload stress[a]	4.502	3.248
Number of job tasks	8.398	2.270
Workplace Experiential Variables		
Co-worker racism experience[b]	.172	.576
Supervisor racism experience[b]	.116	.465
Resident racism experience[b]	.483	.875
Resident family racism experience[b]	.078	.368
Employee feels valued[c]	7.235	2.733

[a] Measured on scale of 1 to 10, ranging from seldom to frequently being pushed to complete one's work.
[b] Measured on a scale of 0 to 3.
[c] Measured on scale of 1 to 10, in which "10" indicates the employee is made to feel extremely valued on the job.

dom to frequently being pushed to complete one's work, has a mean response of 4.5 as participants undertake an average of about 8 tasks in their normal work routine. Respondents' mean salary is $8.38 per hour. The mean values of the racism experiential variables, on a scale of 0 to 3, are .078 for resident family experiences, .116 for supervisor experiences, .172 for co-worker experiences, and .483 for resident experiences. These data indicate that the most frequent workplace experiences involving racism occur with the residents.

Table 8.2 Regression Analysis with Corrected Standard Errors of Job Satisfaction in Assisted Living Facilities

	Model 1 Socio-demographic Factors	Model 2 Human Capital Measures	Model 3 Job Content	Model 4 Work-place Experiences	Model 5 Black Staff Only
Age	.080	.063	.052	.012	.101
	(.049)	(.050)	(.053)	(.050)	(.073)
Marital status (married)	−.604	−.512	−.230	−.554	−1.342
	(1.349)	(1.390)	(1.350)	(1.119)	(2.113)
Number of dependents	.036	.006	−.058	−.030	.083
	(.245)	(.245)	(.233)	(.208)	(.313)
Native-born black[a]	−5.217**	−5.145**	−5.276**	−2.125	n/a
	(1.716)	(1.759)	(1.577)	(1.521)	
Foreign-born black[a]	−10.013**	−9.479**	−10.078***	−6.072**	n/a
	(3.319)	(3.449)	(2.920)	(2.398)	
Current salary		.143	.541	.521	.316
		(.428)	(.389)	(.384)	(.583)
Education		−.289	−.360	−.068	.700
		(.408)	(.406)	(.332)	(.596)
Tenure in current job		−.014	−.012	−.014	−.004
		(.020)	(.021)	(.025)	(.015)
Tenure in profession		.007	.005	.007	.002
		(.007)	(.007)	(.006)	(.007)
Specialized training (training)		−.513	−.625	−.350	.508
		(1.117)	(1.022)	(.890)	(1.613)
Job status (full-time)			−4.186	−2.434	−2.923
			(1.759)	(1.664)	(2.144)
Hours worked per week			.271*	.192**	.220*
			(.089)	(.064)	(.096)
Shift (day shift)			1.632	.587	1.840
			(1.157)	(1.027)	(2.089)
Workload stress			−1.058***	−.670***	−.374
			(.175)	(.155)	(.223)
Number of job tasks			.235	.233	−.187
			(.313)	(.260)	(.392)
Co-worker racism experience				−1.725	n/a
				(1.045)	
Supervisor racism experience				−4.024	n/a
				(2.252)	
Resident racism experience				−1.446*	−1.782*
				(.655)	(.786)
Resident family racism experience				−.037	n/a
				(1.317)	

Table 8.2   (continued)

	Model 1 Socio-demographic Factors	Model 2 Human Capital Measures	Model 3 Job Content	Model 4 Work-place Experiences	Model 5 Black Staff Only
Employee feels valued				1.445*** (.227)	1.563*** (.337)
R^2	.112**	.117*	.231***	.418***	.366***
Sample Size	319	319	319	319	145

[a]Native-born white is reference category.
*p < .05; **p < .01; ***p < .001 (two-tailed tests). Standard errors in parentheses.

Multivariate Results

In Table 8.2, we move to predicting job satisfaction with the JIG as our dependent variable. We present four nested models beginning with sociodemographic predictors and end with a full model that includes workplace experiences (we also include a fifth model for the black staff only). In model 1, race clearly stands out as an important predictor of job satisfaction. The results indicate that compared with native-born whites, native- and foreign-born blacks are less satisfied working in AL. None of the coefficients for the other sociodemographic predictors (i.e., age, marital status, and number of dependents) is statistically significant. In model 2 we control for human capital characteristics such as education, specialized training, and salary, but none of the coefficients is statistically significant. Again, the importance of race is apparent; the coefficients still indicate that native- and foreign-born blacks are less satisfied than native-born whites, with minor attenuation of the coefficients across the two models.

The statistical and substantive importance of race remains in model 3, in which we add job content variables to the equation. In fact, the coefficients for native- and foreign-born blacks actually increase in size compared with model 2. In addition, the coefficients for two other covariates are statistically significant: hours worked per week and whether or not the worker feels pushed to get work done. The positive coefficient for hours worked per week suggests that in workplaces like ALFs, where pay is relatively low, workers are more satisfied when they are able to obtain more work hours in a week. In contrast, when workers feel stress to get their work done, they feel less satisfied with their job.

In model 4, workplace experiences complete our models. First, the coefficients for hours worked per week and feeling stressed to get work done remain statistically significant and in the same direction as described above. Second, the results in model 4 indicate that when workers feel valued as an employee, they have more job satisfaction. Third, and perhaps most important, although the negative coefficient remains negative and significant for the foreign-born black dummy variable, the one for native-born black does not. That is, with the introduction of experiences of racism into the equation, the coefficient for native-born blacks is no longer statistically significant. This is a robust finding across a number of measurement strategies and suggests to us that racism—in this case, experiences with resident racism—is a compelling factor in understanding job satisfaction among native-born blacks. Specifically, in supplementary analyses multiple model specifications indicated that it is the racism variables (and especially the resident racism variable), not the employee-feels-valued variable, that reduces the native-born black coefficient to nonsignificance.

Race in and of itself may be important, but *racism* is essential to understanding job satisfaction in AL. In supplementary analyses in which we compute race-specific models, none of the coefficients for the racism variables is statistically significant in the native-born white models.[6] However, resident racism remains a significant and negative predictor of job satisfaction for native-born blacks (see model 5).[7] Our results strongly suggest that the key to unlocking the door to job satisfaction and race relations in the workplace lies with experiences of racism.

Discussion

A substantive finding from this study is that the dimension of racism that affects black workers' job satisfaction is that which occurs between caregiver and resident, between service provider and customer/client. Low-wage, demanding service work, like that found among care workers in ALFs, is increasing as the U.S. economy continues to bifurcate (Grodsky & Pager, 2001). Often, blacks and other minority workers perform this kind of work in a racialized environment because their customers and clients are usually white. This tension around race encapsulates the work experience and has an impact on job satisfaction. Our findings suggest that increasingly the jobs that are available to a large proportion of the black working population are jobs that, in addition to offering low intrinsic and extrinsic rewards, involve a dimension of racism that surfaces in performing the basic requirements of the job.

Our results show that in the AL setting, in addition to the positive effects of more hours worked per week (resulting in more income) and feeling valued and the negative effect of feeling pushed to get the job done, everyday racism, in this case coming from an older generation of typically white southerners, has a negative impact on job satisfaction. Although other findings (Ball et al., 2009; Berdes & Eckert, 2001) have shown that long-term care DCWs, including black AL workers who experience racism, often view their relationship with residents to be good and rate these relationships as a positive part of their work experience, our findings uncover a problematic aspect in the relations between white AL residents and black AL staff.

Feagin (1991, p. 103) suggests that blacks generally use strategies to avoid, rather than confront, racism when possible. Feagin contends that blacks carefully "evaluate a situation before judging it discriminatory," ignore a discriminatory situation if possible, or respond with "resigned acceptance." Feagin also finds that the effects of racism are cumulative at both the individual and the group level. The negative effects individuals experience as a result of racist behavior, including awareness of racism experienced by other members of the black community, accrue over time. This cumulative effect may change the way blacks internalize racism and, ultimately, the way they respond to experiences that they interpret as discriminatory. An area for further study, then, involves the extent to which experiences with service recipients affect service providers over time.

Another possible research initiative based on our findings in AL, but also applicable to other service-sector settings, might be to investigate whether customer/client racism affects black staff who are aware of negative experiences that they themselves have not encountered as individuals. In this case, perceptions of racism might emerge out of group experience. The AL setting, which is racially, ethnically, and culturally diverse, is an important environment to delve into the complexities of how racism is internalized and how it affects behavior, but further research is required to determine the extent to which our results can be replicated in other workplaces. In light of our findings, more investigation into cultural differences that may exist in these race-related experiences is warranted.

Evidence indicates that in most cases black DCWs do not have the option of avoiding residents who are perceived as exhibiting discriminatory behavior. Unless the situation is particularly malicious, black staff generally must decide between ignoring and confronting the behavior (Ball et al., 2009; Berdes & Eckert, 2001). Without an avoidance strategy, the effects of racism may be more detrimental. According to identity theory, people take active steps to protect their self-concept, which is shaped by the perceptions they have of how others view them (Gecas, 1986; Stryker & Burke, 2000). In line with this perspective, research shows that individuals tend to interact with those who reflect more positively on their self concept and avoid those who may have a negative impact (Felson, 1993). When interacting with residents in AL, DCWs may have fewer ways to selectively protect their self-concept, perhaps hindering their ability to avoid the negative effects of racism.

Hochschild (1983, 1979) frames the issue of identity in terms of emotional work that has been commoditized in situations such as the AL customer/client relationship. Emotional labor has been shown to have negative effects on work stress and job satisfaction (Pugliesi, 1999) and psychological well-being (Bulan, Erickson, & Wharton, 1997). Service interactions have been examined including hairstylists, auto mechanics, physicians (Gutek et al., 2000), fast-food workers (Leidner, 1993), and nursing home caregivers (Lopez, 2006). Although there has been a call for more research in this area (Gutek, 1999), little attention has been given to service interactions and emotional work within the context of race. AL provides a key setting for research on racial identity based on our finding that links resident racism with job dissatisfaction. Additional work is necessary to examine other work settings in the service sector where the service provider has few options, without losing her or his job, regarding racialized interactions with the customer/client.

AL workers provide intimate care to people, people who often express, even if unintentionally, hostility or belittling actions. This behavior seems likely to contribute to dissatisfaction in any interaction, but the effects may be exacerbated when considered in the context of the history of black-white relations in the United States (Bonilla-Silva, 2001; Marx, 1998; Massey & Denton, 1993), which support findings from this study showing that the effects of resident racism may be more poignant for native-born blacks compared with foreign-born blacks.

If job satisfaction is mediated by the behavior of those who are being served, it has implications for a significant portion of the jobs in a service economy.

Specifically within the health care industry, the number of respondents reporting discriminatory behavior in our study of AL is similar to previous qualitative research in nursing homes, in which researchers found comparable levels of workers experiencing resident racism (Berdes & Eckert, 2001, p. 117; see also Mercer et al., 1993). In contrast to findings from the current study, Berdes and Eckert found that black immigrant workers had a greater tendency than African American workers to perceive racial discrimination in their workplace. Findings showed that immigrant workers felt doubly stigmatized, both as immigrants and as people of color. Clearly, more research is needed to disentangle these cultural complexities.

Conclusion

Our results, which clearly link resident racism to dissatisfaction among black workers, are likely indicative of a problem that is pervasive within various types of health care work and in service work more generally. Addressing the effects of routine relationships between care recipients and caregivers that involve dimensions of racism seems essential in this growing industry, characterized by an increasingly diverse workforce. Despite the increasing racial and ethnic diversity of the older population, the contrast between the number of black workers providing care and the number of whites receiving AL care is expected to increase, based on current trends (Ball et al., 2005; Mutran et al., 2001). Our study identifies a problematic consequence of this relationship that likely has ramifications in a substantial and growing number of jobs in today's economy.

NOTES

1. For purposes of this review, the structural effects of institutional racism on class and position in the workplace are included in the section above on race as a sociodemographic predictor of job satisfaction. This section emphasizes the ways in which racism is experienced by black workers.

2. Co-worker and organizational racism are also relevant components of perceived discrimination (Ensher et al., 2001).

3. Blacks use nursing homes at a significantly lower rate than whites (Belgrave, Wykle, & Choi, 1993; Wallace et al., 1998) and have a preference for home care (Morrow-Howell et al., 1996); in addition, there are socioeconomic and discriminatory factors that contribute to disproportionately lower black resident populations.

4. The tenure variables are positively skewed. Supplementary analysis transforming these variables by taking their natural log indicated no effect due to asymmetrical non-normality.

5. We selected out the small number of foreign-born white respondents (N=6) and include only those respondents who have usable data for the variables in our analyses. Also, 99% of our sample is composed of women, with only four men represented in our analytic sample.

6. Supplementary analyses indicated that the negative association of the racism variables with the JIG is a phenomenon primarily due to native-born black staff. First, only 2 (1.7%) white workers reported experiences with racism compared with 62 (43.1%) of native-born black workers. Second, adding multiplicative terms to model 4 showed that there is a significantly different relationship between race and the JIG for those that experienced racism from residents (p = .000) and racism from supervisors (p = .007). Third, when separate models were run for native-born white, native-born black, and foreign-born black staff, resident racism was significant only for native-born black workers, and supervisor racism was significant only for foreign-born black workers.

7. Resident racism is the only racism variable, when these four variables are included in the model, that is significant for native-born blacks. This is also the case if each of the racism variables is independently entered into the model. We show resident racism alone in model 5 to convey this finding while maintaining an acceptable ratio of sample size to the number of independent variables.

APPENDIX

Dependent Variable: Our dependent variable, overall job satisfaction, is measured using the 18-item JIG scale. The JIG was developed by the authors of the Job Descriptive Index (JDI) to be administered with the JDI and to provide a "global, long-term evaluation of the job" (Balzer et al., 2000). The scale ranges from 0 to 54.

Independent Variables: The sociodemographic measures that constitute the independent variables in model 1 include:

Age: measured in single years

Marital status: coded as a dummy variable with married individuals as the reference category

Number of dependents: measured as the number of people who are financially dependent on the respondent

Race and nativity: a set of dummy variables indicating respondents classified as native-born white, native-born black, and foreign-born black. Native-born white serves as the reference category.

The second group of variables, added to model 2, relate to respondents' human capital characteristics and measures:

Current salary: measured in dollars earned per hour

Education: measured as the number of years of schooling completed

Tenure with current job: measured in months that an individual has been employed by the current employer

Tenure in care-giving jobs: measured as the number of months that the respondent has been employed in caregiving positions

Specialized training: coded as a dummy variable in which the reference category includes individuals that have been trained in caregiving, nursing, or other medical specialty versus those who have not been trained

The indicators for current job content, added in model 3, include:

Job status: full- or part-time coded as a dummy variable with individuals employed on a full-time basis as the reference category

Average hours worked per week: measured as an individual's typical workweek hours

Shift: coded as a dummy variable with the day shift as the reference category versus those who work during the afternoon and evening

Workload stress: measured on a scale of 1 to 10 with "1" indicating that the individual is frequently pushed to complete her or his work

Number of job tasks: a measure of the number of identifiable tasks required to be performed by the respondent on a regular basis

A fourth set of variables related to respondents' workplace experiences, in model 4, include:

Co-worker racism: measures the presence and frequency of experiences with racism from co-workers on a scale of 0 to 3 in which "0" is no experience and "3" is frequent experiences

Supervisor racism: measures the presence and frequency of experiences with racism from supervisors on a scale of 0 to 3 in which "0" is no experience and "3" is frequent experiences

Resident racism: measures the presence and frequency of experiences with racism from residents on a scale of 0 to 3 in which "0" is no experience and "3" is frequent experiences

Resident family racism: measures the presence and frequency of experiences with racism from residents' families on a scale of 0 to 3 in which "0" is no experience and "3" is frequent experiences

Employee feels valued: measured on a scale of 1 to 10 in which "10" indicates the employee is made to feel extremely valued on the job

REFERENCES

Anderson, K. 1985. College characteristics and change in students' occupational values. *Work and Occupations* 12, 307–28.

Austin, R., & Dodge, H. 1992. Despair, distrust and dissatisfaction among blacks and women. *Sociological Quarterly* 33, 579–98.

Ball, M. M., Lepore, M., Perkins, M. M., Hollingsworth, C., & Sweatman, M. 2009. "They are the reason I come to work": The meaning of resident-staff relationships in assisted living. *Journal of Aging Studies* 23, 27–47.

Ball, M. M., Perkins, M. M, Whittington, F. J., Hollingsworth, C., King, S. V., & Combs, B. L. 2005. *Communities of care: Assisted living for African American elders*. Baltimore: Johns Hopkins University Press.

Balzer, W., Kihm, J., Smith, P., Irwin, J., Bachiochi, P., Robie, C., et al. 1997. In J. Stanton & C. Crossley (Eds.), *Users' manual for the Job Descriptive Index (JDI; 1997 revision) and the Job in General scales*. Bowling Green, OH: Bowling Green State University.

———. 2000. In J. Stanton & C. Crossley (Eds.), *Users' manual for the Job Descriptive Index (JDI; 1997 revision) and the Job in General scales*. Bowling Green, OH: Bowling Green State University.

Barfield, R., & Morgan, J. 1969. *Early retirement: The decision and the experience*. Ann Arbor: Institute for Social Research, University of Michigan.

Belgrave, L., & Bradsher, J. 1994. Health as a factor in institutionalization disparities between African Americans and whites. *Research on Aging* 16, 115–41.

Belgrave, L., Wykle, M., & Choi, J. 1993. Health, double jeopardy, and culture: The use of institutionalization by African-Americans. *The Gerontologist* 33, 379–85.

Berdes, C., & Eckert, J. 2001. Race relations and caregiving relationships: A qualitative examination of perspectives from residents and nurse's aides in three nursing homes. *Research on Aging* 23, 109–26.

Binstock, R. 1999. Public policies and minority elders. In M. L. Wykle & A. B. Ford (Eds.), *Serving minority elders in the 21st century* (pp. 5–24). New York: Springer.

Blank, R. 2001. An overview of trends in social and economic well-being, by race. In N. J. Smelser, W. J. Wilson, & F. Mitchell (Eds.), *America becoming: Racial trends and their consequences* (Vol. 1, pp. 21–39). Washington, DC: National Academies Press.

Blau, P., & Duncan, O. 1967. *The American occupational structure*. New York: John Wiley and Sons.

Bonilla-Silva, E. 2001. *White supremacy and racism in the post–civil rights era*. Boulder: Lynne Rienner Publishers.

Brooks, S. 1996. Separate and unequal: Long term care is failing to meet the needs of many black elderly. *Contemporary Long Term Care* 19, 40–49.

Bulan, H., Erickson, R., & Wharton, A. 1997. Doing for others on the job: The affective requirements of service work, gender, and emotional well-being. *Social Problems* 44, 235–56.

Crown, W. 1994. A national profile of homecare, nursing home, and hospital aides. *Generations* 18 (3), 29–33.

Deitch, E., Barsky, A., Butz, R., Chan, S., Brief, A., & Bradley, J. 2003. Subtle yet significant: The existence and impact of everyday racial discrimination in the workplace. *Human Relations* 56, 1299–1324.

Ensher, E., Grant-Vallone, E., & Donaldson, S. 2001. Effects of perceived discrimination on job satisfaction, organizational commitment, organizational citizenship behavior, and grievances. *Human Resource Development Quarterly* 12, 53–72.

Feagin, J. 1991. The continuing significance of race: Antiblack discrimination in public places. *American Sociological Review* 56, 101–16.

Felson, R. 1993. The (somewhat) social self: How others affect self-appraisals. In J. Suls (Ed.), *Psychological perspectives on the self: The self in social perspective* (1–26). Hillsdale, NJ: Lawrence Erlbaum Associates.

Firebaugh, G., & Harley, B. 1995. Trends in job satisfaction in the U.S. by race, gender, and type of occupation. *Research in the Sociology of Work* 11, 87–104.

Foner, N. 1994. *The caregiving dilemma: Work in an American nursing home.* Berkeley: University of California Press.

Friedland, R. 2004. *Caregivers and long-term care needs in the 21st century: Will public policy meet the challenge?* Long-term Care Financing Project, Georgetown University.

Galloro, V. 2001. Staffing outlook grim. *Modern Healthcare* 31, 64.

Gaugler, J., Keith A., & Leach, C. 2003. Predictors of family involvement in residential long-term care. *Journal of Gerontological Social Work* 42, 2–26.

Gecas, V. 1986. The motivational significance of self-concept for socialization theory. *Advances in Group Processes* 3, 131–56.

Gilbert, D., & Kahl, J. 1987. *The American class structure: A new synthesis.* Chicago: Dorsey.

Glenn, N., & Weaver, C. 1982. Further evidence on education and job satisfaction. *Social Forces* 61, 46–55.

Grodsky, E., & Pager, D. 2001. The structure of disadvantage: Individual and occupational determinants of the black-white wage gap. *American Sociological Review* 66, 542–67.

Gutek, B. 1999. The social psychology of service interactions. *Journal of Social Issues* 55, 603–17.

Gutek, B., Bennett, C., Bhappu, A., Schneider, S., & Woolf, L. 2000. Features of service relationships and encounters. *Work and Occupations* 27, 319–51.

Hawes, C., Mor, V., Wildfire, J., Iannacchione, V., Lux, L., Green, R., et al. 1995. *Analysis of the effect of regulation on the quality of care in board and care homes.* Research Triangle Park, NC: Research Triangle Institute and Brown University.

Hawes, C., Phillips, C. D., & Rose, M. 2000. *High service or high privacy assisted living facilities, their residents and staff: Results from a national survey.* Washington, DC: U.S. Department of Health and Human Services.

Hawes, C., Rose, M., & Phillips, C. 1999. *A national study of assisted living for the frail elderly: Results of a national survey of facilities.* Beachwood, OH: Myers Research Institute.

Heaney, C., Israel, B., & House, J. 1994. Chronic job insecurity among automobile workers: Effects on job satisfaction and health. *Social Science and Medicine* 38, 1431–37.

Herzberg, F., Mausner, B., & Snyderman, B. 1959. *The motivation to work*. New York: John Wiley and Sons.

Hochschild, A. 1979. Emotion work, feeling rules, and social structure. *American Journal of Sociology* 85, 551–75.

———. 1983. *The managed heart: Commercialization of human feeling*. Berkeley: University of California Press.

Hughes, D., & Dodge, M. 1997. African American women in the workplace: Relationships between job conditions, racial bias at work and perceived job quality. *American Journal of Community Psychology* 25, 581–89.

Janson, P., & Martin, J. 1982. Job satisfaction and age: A test of two views. *Social Forces* 60, 1089–1102.

Jervis, L. 2001. Pollution of incontinence and the dirty work of caregiving in a U.S. nursing home. *Medical Anthropology Quarterly* 1, 84–99.

Johnson, G., & Johnson, W. 2000. Perceived overqualification and dimensions of job satisfaction: A longitudinal analysis. *Journal of Psychology* 134, 537–55.

Johnson, M., Mortimer, J., Lee, J., & Stern, M. 2007. Judgments about work: Dimensionality revisited. *Work and Occupations* 34, 290–317.

Kalleberg, A. 1974. A causal approach to the measurement of job satisfaction. *Social Science Research* 3, 299–322.

———. 1977. Work values and job rewards: A theory of job satisfaction. *American Sociological Review* 42, 124–43.

Kalleberg, A., & Loscocco, K. 1983. Aging, values, and rewards: Explaining age differences in job satisfaction. *American Sociological Review* 48, 78–90.

Lareau, A. 2003. *Unequal childhoods: Class, race, and family life*. Berkeley: University of California Press.

Leidner, R. 1993. *Fast food, fast talk: Service work and the routinization of everyday life*. Berkeley: University of California Press.

Lim, V. 1996. Job insecurity and its outcomes: Moderating effects of work-based and non-network-based social support. *Human Relations* 49, 171–94.

Lopez, S. 2006. Emotional labor and organized emotional care: Conceptualizing nursing home care work. *Work and Occupations* 33, 133–60.

Martin, J., & Tuch, S. 1993. Black-white differences in the value of job rewards revisited. *Social Science Quarterly* 74, 884–901.

Marx, A. 1998. *Making race and nation: A comparison of the United States, South Africa, and Brazil*. Cambridge: Cambridge University Press.

Maslow, A. 1954. *Motivation and personality*. New York: Harper.

Massey, D., & Denton, N. 1993. *American apartheid: Segregation and the making of the underclass*. Cambridge: Harvard University Press.

Mercer, S., Heacock, P., & Beck, C. 1993. Nurse's aides in nursing homes: Perception of training, work loads, racism, and abuse issues. *Journal of Gerontological Social Work* 21, 95–112.

Miller, J. 1980. Individual and occupational determinants of job satisfaction. *Work and Occupations* 7, 337–66.

Mirage, L. 1994. Development of an instrument measuring valence of ethnicity and perception of discrimination. *Journal of Multicultural Counseling and Development* 22, 49–59.

Morrow-Howell, N., Chadiha, L., Proctor, E., Hourd-Bryant, M., & Dore, P. 1996. Racial differences in discharge planning. *Health and Social Work* 21, 131–39.

Mortimer, J., & Lorence, J. 1979. Work experience and occupational value socialization. *American Journal of Sociology* 84, 1361–85.

Mui, A., & Burnette, D. 1994. Long term care service use by frail elders: Is ethnicity a factor? *The Gerontologist* 34, 190–98.

Murtaugh, C., Kemper, P., Spillman, B., & Carlson, B. 1997. The amount, distribution, and timing of lifetime nursing home use. *Medical Care* 35, 204–18.

Mutran, E. J., Sudha, S., Reed, P. S., Menon, M., & Desai, T. 2001. African American use of residential care in North Carolina. In S. Zimmerman, P. Slone, & K. Eckert (Eds.), *Assisted living: Needs, practices, and policies in residential care for the elderly* (pp. 92–114). Baltimore: Johns Hopkins University Press.

Phelan, J., Bromet, E., Schwartz, J., Drew, M., & Curtis, E. 1993. The work environment of male and female professionals. *Work and Occupations* 20, 68–89.

Pugliesi, K. 1999. The consequences of emotional labor: Effects on work stress, job satisfaction, and well-being. *Motivation and Emotion* 23, 125–54.

Quinn, R., & Baldi de Mandilovitch, M. 1975. *Education and job satisfaction: A questionable payoff.* Ann Arbor: Survey Research Center, University of Michigan.

Redfoot, D., & Houser, A. 2005. *We shall travel on: Quality of care, economic development, and the international migration of long-term care workers.* Washington, DC: AARP Public Policy Institute.

Riley, A. 2000. The quality of work life, self-evaluation and life satisfaction among African Americans. *African American Research Perspectives* (Vol. 6). Retrieved from www .rcgd.isr.umich.edu/prba.

Rosenberg, M. 1957. *Occupations and values.* New York: Free Press.

Salmon, J., Crews, C., Reynolds-Scanlon, S., Jang, Y., Wever, S., & Oakley, M. 1999. *Nurse aide turnover: Literature review of research, policy and practice.* Florida Policy Exchange Center on Aging, University of South Florida, Tampa.

Schneider, K., Hitlan, R., & Radhakrishnan, P. 2000. An examination of the nature and correlates of ethnic harassment: Experiences in multiple contexts. *Journal of Applied Psychology* 85, 3–12.

Shapiro, E. G. 1977. Racial differences in the value of job rewards. *Social Forces* 56, 21–30.

Shields, M., & Price, S. 2002. Racial harassment, job satisfaction and intentions to quit: Evidence from the British nursing profession. *Economica* 69, 295–326.

Sikorska-Simmons, E. 2005. Predictors of organizational commitment among staff in assisted living. *The Gerontologist* 45, 196–205.

Spector, P. 1997. *Job satisfaction: Application, assessment, causes, and consequences.* Thousand Oaks, CA: Sage Publications.

Spilerman, S. 1977. Careers, labor market structures and socioeconomic achievement. *American Journal of Sociology* 83, 551–93.

StataCorp. 2007. *Stata Statistical Software: Release 10.* College Station, TX: StataCorp LP.

Stone, R. 2001. Research on frontline workers in long-term care. *Generations* 25 (1), 49–57.

Stryker, S., & Burke, P. 2000. The past, present, and future of an identity theory. *Social Psychology Quarterly* 63, 284–97.

Toffler, A., & Toffler, H. 2006. *Revolutionary wealth.* New York: Alfred A. Knopf.

Tuch, S., & Martin, J. 1991. Race in the workplace: Black/white differences in the sources of job satisfaction. *Sociological Quarterly* 32, 103–16.

U.S. General Accounting Office. 2001. Nursing workforce: Recruitment and retention of nurses and nurse aides is a growing concern. Testimony statement of William J. Scanlon, Director Health Care Issues.

Wallace, S., Levy-Storms, L., Kington, R., & Anderson, R. 1998. The persistence of race and ethnicity in the use of long-term care. *Journals of Gerontology: Social Sciences* 53B, S104–12.

Wharton, A. 1993. The affective consequences of service work. *Work and Occupations* 20, 205–32.

Wharton, A., Rotolo, T., & Bird, S. 2000. Social context at work: A multilevel analysis of job satisfaction. *Sociological Forum* 15, 65–90.

Wilson, G., Eitle, T., & Bishin, B. 2006. The determinants of racial disparities in perceived job insecurity: A test of three perspectives. *Sociological Inquiry* 76, 210–30.

Wright, J., & Hamilton, R. 1978. Work satisfaction and age: Some evidence for the job change hypothesis. *Social Forces* 56, 1140–58.

CHAPTER NINE

Staff Turnover in Assisted Living

A Multilevel Analysis

Molly M. Perkins, Ph.D.
Robert M. Adelman, Ph.D.
Carolyn Furlow, Ph.D.
W. Mark Sweatman, M.B.A.
Jim Baird, Ph.D.

The growing shortage of frontline workers is one of the most significant challenges facing long-term care service providers. Unless providers develop more effective ways of recruiting and retaining staff, current projections indicate that this problem will continue to escalate. The long-term care population is increasing faster than the population as a whole, and estimates show that at least 1 million additional care workers will be needed by the year 2016, an increase of 34 percent over the year 2006 (U.S. Bureau of Labor Statistics, 2008–2009). Currently, not enough workers are entering or remaining in the direct care workforce to meet this growing demand, and the recent downturn in the economy and related rise in unemployment rates are not expected to alleviate this crisis (Harris-Kojetin et al., 2004). Although turnover from job to job is a challenging issue, recent findings suggest that many direct care workers (DCWs) are leaving the field altogether (Smith & Baughman, 2007). In addition, the pool of workers who have traditionally filled these positions, which is composed primarily of middle-aged women with generally low levels of education, is projected to decline as the need for these workers continues to increase (Stone, 2004).

High turnover negatively affects residents, providers, and DCWs who remain on the job. Low staff retention and high turnover rates produce staff shortages and disrupt continuity of care, both of which directly affect residents' quality of care and overall quality of life. High turnover also substantially increases providers' costs related to recruitment and training of new staff, overtime pay, and use of temporary staff. Estimates indicate that the total cost of turnover per employee is at least $2,500 (Seavey, 2004). DCWs who remain on the job experience increased workloads, added stress, frustration, and an increased risk of on-the-job injuries, factors that also can increase turnover (Wright, 2005).

Conceptual Model

Over the past three decades, a variety of conceptual models of the turnover process in long-term care have been proposed, many employing job satisfaction as a principal explanatory factor (see, for example, Castle, Engberg, Anderson, & Men, 2007; Kiyak, Namazi, & Kahana, 1997; Price & Mueller, 1981). These studies have led to inconsistent findings regarding the relationship between job satisfaction and staff turnover. In addition, despite the continued growth of assisted living, few studies have addressed the growing shortage of DCWs in this setting. Recognizing the complexity of predicting who will stay or leave a job, researchers have recently proposed more comprehensive models that consider both direct and indirect effects of multiple factors, including job satisfaction and intent to leave, on employee turnover. In addition, few previous studies investigating these relationships have accounted for the hierarchical nature of the data, failing to acknowledge the interdependence that exists among DCWs within the same facility and leading to biased estimates.

Throughout this book, we explore a variety of factors hypothesized to influence satisfaction and retention of assisted living DCWs. Much of this work is qualitative in nature and focuses on DCWs' perceptions, attitudes, motivations, and day-to-day experiences. An aim of the analysis presented in this chapter is to identify structural and workplace factors that influence actual turnover, which will provide context for the qualitative findings. Another key aim is disentangling the complex relationships known to exist between job satisfaction, intent to leave, and actual turnover, the nature of which is not yet well understood, as well as identifying factors at the individual and macro levels that influence each of these outcomes. An innovation of the current study is the multilevel statistical approach we use to address these aims.

Building on a model proposed by Kiyak and colleagues (1997) for nursing home staff and on other recent research (see, for example, Castle & Engberg, 2006; Castle et al., 2007), we propose that staff turnover in assisted living is a function of (1) personal characteristics; (2) employment characteristics; and (3) facility and community characteristics. As our conceptual model indicates (see Figure 9.1), we assess the direct effects of these three types of independent variables on actual turnover, as well as their indirect effects mediated through overall job satisfaction and intent to leave. Although we acknowledge that individual and contextual factors may affect actual turnover directly, we hypothesize that their main effect is through one's satisfaction with the job and then based on the likelihood that an individual plans to remain (or leave) a position. Thus, in the various analyses, satisfaction and intent to leave serve as independent, mediating, and dependent variables. The measures used in these analyses are described below.

Methods

This analysis is based on data from 370 staff from 45 assisted living facilities (ALFs) who completed Type 1 interviews. Most (99%) are female, and more than half (61%) are nonwhite. As noted in the previous chapter, 18 percent of nonwhite staff are foreign-born. The mean age of staff is 40 (range = 18–75, SD = 12.93). Most (95%) have at least a high school degree or the equivalency. A detailed description of the participants and sample facilities is provided in Chapter 3 of this volume. Table 9.1 provides descriptive statistics for study variables included in the current analysis.

Measures
Dependent and Mediating Variables

Actual turnover (dependent), the final outcome measure in this analysis, is a dichotomous variable (0 = no, 1 = yes), indicating whether a respondent terminated the job or did not terminate the job during the year following her or his interview. *Intent to leave* (dependent and mediating) is a continuous measure, ranging from 1, "very unlikely to leave," to 10, "very likely to leave." *Overall job satisfaction* (dependent and mediating) is measured using the 18-item Job in General (JIG) scale (Balzer et al., 1997, 2000). The measure has a simple "yes," "no," and "uncertain" response format, and possible scores range from

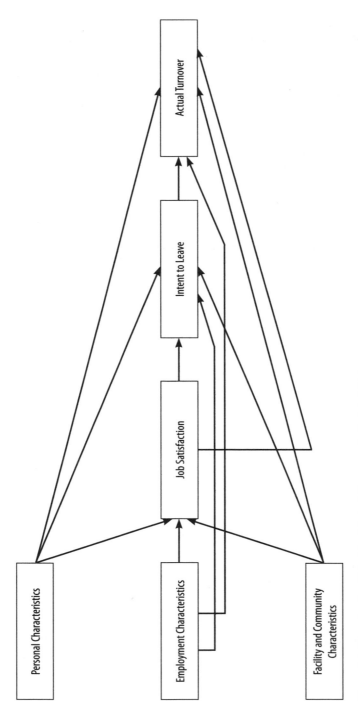

Figure 9.1. Hypothesized Model of Actual Turnover in Assisted Living

Table 9.1   Correlations, Means, and Standard Deviations among Study Variables (N=370)

	Mean	SD	Job Satisfaction	Intent to Leave	Actual Turnover
Personal Characteristics					
Age	40.19	12.93	0.12*	−0.14**	−0.21***
Race (nonwhite)	0.61	0.49	−0.30***	0.26***	0.01
Education	12.69	1.77	−0.13**	0.25***	0.15**
Number of dependents	1.81	2.07	−0.12*	0.02	0.04
Employment Characteristics					
Hours worked per week	38.95	7.65	0.09†	−0.07†	−0.12**
Perceived workload	4.52	3.21	−0.24***	0.17***	−0.01
Hourly wage	8.38	1.64	−0.03	−0.03	−0.10*
Employee tenure (in months)	29.25	31.29	0.03	−0.07	−0.28***
Facility Characteristics					
Facility location (urban)	0.76	0.43	−0.27***	0.22***	0.07†
County unemployment rate	5.20	1.06	0.04	−0.01	−0.13**
Facility size (number of occupied beds)	38.02	22.37	−0.15**	0.09**	0.01
Facility ownership (corporate)	0.69	0.47	−0.15**	0.09†	0.01
Dependent variables					
Job satisfaction	41.74	11.41	—	−0.47***	−0.14**
Intent to leave	4.19	3.41	−0.47***	—	0.20***
Actual turnover	0.42	0.49	−0.14**	0.20***	—

Note: Findings show that employee tenure is positively skewed, indicating more employees at the lower end of the distribution. Therefore, we transformed this variable using the natural logarithm to bring the distribution closer to normal before conducting subsequent analyses.
† $p < .10$; *$p < .05$; **$p < .01$; ***$p < .001$.

0 to 54, with higher scores indicating higher levels of overall job satisfaction. In the present study, the Cronbach's alpha coefficient for the scale is .88. A detailed description of this measure is provided in Chapter 3 of this volume.

Independent Variables

We included three groups of predictors in this analysis: (1) personal characteristics; (2) employment characteristics; and (3) facility characteristics. Because we did not have enough facilities in each of the 25 counties represented in this study to analyze data at the individual, facility, and community level, we operationalized community-level characteristics (i.e., geographic location and county unemployment rate) as facility-level (level-2) predictors in this analysis.

Personal characteristics include *age* (continuous), *race* (0 = white, 1 = nonwhite), *education* (years in school, continuous), and *number of dependents* (total number of dependents, including children, spouses, and elderly family members, both within and outside the home, continuous).[1]

Employment characteristics include hours worked per week, perceived workload, hourly wage, and employee tenure. *Hours worked per week* is a continuous measure. *Perceived workload* is measured on a scale ranging from 1 to 10, with higher scores indicating higher perceived workload. *Hourly wage* is a continuous measure, based on an hourly rate. *Employee tenure* is a continuous measure, based on the number of months a participant was employed in her or his current facility at the time of the interview.

Facility characteristics include facility location, county unemployment rate, facility size, and facility ownership category. *Facility location* is a dichotomous measure (0 = rural, 1 = urban), based on a classification system commonly referred to as the "Beale codes," which measures degree of urbanization along a nine-point continuum (1 = metropolitan counties with an urban population of 1 million or more; 9 = completely rural areas with populations of 2,500 or less). For purposes of this analysis, we coded populations with 20,000 or more as "urban." *County unemployment rate* is based on Georgia Department of Labor statistics collected for each facility at the time that interviews were conducted and is calculated as the total number of unemployed workers times 100 divided by the number of persons in the labor force. Facility location and county unemployment rate both serve as proxy measures of local economic conditions and an indication of the availability of local jobs. *Facility size* is a continuous measure, based on number of occupied beds, and serves as an indicator of facility resources and economies of scale.[2,3] *Facility ownership* is a dichotomous measure, representing facility ownership category (0 = independent, 1 = corporate).

Analytic Strategy

We used hierarchical linear modeling (HLM) and hierarchical generalized modeling (HGLM) techniques available in HLM software version 6.02 (Raudenbush, Bryk, & Congdon, 2004) to estimate a series of two-level random-intercept, fixed slope models, predicting three separate outcomes: actual turnover, intent to leave, and overall job satisfaction. The primary purpose of random-intercept models is to assess the degree to which the mean value of a given dependent variable (the intercept) varies across level-2 units (e.g., facilities) and to determine whether a set of explanatory variables contributes to that variation. To predict actual turnover, a dichotomous outcome, we used the HGLM Bernoulli model with Laplace approximations. We estimated HLM models using full maximum likelihood estimation to predict the two continuous outcomes. Both of these estimation procedures provide deviance statistics that may be used to compare nested models. For ease of interpretation, we grand mean center all continuous individual-level variables.

These multilevel modeling techniques address the fact that staff members working within the same facility may have experiences that are similar to one another, compared with staff members working in other facilities, and therefore may not constitute independent observations. Failure to adjust for nonindependence of observations can result in standard errors that are biased downward, resulting in invalid estimates (Kreft & de Leeuw, 2006; Raudenbush & Bryk, 2002). In addition, these methods allow us to simultaneously investigate individual- and facility-level variance in the outcome variables while still maintaining the appropriate level of analysis for the independent variables. In the current analysis, individual staff members constitute the first level of analysis (level 1), and facilities constitute the second level (level 2).

The first step in estimating these models is to investigate whether systematic within- and between-group variance exists in the criterion variables (actual turnover, intent to leave, and overall job satisfaction) by estimating an unconditional model for each outcome. The unconditional model partitions the total variance of a dependent variable into within- and between-group components, and the intercept for each unconditional model represents the average level of that variable (e.g., actual turnover) across individuals. To determine whether significant between-group variance is present in the outcome variables, we calculated the intraclass correlation coefficient (ICC), which is calculated as $[V_f] / [V_f + V_i] \times 100\%$, where V_f = facility-level variance and V_i = individual variance. Because the HGLM method does not incorporate a level-1 variance component in the conventional way, we used a formula suggested by Snijders and Bosker (1999) to estimate an approximate ICC for the dichotomous turnover outcome, which is calculated with $V_i = \Pi^2 / 3$ (i.e., 3.29).

Because we had only 45 units at level 2, to conserve available degrees of freedom, we used a model-fitting process in which each of the four level-2 variables was entered into the regression equations individually and its significance level and effect on facility-level variance assessed (Snijders & Bosker, 1999). Variables that do not decrease facility-level variance (i.e., explain variance in the outcome variables) were eliminated before fitting the final models.

Based on results from the HLM analyses, we used a structural equation modeling (SEM) approach to estimate a final path model, which allowed us to test each hypothesized single mediated effect and also assess the effects of multiple mediators simultaneously (MacKinnon, 2008). To account for the complexity of our research design (i.e., a model with a hierarchical data structure that includes both a binary and continuous outcomes), we used the "type = complex" feature available within Mplus 5.1 software (Muthen & Muthen, 1998–2007) that adjusts standard errors for nonindependence using a Taylor expansion of the Huber-White sandwich estimator (Muthen & Satora, 1995) in combination with a mean- and variance-adjusted weighted least squares (WLSMV) estimation method.

To evaluate mediated relations suggested by our conceptual model (Figure 9.1), we used four criteria for establishing mediation outlined by Baron and Kenny (1986): (1) establish that an independent variable X has an effect on the dependent variable Y; (2) establish that the independent variable X has an effect on the mediator (M); (3) show that M has an effect on Y; and (4) show that the strength of the direct effect that X has on Y is reduced when M is added to the model. When making these assessments, we relied on findings from the HLM analyses, as well as results from the path analysis, where we examined all potential mediators simultaneously in the same model. We tested mediated effects for statistical significance using the Sobel test (Sobel, 1982), which yields a statistic that is approximately distributed as Z.

Before conducting multivariate analyses, we computed descriptive statistics and Pearson correlations for the variables included in this analysis. Findings show that none of the independent variables included in these analyses is highly correlated ($r > .47$). We also used the variance inflation factor (VIF) test to rule out multicollinearity and eliminate some variables assessed in preliminary analyses based on these tests. The mean VIF for the predictor variables used in the current analyses is 1.34, with a range from 1.09 to 1.72, indicating no problem with multicollinearity. We excluded gender and marital status because most (99%) staff are female and marital status shows no association with any of the three outcome measures in preliminary analysis. We note that more than half of staff (61%) are unmarried.

To address a small amount of missing data (1.17%) among individual-level variables, we used a multiple imputation procedure in Prelis (Joreskog & Sorbom, 2003), which employs an estimation-maximization (EM) algorithm. This procedure is more efficient than traditional methods, such as listwise deletion or mean substitution, in that it provides more accurate standard error and test statistics and performs well with small sample sizes (Allison, 2002; Tomarken & Waller, 2005).

Findings

Descriptive Statistics and Correlations

Table 9.1 presents the descriptive statistics and correlations for the study variables. The mean number of occupied beds (facility size) is about 38 (range = 13–96, SD = 22.37). Most (76%) facilities are located in urban areas, and a large percentage (69%) are corporate-owned. The mean unemployment rate is 5.20 (range = 3.40–7.40, SD = 1.06), with the highest rates found in rural south Georgia, an area characterized by persistent poverty and a large African American population (Wimberly & Morris, 2002).

With regard to actual turnover, these findings show that close to half (42%) of staff interviewed in this study left their jobs within the subsequent year. Available information on reason for leaving shows that about 66 percent of those who actually left resigned, compared with 34 percent who were terminated.[4] On a scale ranging from 1 to 10, the mean intent-to-leave score is 4.19 (range = 1–10, SD = 3.41), indicating a relatively low level of intent to leave. Supplementary analyses (not shown) indicate that more than half (56%) of staff who scored at the high end (scores ranging from 6 to 10) of intent to leave actually left their jobs, compared with 34 percent of staff who scored lower on this measure (scores ranging from 1 to 5). The mean overall job satisfaction score is 41.74 (range = 3.00–54.00, SD = 11.41), indicating that on average staff members in this study are satisfied with their jobs.

The correlations show support for several of the relationships proposed in our conceptual model (see Figure 9.1). As expected, intent to leave and lower levels of job satisfaction are significantly associated with actual turnover. In addition, overall job satisfaction is negatively correlated with intent to leave. With the exception of a significant correlation between actual turnover and county unemployment rate, these findings show little association between actual turnover and any of the other facility-level predictors. This finding indicates that staff members living in areas with fewer employment options may be less inclined to leave their job. To investigate these relationships further, we focus on findings from multivariate analyses.

Multivariate Analyses

Before testing the relationships hypothesized in our conceptual model, we estimated unconditional models for each of the three outcome variables. Results show statistically significant variation ($p < .001$) in satisfaction and intent to leave across facilities and marginally significant variation ($p < .10$) in actual turnover across facilities. These findings indicate that a substantial proportion of the total variance in these three outcomes is explained by differences among individuals as opposed to facility-level differences. Specifically, 97 percent of the variance in actual turnover is at the individual level, 91 percent of the variance in intent to leave is at the individual level, and 81 percent of the variation in overall job satisfaction is at the individual level. In interpreting the ICC for actual turnover, we note that a liberal alpha level may be preferred because it is possible that group effects may emerge only after controlling for covariates (Snijders & Bosker, 1999).[5]

Next, we estimated a series of multilevel regression models to test the hypothesized main effects associated with each of the three outcome variables depicted in Figure 9.1: (1) overall job satisfaction; (2) intent to leave; and (3) actual turnover. These findings are presented in Tables 9.2, 9.3, and 9.4. The fully unconditional model is represented in model 1 in each of these tables.

Prediction of Overall Job Satisfaction

In the first series of regression analyses, we assessed the relative influence of employment characteristics versus facility characteristics on overall job satisfaction, net of personal characteristics. These findings are presented in Table 9.2. When tested individually, only two level-2 variables, facility location and county unemployment rate, lead to a decrease in level-2 variance (i.e., explain variance in overall job satisfaction) (see model 3). As model 3 shows, the addition of these variables increases the significance of age, indicating a possible suppressor effect.

Deviance statistics[6] show that model 4, which combines personal characteristics with employment characteristics and facility-level characteristics, is an improvement over model 2 (personal characteristics and employment characteristics only) and model 3 (personal characteristics and facility-level characteristics only). In combination, these variables account for 70 percent of the original between-group variance and 13 percent of the original within-group variance in overall job satisfaction.[7] Although relatively small, the amount of

Table 9.2 Multilevel Regression Models Predicting Job Satisfaction with Personal Characteristics, Employment Characteristics, and Facility Characteristics (N=370)

	Model 1	Model 2	Model 3	Model 4
	coefficient (SE)	coefficient (SE)	coefficient (SE)	coefficient (SE)
Intercept $y_{.00}$	42.38*** (0.94)	46.24*** (0.87)	42.93*** (3.67)	44.23*** (3.66)
Personal Characteristics				
Age		0.07† (0.05)	0.08* (0.04)	0.06† (0.04)
Race (nonwhite)		−7.09*** (1.23)	−6.04*** (1.64)	−6.66*** (1.39)
Education		−0.31 (0.36)	−0.19 (0.33)	−0.22 (0.35)
Number of dependents		−0.16 (0.24)	−0.01 (0.24)	−0.15 (0.24)
Employment Characteristics				
Hours worked per week		0.09 (0.08)		0.08 (0.07)
Perceived workload		−0.97*** (0.18)		−0.94*** (0.17)
Hourly wage		0.16 (0.43)		0.49 (0.51)
Employee tenure (in months)		0.19 (0.59)		−0.06 (0.62)
Facility Characteristics				
Facility location (urban)			−5.79*** (1.14)	−5.61*** (1.09)
County unemployment rate			1.43† (0.76)	1.22† (0.80)
Variance Components				
Between facility (τ_{00})	24.26***	11.44***	10.28***	7.23***
Within facility (σ^2)	107.67	93.93	100.66	93.55

†p < .10; *p < .05; **p < .01; ***p < .001.

between-group variance remaining is statistically significant, indicating that other facility-level factors yet to be identified contribute to staff satisfaction levels. Also, as previously noted, most (81%) of the variability in overall satisfaction is attributed to differences among individuals. Yet only 13 percent of this variance is explained by covariates in the final model (model 4). Consistent with findings presented in the previous chapter, race is a highly significant predictor of overall job satisfaction, indicating that nonwhite staff are less satisfied compared with white staff. Other highly significant predictors of satisfaction include a lower perceived workload and rural facility location. Net of other variables in the final model, age and county unemployment rate are marginally significant, indicating some association between overall job satisfaction and these variables.

Prediction of Intent to Leave

Table 9.3 presents results from analyses predicting intent to leave. As shown in Table 9.3, facility location is the only facility-level variable that attains statistical significance, and findings show that this variable accounts for a large proportion of facility-level variance in intent to leave. With the addition of this variable, findings show that no residual variance in the intercept remains to be explained, indicating that facility location plays an important role in explaining an individual's intent to leave. However, this effect is reduced when job satisfaction is included in model 5, indicating a possible mediating effect. Deviance statistics show that the final model (model 5) is a significant improvement over all previous models, lending additional support for the relationships hypothesized in Figure 9.1. These results show that dissatisfaction with the job is a highly significant predictor of intent to leave. Race (nonwhite), higher levels of education, a higher perceived workload, and a lower hourly wage also are significant predictors of intent to leave. Variables included in model 5 account for 82 percent of the original between-group variance and 25 percent of the original within-group variance in intent to leave.

Prediction of Actual Turnover

Table 9.4 presents results from multilevel regression analyses, predicting the final outcome variable, actual turnover. In model 1, the significance of the grand mean intercept (-0.32) corresponds to a mean level (0.42) of turnover risk across facilities ($0.42 = \exp(-0.32) / 1 + \exp(-0.32)$). However, as we previously note, subsequent analysis reveals little evidence of between-group variability (i.e., with the addition of covariates, intercept variance at level 2 remains only marginally significant). As indicated in Table 9.3, county unemployment rate is a significant predictor of actual turnover, net of personal characteristics. Interestingly, the inclusion of this variable substantially increases the significance of age, indicating that its effect may have been suppressed by not controlling for county unemployment rate.

Table 9.3 Multilevel Regression Models Predicting Intent to Leave with Personal Characteristics, Employment Characteristics, Facility Characteristics, and Job Satisfaction (N=370)

	Model 1	Model 2	Model 3	Model 4	Model 5
	coefficient (SE)	coefficient (SE)	coefficient (SE)	coefficient (SE)	coefficient (SE)
Intercept $y_{.00}$	4.03*** (0.24)	3.10*** (0.23)	2.38*** (0.29)	2.21*** (0.24)	3.15*** (0.29)
Personal Characteristics					
Age		−0.02† (0.01)	−0.02† (0.01)	−0.02† (0.01)	−0.01 (0.01)
Race (nonwhite)		1.71*** (0.29)	1.35*** (0.32)	1.49*** (0.33)	0.78** (0.31)
Education		0.40*** (0.09)	0.36*** (0.08)	0.38*** (0.09)	0.35*** (0.08)
Number of dependents		−0.06 (0.07)	−0.09† (0.07)†	−0.07 (0.06)	−0.09† (0.06)
Employment Characteristics					
Hours worked per week		−0.01 (0.03)		−0.01 (0.03)	−0.01 (0.03)
Perceived workload		0.24*** (0.05)		0.23*** (0.05)	0.12** (0.05)
Hourly wage		−0.21** (0.08)		−0.26** (0.08)	−0.22** (0.08)
Employee tenure (in months)		0.06 (0.17)		0.07 (0.16)	0.09 (0.14)
Facility Characteristics					
Facility location (urban)			1.15** (0.38)	1.23** (0.36)	0.64† (0.37)
Job satisfaction					−0.11*** (0.02)
Variance Components					
Between facility (τ_{00})	1.05***	0.36*	0.08	0.26†	0.19†
Within facility (σ^2)	10.74	9.29	10.00	9.23	7.99

†p < .10; *p < .05; **p < .01; ***p < .001.

When combined with employment characteristics in model 4, the effect of county unemployment rate is reduced to nonsignificance, indicating a possible mediating effect. The effect of age also is reduced. Deviance statistics show that model 4 is a significant improvement over model 2 (personal characteristics and employment characteristics only) and model 3 (personal char-

Table 9.4 Multilevel Regression Models Predicting Actual Turnover with Personal Characteristics, Employment Characteristics, Facility Characteristics, Job Satisfaction, and Turnover Intent (N=370)

	Model 1		Model 2		Model 3	
	co-efficient (SE)	Exp(b)	co-coefficient (SE)	Exp(b)	co-efficient (SE)	Exp(b)
Intercept y_{00}	−0.32** (0.12)	0.75	−0.32† (0.22)	0.72	0.98 (0.56)	2.67
Personal Characteristics						
Age			−0.02† (0.01)	0.98	−0.03*** (0.01)	0.97
Race (nonwhite)			−0.07 (0.28)	0.93	−0.06 (0.25)	0.94
Education			0.16* (0.07)	1.17	0.15* (0.07)	1.16
Number of dependents			0.02 (0.07)	1.02	0.02 (0.06)	1.02
Employment Characteristics						
Hours worked per week			−0.02 (0.02)	0.98		
Perceived workload			0.02 (0.04)	1.01		
Hourly wage			−0.06 (0.10)	0.94		
Employee tenure (in months)			−0.60*** (0.13)	0.55		
Facility Characteristics						
County unemployment rate					−0.25* (0.11)	0.78
Job satisfaction						
Turnover Intent						
Variance Component						
Between facility (τ_{00})	0.10†		0.14†		0.06†	

†p < .10; *p < .05; **p < .01; ***p < .001.

	Model 4		Model 5		Model 6	
	co-efficient (SE)	Exp(b)	co-efficient (SE)	Exp(b)	co-efficient (SE)	Exp(b)
	0.44 (0.68)	1.56	0.51 (0.64)	1.67	0.50 (0.68)	1.65
	−0.02* (0.01)	0.98	−0.02† (0.01)	0.98	−0.02† (0.01)	0.98
	−0.01 (0.28)	0.99	−0.18 (0.29)	0.83	−0.28 (0.30)	0.76
	0.15* (0.07)	1.17	0.15* (0.07)	1.16	0.11† (0.07)	1.12
	0.02 (0.07)	1.02	0.02 (0.07)	1.02	0.03 (0.07)	1.03
	−0.02 (0.02)	0.98	−0.02 (0.02)	0.98	−0.02 (0.02)	0.98
	0.01 (0.04)	1.01	0.01 (0.04)	0.99	−0.02 (0.04)	0.98
	−0.08 (0.10)	0.92	−0.09 (0.10)	0.92	−0.07 (0.11)	0.94
	−0.57*** (0.13)	0.57	−0.56*** (0.13)	0.57	−0.59*** (0.13)	0.56
	−0.16 (0.13)	0.86	−0.15 (0.13)	0.86	−0.14 (0.14)	0.87
			−0.02† (0.01)	0.98	−0.01 (0.01)	0.99
					0.10** (0.04)	1.11
	0.10†		0.04†		0.08†	

acteristics and county unemployment rate only), providing additional support for the relationships proposed in our conceptual model.

Inclusion of job satisfaction in model 5 significantly improves model fit, but its coefficient is only marginally significant. The addition of intent to leave in model 6 also significantly improves model fit and, as hypothesized, results in a reduction in the effect of job satisfaction, indicating another possible mediating effect. Controlling for all other modeled variables, these findings show that for each additional month of employment a staff person is 44 percent less likely to leave the job. Consistent with our predictions, findings also show that intent to leave is a significant factor in actual turnover. In particular, a one-unit increase in intent to leave is associated with an 11 percent increase in the odds that a staff person will leave the job. Age and education are only marginally significant predictors, indicating some association between actual turnover and having a higher level of educational attainment and being younger in age.

Evaluation of Potential Mediated Effects

To evaluate potential mediated effects, we used SEM techniques to estimate a reduced model of actual turnover, based on findings from the analyses described above. Standardized estimates for the final turnover model are shown in Figure 9.2. Model fit statistics show a good fit of the model to the data, χ^2 (2,[8] N=370) = 1.01, ns; comparative fit index (CFI) = 1.00; Tucker-Lewis index (TLI) = 1.09; weighted root mean square residual (WRMR)[9] = 0.24. As Figure 9.2 shows, variables retained in the final model account for 27 percent of the variance in actual turnover, with only two variables having direct effects.

These findings show that, compared with other variables in the model, employment tenure has the strongest direct effect on actual turnover ($\beta = -.41$, $p < .001$). As hypothesized, intent to leave also has a significant direct effect on actual turnover ($\beta = .18$, $p < .01$). We find that none of the other variables retained in the final model, including overall job satisfaction, influence actual turnover directly.

As hypothesized, we find that intent to leave significantly mediates the association between overall job satisfaction and actual turnover ($z = -2.75$, $p < .01$). Results show that overall job satisfaction has a strong direct effect on intent to leave ($\beta = -.45$, $p < .001$), which in turn increases the likelihood of actual turnover. This analysis shows that intent to leave also significantly mediates the effect of education on actual turnover ($z = 2.43$, $p < .01$). Although we

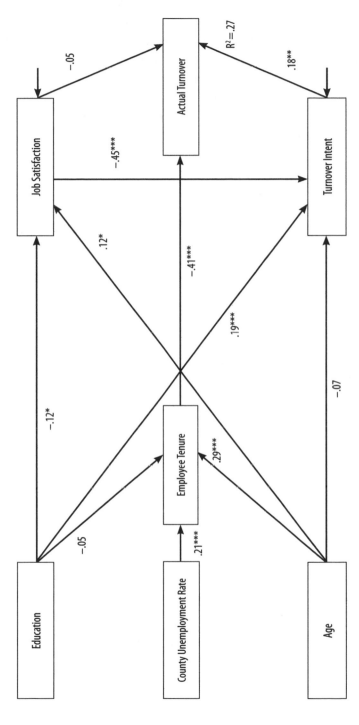

Figure 9.2. Standardized Estimates for the Final Model Predicting Actual Turnover in Assisted Living (*p < .05; **p < .01; ***p < .001)

find no direct effect of county unemployment rate on actual turnover, we find that its indirect path through employment tenure is statistically significant (z = −3.25, p < .001). These findings show that county unemployment rate has a strong direct effect on employee tenure (β = −.21, p < .001), which in turn has an important influence on actual turnover. If county employment rate is indeed a good proxy of the availability of local jobs, this finding indicates that those who perceive more limited opportunity are more likely to stay longer in their current job. Findings also show that employee tenure significantly mediates the effect of age on actual turnover (z = −4.48, p < .001), indicating that an increase in age is associated with a longer length of employment, which in turn is associated with a lower likelihood of leaving the job. Overall, these findings provide mixed support for the relationships hypothesized in our conceptual model (Figure 9.1). These implications are discussed below.

Discussion

Although our findings show that on average staff in this study were relatively satisfied with their jobs and expressed relatively low levels of intent to leave, information collected a year after interviews were completed show that close to half (42%) of DCWs interviewed in this study actually left their jobs. This finding is consistent with national trends showing a high level of turnover across long-term care settings. Available information we have on reason for leaving shows that a large percentage (about 66%) of turnover is voluntary. Unfortunately, owing to a large amount of missing data on this variable, we were unable to control for it in our analyses. Future studies should attempt to discriminate between employees who leave voluntarily and those who are terminated. However, as we noted previously, turnover has substantial negative consequences for residents, providers, and the staff who stay on the job, regardless of the reason. Turnover in administrators and changes in facility management, factors that prevented us from collecting more complete information on staff turnover, also are factors that may influence staff turnover and should be considered in future related studies.

Our findings show that facility-level factors explain little, if any, variation in staff turnover. However, as Banaszak-Holl and Hines (1996, p. 516) noted, the decision to leave a job is "a highly individualized process," which may be influenced by a host of other factors not included in the present analysis. Our final model of turnover (Figure 9.2) does, however, provide some insight into macro-level influences that may affect turnover. In particular, the findings show that the county unemployment rate has an important influence on employee tenure, a factor that has a strong direct effect on the decision to leave, thus providing support for previous research showing a significant association between local economic conditions and turnover (Banaszak-Holl & Hines, 1996). Interestingly, this analysis shows no association between employee tenure and job satisfaction or intent to leave.

As we hypothesized, intent to leave has a significant direct effect on turnover and also is an important mediator in the relationship between turnover and satisfaction. However, we find no support for our hypotheses that intent to leave and job satisfaction would be important mediators in the relationship between turnover and the other hypothesized predictors. As shown in our revised turnover model (Figure 9.2), employee tenure emerges as the most important determinant of turnover in this study. This variable also is an important mediator in the relationship between turnover and local economic conditions, as well as in the relationship between turnover and age.

With regard to overall job satisfaction and intent to leave, our findings show that these outcomes vary significantly across facilities, supporting the need for a multilevel statistical approach. In the present study, much of the facility-level variance in satisfaction is unaccounted for, indicating that other factors at the facility or community level not captured here are determinants of this outcome. Interestingly, in this study, we found that facility location, another indicator of local economic conditions, accounts for most, if not all, of the facility-level variance in intent to leave. These findings indicate that staff who reside in rural areas are less likely to express an intent to leave the job, providing further evidence that opportunity plays an important role in individuals' decision-making process when deciding whether to leave a job.

Based on the relationships hypothesized in our conceptual model and the need to conserve available degrees of freedom, we did not test whether the effects of any of the individual-level predictors vary across facilities in this study (e.g., testing for cross-level interactions). However, based on the findings presented here and in the previous chapter, an important focus of future research should be on possible facility-level variations in the effects of race, age, and education. Supplementary analysis (not shown) indicates that certain relationships, such as the effect of race on satisfaction, may indeed vary across facility.

Findings from the current study show variations in mean levels of staff satisfaction and retention across different types of communities (e.g., rural versus urban), indicating that strategies to address these issues may need to be tailored to the community. Of some concern are the implications of retention resulting from lack of opportunity. Other findings presented elsewhere in this book show that DCWs in rural areas (i.e., areas with higher unemployment rates and fewer employment opportunities) tend to be older on average and have relatively lower levels of education, compared with staff working in urban areas. In addition, rural DCWs receive lower wages and have less access to facility health benefits, compared with DCWs in urban areas.

For decades, the rural South has been characterized as a region of acute poverty. Analysis of data from the 2000 U.S. Census shows that, of the four regions in the United States, poverty rates continue to be disproportionately concentrated in nonmetropolitan counties in the 16-state census-defined southern states, including Georgia (Wimberly & Morris, 2002). These figures show that a rural subregion known as the southern Black Belt, which extends through most of south Georgia, contains a higher percentage of the nation's total poor population than any other region in the United States. The Black Belt, which originally obtained its name from the dark fertile soil that distinguishes the region and was the site of the South's profitable slave-based cotton plantations, is more often noted today for its disproportionately large representation of African Americans and its persistent poverty. Nonmetropolitan counties in Appalachia, another rural subregion that includes the north Georgia mountains, despite significant economic gains made over the past 30 years, also carries the distinction of being among one of the nation's poorest regions (Applied Population Laboratory, 2000; Wimberly & Morris, 2002). Geographic isolation, inadequate provision of infrastructure, a lack of investment in human capital (i.e., education and occupational and vocational training), limited industrial development, outsourcing of low-skill manufacturing jobs to foreign markets, and the decline in the small farm economy limit employment opportunities and contribute to the persistent poverty found in these areas. Although racial segregation is no longer legally sanctioned, de facto racial segregation and discrimination remain a part of the culture in many of these rural areas and contribute to employment difficulties experienced by African Americans and other racial and ethnic minorities (Annie E. Casey Foundation, 2006; Lichter, Parisi, Taquino, & Beaulieu, 2008; see also Chapter 6, this volume).

As individuals living and working in these economically deprived areas, these DCWs represent an especially vulnerable segment of the low-wage assisted living workforce. What is not known is what effect these conditions have on resident care or the health and well-being of these DCWs and their families. More attention needs to be directed at the needs of these DCWs and the residents they care for.

In focusing on the needs of rural workers, we acknowledge that some of the same factors affecting these DCWs, such as a lack of education and limited access to transportation, also can limit employment opportunities among DCWs living in more urbanized areas, where low-wage jobs are more plentiful. With regard to this group of DCWs, many of whom may perceive their work as a job of last resort, the link between lack of opportunity and motivation for entering and remaining in this line of work and its implications are addressed to some extent in Chapter 4 in this volume but also require further attention. Previous research has shown that under certain conditions and without adequate safeguards in place (e.g., proper training and supervision) residents' care may be compromised at the hands of some of these less professionally and altruistically motivated DCWs (Ball et al., 2005; Perkins, Ball, Whittington, & Combs, 2004). Based on our previous research (Ball et al., 2004), we believe that outreach efforts should include improving access to training, which can promote better resident care, increase employee morale and organizational commitment, and help prevent workplace injuries.

Conclusion

Assisted living DCWs are nested within multiple levels, including facility, structural, and cultural contexts. A key aim of future research should be disentangling effects that occur within different contexts. Findings from the current research indicate the need for at least three levels of analysis (i.e., individual, facility, and community).The development of increasingly sophisticated statistical techniques and software packages over the past several years should contribute to advances in this area. More mixed-method approaches, such as the one reported in this book, also will help address this need. The final model of turnover we present provides an analytic framework that may guide some of these efforts.

Our findings show that facility-level factors explain little, if any, variation in DCW turnover, which suggests that decision making regarding turnover is highly individualized and may be influenced by other individual-level factors not included in the present analysis. Based on findings from Chapter 8 in this volume and results from qualitative analysis presented throughout this book, future studies should investigate the influence of cultural attitudes and beliefs, as well as perceptions of various workplace experiences, such as racial discrimination.

Data used in this study constitute a representative sample of DCWs in Georgia, and, as noted in Chapter 3 in this volume, the demographic profile of these study participants is similar to that of frontline care workers in other states. Therefore, we expect that the current findings, based on our conceptual framework, are generalizable to other states in the southern United States and perhaps beyond. Future studies should include additional states and regions in the United States and investigate the potential for regional and cultural differences that may exist both within and across states. Because this study is cross-sectional in nature, we proposed and tested some directional links but could not determine causal relations among variables. Future studies also should examine these relations over time. Another aim should be to investigate what effect these relationships have on resident care.

NOTES

1. A number of DCWs in this study, about one-third (33%), report that they provide care or material support to someone outside the home. Of those, 11% are foreign-born staff, many of whom report supporting family members back in their native countries.

2. Because of its influence on staff wages and facility staffing ratios, we use number of occupied beds as opposed to facility licensing capacity as an indicator of facility size. Facility occupancy rate, which was not a significant predictor of any of the three outcome measures in preliminary analyses, ranges from 50% to 100%, with a mean of 81%.

3. In the current study, facility size is significantly and positively correlated with resident fees ($r = .65$), which is calculated as the midpoint between the lowest and highest resident fees charged by each of the 45 facilities. All 14 large facilities (homes with more than 50 occupied beds) and close to half (N=6) of the 13 medium-sized facilities (homes with 26 to 50 occupied beds) charged fees that were above the median rate of $2,250.00 (range = $772–$4,545, SD = 750). Only 1 of 15 small homes, a home with 20 occupied beds, charged fees that fell above the median. For purposes of this analysis, we used facility size as an indicator of these two closely related predictors.

4. Owing to administrator turnover and other changes in facility management that occurred within the year following staff interviews, we were unable to collect information on reason for leaving for all staff. The figures we report are based on data from 84% of the staff who left.

5. Consistent with findings from the unconditional model for actual turnover, we found little evidence of between-group variability in subsequent analysis, and results were nearly identical to those obtained from a conventional logistic regression analysis with a Huber-White correction for clustering, indicating that less computationally in-

tensive statistical methods may have been used to predict this outcome. However, for consistency, we report results from HLM analyses for all three outcomes.

6. For brevity, we report results of model fit in the text but do not include deviance statistics in the tables.

7. We calculate variance explained at level 1 as σ^2 (unconditional model) $- \sigma^2$ (conditional model) $/ \sigma^2$ (unconditional model). Variance explained at level 2 is calculated as τ_{00} (unconditional model) $- \tau_{00}$ (conditional model) $/ \tau_{00}$ (unconditional model).

8. When using the WLSMV estimator, the degrees of freedom are not calculated in the customary way (see Muthen, 1998–2004).

9. Yu and Muthen (2001) developed the weighted root mean square residual (WRMR) to identify good-fitting models with categorical outcomes. They suggest a cutoff value of less than or equal to 1.00 for models with categorical outcomes.

REFERENCES

Allison, P. D. 2002. *Missing data*. Thousand Oaks, CA: Sage.
Annie E. Casey Foundation. 2006. *Race matters: Unequal opportunities for rural family economic success*. Online Knowledge Center Publication Series. Retrieved May 19, 2009, from www.aecf.org/upload/publicationfiles/factsheet_ruralfes.pdf.
Applied Population Laboratory. 2000. *Recent trends in poverty in the Appalachian Region: The implications of the U.S. Census Bureau small area income and poverty estimates on the ARC distressed counties designation*. Report Presented to: The Appalachian Regional Commission. Retrieved May 23, 2009, from www.arc.gov/images/reports/poverty/ARC-APLFinal.pdf.
Ball, M. M., Perkins, M. M., Whittington, F. J., Connell, B. R., Hollingsworth, C., King, S. V., et al. 2004. Managing decline in assisted living: The key to aging in Place. *Journals of Gerontology: Social Sciences* 59, S202–12.
Ball, M. M., Perkins, M. M., Whittington, F. J., Hollingsworth, C. King, S. V., & Combs, B. L. 2005. *Communities of care: Assisted living for African American elders*. Baltimore: Johns Hopkins University Press.
Balzer, W. K., Kihm, J. A., Smith, P. C., Irwin, J. L., Bachiochi, P. D., Robie, C., et al. 1997. In J. Stanton & C. Crossley (Eds.), *Users' manual for the Job Descriptive Index (JDI; 1997 Revision) and the Job in General scales*. Bowling Green, OH: Bowling Green State University.
———. 2000. In J. Stanton & C. Crossley (Eds.), *Users' manual for the Job Descriptive Index (JDI; 1997 Revision) and the Job in General scales*. Bowling Green, OH: Bowling Green State University.
Banaszak-Holl, J., & Hines, M. A. 1996. Factors associated with nursing home staff turnover. *The Gerontologist* 36, 512–17.
Baron, R., & Kenny, D. 1986. The moderator-mediator variable distinction in social psychological research: conceptual, strategic, and statistical considerations. *Journal of Personality and Social Psychology* 51, 1173–82.
Castle, N. G., & Engberg, J. 2006. Organizational characteristics associated with staff turnover in nursing homes. *The Gerontologist* 46, 62–73.
Castle, N. G., Engberg, J., Anderson, R., & Men, A. 2007. Job satisfaction of nurse aides in nursing homes: Intent to leave and turnover. *The Gerontologist* 47, 192–204.

Harris-Kojetin, L., Lipson, D. Fielding J., Kiefer, K., & Stone, R. L. 2004. *Recent findings on frontline long-term care workers: A research synthesis 1999–2003*. U.S. Department of Health and Human Services, Office of Disability, Aging, and Long-Term Care Policy, and the Institute for the Future of Aging Studies. Retrieved October 9, 2008, from www.ohca.com/workforce_center/docs/Recent_Findings_on_Frontline_LTC_Workers.pdf.

Joreskog, K. G., & Sorbom, D. 2003. *Lisrel (Version 8.5)* [Computer software]. Lincolnwood, IL: Scientific Software International.

Kiyak, H. A., Namazi, K. H., & Kahana, E. F. 1997. Job commitment and turnover among women working in facilities serving older persons. *Research on Aging* 19, 223–46.

Kreft, I. G. G., & de Leeuw, J. 2006. *Introducing multilevel modeling*. Thousand Oaks, CA: Sage Publications.

Lichter, D. T., Parisi, D., Taquino, M. C., & Beaulieu, B. 2008. Race and the micro-scale spatial concentration of poverty. *Cambridge Journal of Regions, Economy and Society* 1, 51–67.

MacKinnon, D. P. 2008. *Introduction to statistical mediation analysis*. New York: Taylor & Francis Group.

Muthen, B. O. 1998–2004. *Mplus technical appendices*. Los Angeles: Muthen & Muthen.

Muthen, B. O., & Satora, A. 1995. Technical aspects of Muthen's LISCOMP approach to estimation of latent variable relations with a comprehensive measurement model. *Psychometrika* 60, 489–503.

Muthen, L. K., & Muthen, B. O. 1998–2007. *Mplus (Version 5.0)* [Computer software]. Los Angeles: Muthen & Muthen.

Perkins, M., Ball, M. M., Whittington, F. J., & Combs, B. L. 2004. Managing the needs of low-income board and care home residents: A process of negotiating risks. *Qualitative Health Research* 14, 478–95.

Price, J. I., & Mueller, C. W. 1981. A causal model of turnover for nurses. *Academy of Management Journal* 24, 543–65.

Raudenbush, S., & Bryk, A. 2002. *Hierarchical linear models: Applications and data analysis methods* (2nd ed.). Thousand Oaks, CA: Sage Publications.

Raudenbush, S., & Bryk, A., & Congdon, R. 2004. *Hierarchical linear and nonlinear modeling (HLM) (Version 6.0)* [Computer Software]. Chicago: SSI Scientific Software International.

Seavey, D. 2004. *The cost of frontline turnover in long-term care*. A Better Jobs Better Care practice and policy report. Washington, DC.

Smith, K., & Baughman, R. 2007. Caring for America's aging population: A profile of the direct care workforce. Monthly Labor Review, U.S. Department of Labor, Bureau of Labor Statistics. Retrieved November 22, 2008, from www.bls.gov/opub/mlr/2007/09/art3full.pdf.

Snijders, T., & Bosker, R. 1999. *Multilevel analysis: An introduction to basic and advanced multilevel modeling*. Thousand Oaks, CA: Sage Publications.

Sobel, M. 1982. Asymptomatic confidence intervals for indirect effects in structural equation models. *Sociological Methodology* 13, 290–312.

Stone, R. I. 2004. The direct care worker: The third rail of home care policy. *Annual Review of Public Health* 25, 521–37.

Tomarken, A. J., & Waller, N. G. 2005. Structural equation modeling: Strengths, limitations, and misconceptions. *Annual Review of Clinical Psychology* 1, 31–65.

U.S. Bureau of Labor Statistics. 2008–2009. Nursing, psychiatric, and home health aides. In *Occupational Outlook Handbook*. Retrieved October 11, 2008, from http://data.bls .gov/cgi-bin/print.pl/oco/ocos165.htm.

Wimberly, R. C., & Morris, L. V. 2002. The regionalization of poverty: Assistance for the Black Belt South? *Southern Rural Sociology* 18, 294–306.

Wright, B. 2005. *Direct care workers in long-term care* (AARP Public Policy Institute Publication No. DD117). Retrieved November 11, 2008, from www.aarp.org/research/ longtermcare/nursinghomes/dd117_workers.html.

Yu, C. Y., & Muthen, B. O. 2001. *Evaluation of model fit indices for latent variable models with categorical outcomes* (Technical Report). Los Angeles: University of California, Los Angeles, Graduate school of Education and Information Studies.

Part III / Lessons Learned

CHAPTER TEN

Hiring and Training Workers

Mary M. Ball, Ph.D.
Carole Hollingsworth, M.A.
Michael J. Lepore, Ph.D.

Owing to high turnover rates of direct care workers (DCWs) across long-term care (LTC) (Banaszak-Holl & Hines, 1996; Seavey, 2004; Wright, 2005), including assisted living (AL) (Institute for the Future of Aging Services [IFAS], 2007), LTC administrators often must recruit, hire, and train new workers. Although few studies address these organizational processes in LTC, persistent and widespread turnover problems indicate that current recruitment, hiring, and training strategies need improvement. Each LTC setting (e.g., AL, nursing home, and private home) and every state defines its own specific criteria for care work employment (Mollica, Johnson-Lamarche, & O'Keeffe, 2005), making hiring and training context-specific. Previous research in various states and LTC settings provides grounding for the examination of AL recruitment, hiring, and training strategies presented here.

Recruitment comes early in the hiring process, and research indicates that social networks are primary conduits to LTC. In a study of home care employment, Howes (2008) found that most DCWs were friends or family members of their care recipients. Eaton (2001) similarly found that word of mouth among friends and family was a common recruitment strategy in nursing homes, particularly those with low DCW turnover rates. No known studies have yet examined worker recruitment in assisted living facilities (ALFs) or the influence of various recruitment strategies on worker outcomes, but previous studies suggest that informal social networks also may play an important role in the AL setting.

State and federal regulations regarding educational and training criteria for hiring DCWs influence applicant pools. In nursing homes, federal regulations require DCWs to have completed preemployment training as a certified nursing assistant (CNA), which entails a minimum of 75 hours of instruction and passing an exam (Mollica et al., 2005). Some states augment these requirements.

Because AL is state-regulated, the criteria for DCW employment are variable. Although most states specify some type of preservice training for AL staff, the majority (35) do not require a set number of hours. For states that do, preservice training hours are fewer than the requirements for nursing home CNAs: 11 states require from 1 to 16 hours, and 4 require 20 or more (Mollica, Sims-Kastelein, & O'Keeffe, 2007). Hawes, Rose, and Phillips (1999), in a national AL study, found that training methods varied across facilities and states, and, overall, DCWs had little formal training. Most preservice training was intended to last just 1 to 16 hours, and few DCWs actually completed this training before working "on the floor." The openness of AL hiring criteria highlights the necessity of taking into account setting contexts when examining hiring processes, as well as the importance of training received on the job.

Similar to preservice training, continuing education requirements for AL staff also vary by state. Twenty-seven states do not specify a required number of hours, 13 states require from 4 to 8 hours, and the remaining 10 states (including Georgia) and Washington, DC, require 10 to 20 hours (Mollica et al., 2007). These requirements indicate that training for DCWs in AL is minimal.

The influence of recruitment, hiring, and training strategies on care worker outcomes, including satisfaction and turnover, has received some attention in the literature, but findings have been inconclusive and are particularly lacking with regard to AL. In one of the few studies to examine training in AL, findings suggest that teaching DCWs to deal with residents' "behavioral distress" promotes job satisfaction and a sense of competence, but these findings were not statistically significant (Teri et al., 2005). Other research also demonstrates an association (not significant) between training and job satisfaction across LTC settings (nursing homes, AL, and home care), with more satisfied DCWs expressing more positive views of their job orientation, their mentors at the time of hire, and the continuing education programs in their facilities (Ejaz, Noelker, Menne, & Bagaka, 2008). However, the study sample was composed mostly of nursing homes, with a limited number of ALFs.

Other research (Grant, Kane, Potthoff, & Ryden, 1996) examined the influence of staff training on turnover in a sample of nursing homes and found that more diversity in training methods was associated with higher turnover among licensed nurses and lower turnover among nursing assistants. This inconsistency from one type of worker to another indicates the importance of addressing training outcomes at the specific level of employment. Furthermore, Aylward, Stolee, Keat, and Johncox (2003) determined that high worker turnover rates in LTC make it difficult to assess the effectiveness of training, thereby identifying an entrenched barrier to unraveling the influence of training on worker outcomes. Adding further complexity to the topic of LTC training, Leon, Marainen, and Marcotte's (2001) research in nursing home and home health care settings ambiguously revealed that providers who demand more training of DCWs face increased recruitment problems but have higher rates of retention. Further, Eaton (2001) found that nursing homes with high turnover rates typically provide new DCWs with scant orientation training, if any at all. Ultimately, the existing literature suggests that training strategies may influence worker outcomes, but the exact nature of this relationship remains unclear.

In addition to worker outcomes, hiring and training strategies also influence care quality. Multiple studies point to poor training as a source of poor quality LTC (IFAS, 2007; Meagher, 2006; Miller & Mor, 2006). For instance, national reports have charged that the minimum requirements for nursing home employment are inadequate (Eaton, 2001; Stone & Wiener, 2001). In her testimony before Congress, Hawes (2003) indicted poor training for nursing home employment as one of the two most significant causes of poor quality in nursing homes. Given the lower training requirements for ALFs compared with nursing homes and the increasing disability levels of AL residents (Miller & Mor, 2006), concerns about the influence of DCW education and training on care quality in AL has received surprisingly little attention.

In this chapter, we examine practices for recruiting, hiring and training DCWs in AL. We also explore the views of administrators and DCWs regarding how these processes relate to various worker and care outcomes. Our specific questions are (1) What strategies do ALFs use to recruit, hire, and train DCWs? (2) What individual-, facility-, and community-level factors influence these processes? and (3) How do these processes influence DCW satisfaction and retention?

Methods

The data for this chapter derive primarily from in-depth, qualitative interviews conducted with 44 administrators. In these interviews we asked administrators to describe the qualities they look for when hiring DCWs as well as their hiring, recruitment, and training procedures. We also asked them to identify the challenges they face in recruiting and hiring desirable workers. Training data also are drawn from qualitative interviews with 41 DCWs, which addressed their perceptions of the training they received at their facilities. In addition, we used data from several questions related to training from the surveys we conducted with 370 DCWs. In analyzing these different types of data, we followed the principles of grounded theory (Strauss & Corbin, 1998; see Chapter 3, this volume, for details of sampling and data collection and analysis).

The Hiring Process
Hiring Criteria

In interviewing administrators we asked them to identify the qualities they look for when hiring DCWs. Hiring criteria include both personal qualities and characteristics related to education and experience. Whereas attitudes regarding personal qualities were somewhat universal, other criteria varied with a facility's size, location, resources, and resident profile.

A Caring Spirit

With few exceptions, administrators look for individuals who are compassionate. They used descriptors such as a "caring spirit" or "a heart for caregiving." Some seek only this trait; others consider it primary; and for still others, it is one of a number of ideal qualities. This sentiment was expressed in a variety of ways but with similar meaning across all size and types of homes. It takes a special kind of person to do this kind of work, and the requisite traits cannot be taught. A small-home administrator articulated a widespread sentiment: "We want people that have a caregiver's heart. . . . There are people out there that just don't get the concept of caregiving. This is just such a unique thing. I don't think it is anything you can teach out of a text book. You just have to have a caregiver's heart and it has to show." The director of a large, urban home expressed this view in another way: "The main quality is a caring spirit. . . . I can teach someone to make a bed, I can teach someone how to change a diaper, but I can't teach someone how to be a good person. You either are or you aren't."

The principal reason given for the need for "heart" is that caregiving involves people, and, specifically, elderly people. As expressed by the manager of a small home: "We are not making widgets. We are serving elderly people, and that is an important job to me. You cannot do that if you are not dedicated and if that sort of work doesn't appeal to you. You just aren't going to put your heart into it." The director of a large, corporately owned home stated a similar view: "That heart for caregiving, when you see the residents as people and not just as patients, not someone you just come in and help and then leave out, not like cattle."

Related to a caring spirit is an aptitude for elder care, people who "like working with elders" or "have an affinity for the elderly." Again, the oft heard view was that such traits are innate. In the words of one administrator, "I think you have to have the gift to work with older people."

In the ideal, a worker's commitment to caregiving goes beyond the need for a paycheck. To many administrators this level of commitment is crucial to lasting in the field, a sentiment articulated by the director of a medium home: "I say this, if a person is coming to work and their only interest is in what they are making, we know that plays a big part, we all work for money, but you cannot be happy just with money. This line of work, if you don't have a caring attitude and you want to take care of residents, you don't last in this business or you don't last with me, I should say." In addition, administrators hope that these "special" people will settle for a small paycheck for the difficult work they do. Many admitted that such low compensation only heightens the need for extra compassion. Another director said, "It is hard to find someone who is willing to work for that [low pay] and do some of the duties that they do. If they didn't have the heart for it, they wouldn't do it."

Fitting In

Another widespread consideration is compatibility with co-workers. The director of a large home said, "We also look for someone who related well with the other RAs [resident assistants] and the staff since they have to work so closely together." Often this quality is couched in terms of "team play." One director said, "We do look for team players. We are a team, and if a person doesn't work within that team it can throw everything off." This criterion may be especially important in smaller homes. The director of three small homes that share a common campus said, "Funny enough we have three houses and each one has its own personality. Some staff when they come in, I just know they will be a perfect fit for house three or that they would fit the personality for house two. If I am looking to fill positions, I do take into account if they are going to be a good fit for that house."

Age, Appearance, and Gender

About a third of administrators consider an applicant's age when hiring. The most common preference is for "mature" or even older workers. For the small-home director quoted above, age is an informal criterion: "We don't like anyone right out of high school. We feel like there is too much immaturity. This is not just a job. We want mature attitudes. Sometimes that is not an age thing so much as a disposition." Some administrators also associate mature age with better work habits and greater retention, as one said: "I love the older person. I rarely or never take a 20-year-old seriously because they don't last."

For one small-home owner, appearance comes first: "First, appearances are number one. I mean, I'm sorry, I don't care what the job is that you are going after, and I'm not looking for them to wear nylons and high heels, but to walk in clean, hair combed, presentable." Only one administrator specified female gender as a criterion. She explained, "My residents will not let us hire men caregivers. When we have hired them in the past they have refused to let them give them baths." Interview data indicate, however, that administrators operate on the premise that applicants by and large are women.

Education and Experience

Georgia has no formal education requirements for AL staff, and education criteria are not stressed by administrators. Only 7 of the 45 homes require workers to have a high school diploma or the equivalency, although 5 others prefer this level. Most of these were large homes. Two types of reasons account for the lack of emphasis on education. One is the notion that formal education simply is not necessary because workers can be trained, the viewpoint of the administrator of a medium home: "We do not have minimum requirements or qualifications on education and training. We hire caregivers and train them to do caregiving." Also noted by one small-home owner is the lack of skill required for the work: "This is unskilled work, really, and you would be crazy to require a high school graduate. I don't think it has anything to do with the ability to do this kind of work." The other reason has to do with the inability to find workers with this level of education. Pay obviously is a factor, but a facility's location, such as being in a rural area, also has influence. The owner of a small home in a mountain area said this: "In a lot of cases it is the older people that come in looking for a job and they are very good and very patient but they didn't graduate. That is not a big requirement."

Only seven administrators specifically mentioned literacy as a requirement, but it is likely that for others this requirement was a given. When noted, literacy had to do with the ability to assist with medications or provide documentation. One low-income home owner with minimal criteria explained, "I have to have you where you can read and write, because sometimes you have to administer medicine. All my medicine comes in a pack, and all they have to do is hand it out. All you need to be able to do is read John Doe." Other administrators specified the need for applicants to be able to read, write, and speak English, primarily because of the necessity to communicate with residents, who with few exceptions are English speaking.

Only 2 homes, both large, require workers to be CNAs, although 12 others prefer CNA training. Attitudes regarding CNA training are similar to those about formal education. Administrators who look upon direct care work as skilled seek better-trained workers. The director of a large home who hires only CNAs said this: "My minimum is that they have CNA, first aid and CPR. Since I have been here there have been some folks who have scooted in without a CNA. Two of them are in the ones I have terminated, just because they did not have the experience. They didn't have any of the qualifications and I just said I greatly appreciate it and I will give you two weeks' severance but I am sorry I just can't put you in this position because this is what I must have. I feel that way because people think there is not a skill to giving care. There is body mechanics and being able to move people and keep yourself safe."

Administrators, though, largely believe that they have the resources to train workers. Another director said, "Definitely, you are looking at the most qualified candidate and you are looking at someone with training and have gone to school for it and has some real life experience. But you do not have to have any experience or skill training to work for [corporation name] because we do provide our own training here." Other administrators stated the reality of whom they can hire given their location and resources. As with education, some administrators in homes with more independent residents believe that CNAs are "overqualified" for the type of care they provide.

Approximately half of administrators, across all home sizes, prefer to hire people with caregiving experience. Some require it. For one director of a medium home, experience is primary: "What I look for is their background, to give them geriatric background. That is the biggest part of what I look for." The importance of experience may vary with the specific job, such as medication assistance, or shift. A common view is that experience is more important for working in dementia care units (DCUs). One large home requires experience only for this area: "Well, in the dementia unit, it is a little bit different. That is where you want to put your best employees. Someone who has experience working with people who have dementia is a plus."

Experience also is more important in homes with heavy-care residents, where more hands-on skill is required. The director of a large home with relatively higher level of resident frailty explained, "We have hired a lot of people that don't necessarily have experience in this, but I think it helps them if they do, just because they have a lot more to get under their belt. You know someone who has never transferred someone or never turned someone in the bed, that is definitely a learning curve for them when they come here."

In many cases, experience taking care of family members is given the same weight as paid care work, even for DCU staff, as the director of a large home indicates: "Individuals who have had experience dealing with Alzheimer [disease] would take precedence. It doesn't mean work experience. Maybe they have had a family member who had the disease. They have seen it and understand it a little bit." Child care is viewed by some administrators as acceptable. The director of a medium home said, "Previous experience in the field, whether it be assisted living or nursing home. Oftentimes daycare workers make good workers. The jobs are basically the same, just different size people."

Only a few administrators view experience as a negative. These viewpoints generally relate to the opportunity to acquire bad habits, as this small-home owner expressed: "I do like for them to have experience, but at the same time I don't want them coming from a nursing home or another AL because they pick up bad habits there. Sometimes it is easier to train someone without experience, because they are fresh and they are going to learn everything that you want them to learn." Possible burnout also was named as the downside of experience. One large-home director believes workers without experience "can be more positive when they come in," particularly if "they have been in a negative experience."

About one-third of administrators specifically mentioned wanting workers with a stable job history, primarily because this quality indicates greater retention potential. One large-home director for whom stability was the number one criterion said, "Job stability in their history would be the first thing. If they work a couple of months here and three months there, they are only going to work a couple of months for us so let's not hire them." Stability in any field serves as an indicator.

Hiring Practices

Identifying desirable qualities for a DCW is only one part of the hiring process. Determining whether applicants possess the qualities is equally important and often more challenging. Hiring practices also are aimed at educating potential workers about the reality of direct care work. Administrators employ a variety of strategies to achieve these aims. Some are more or less universal; others are unique. A particular home's locale, which has considerable influence on the potential applicant pool, is a major factor influencing hiring strategies as well as hiring criteria. The goal of the hiring process is not only to hire the workers who will do a quality job but also to hire workers who will be satisfied and stay employed. We found variability across homes in the hiring process, but certain components were common to all.

The Application and the Interview Process

Some administrators use an applicant's performance in completing an application to assess literacy, English language skills, and the ability to follow instructions. The strategy of requiring workers to complete the application on site acts as an initial screen in some facilities. One administrator explained, "We do have them fill out their applications on site so then we can see a little bit of the literacy because in order to communicate they have to be able to read and write in English."

For most administrators, the interview process is a critical component of hiring. All conduct at least one interview with an applicant. In some homes, of all size categories, multiple interviews are used, typically to gain multiple perspectives. The director of a large corporate home explained, "Generally we like at least two people to interview. It might be the assisted living coordinator and the ED [executive director]. It might be the assisted living coordinator and the DCU coordinator or the health care coordinator, just to have more than one viewpoint on them." Several homes, all large, also employ group interviews. This practice can screen for compatibility or "fit," as articulated by this director: "We have a group of applicants in and see how they mesh and invite some of our care managers in and we sit around after and discuss."

Administrators use a variety of interviewing techniques for determining whether applicants possess the desired qualities. The number one quality, "heart," may be the most difficult to establish. A typical practice is to observe how an applicant interacts with residents and staff in the facility. Some administrators also ask specific questions to judge this quality. A director of a large corporate facility described his method: "We look for the heart. Since you can't see the heart, we look for the smile on the face and the interaction when they are sitting and waiting for the interview. Our concierge plays a huge role, they watch how they interact with the residents who come by, how they interact with the staff that come by, how they interact with anybody they brought with them. We see heart through volunteerism, giving of their time to causes, whatever they may be. We see heart in the interview process by the way they answer certain questions. We have a list of questions we can pull from to try to gauge where they are in that process, where their heart is leaning."

Another strategy is to see how applicants "present themselves" during an interview, including their appearance. One small-home owner said, "I want to see how you'll speak to me. Then I'll figure out how you'll speak to the residents and how they act when I'm talking to them, if they look at me and talk back to me, answer my questions directly, without going all around the bush and all that." During the initial interview, one medium-home owner looks at whether applicants are "being professional" or "are getting into their language that they talk on the street." A large-home director noted the importance of appearance: "That is important. I have had people come in and I ask them, 'You want me to interview you right now?' Appearance, that is just how important it is." The owner of a home in a rural locale finds the interview process useful to judge stability: "I meet a lot of very unstable girls in this community, a lot of boyfriend problems, a lot of husband problems, a lot of personal problems. What I find is they are very vocal about it in the interview. They don't hold back, and you can get a sense right away of where they are and I don't like to bring people into the house with those types of problems because they tend to follow them."

Other administrators create typical work scenarios to see whether applicants respond appropriately. One director explained her tactic for assessing compassion: "In the interview process I have, in the targeted selection process, I will ask them to give me some example. I will create scenarios as well. If I can't establish in my mind a high level of compassion for our residents, I would probably pass on them." Another corporation employs a new technique of asking past behavior questions. A director explained, "Give me an example when you dealt with a difficult person. Past behavior predicts future behavior. Most people ask the general interview questions, but that usually causes people to predict what they would do."

One goal of the interview process is to educate potential workers, especially those who are first-time caregivers, about the true nature of the work to assess their appropriateness for the job and retention potential. One small-home director explained her procedure: "I talk a lot about working with bodies, senior bodies, if they haven't had the experience with that. I like to talk about incontinence and bathing to get a sense of whether they have the stomach for that. We talk a lot about that. I like to give them scenarios. You can tell by talking to someone if they are going to grimace."

It is also important to ensure that potential workers understand up front the universal worker concept, the "biggest challenge" for one large-home director: "Staff are expected to work with residents not only in their ADL care but in dining and activities and light housekeeping. We need to make sure that from the moment we interview and hire, through the process, that they completely understand the process and buy into it. People who have worked in a nursing home are in a completely different environment now. Generally a nursing home has a very delineated job description. If I am a housekeeper, I am a housekeeper. It is an effort to change that mind-set, to the point that it shows through the job performance."

Another technique aimed at increasing job satisfaction is to match task preferences with the job configuration of a particular shift. The director of a large home explained, "I was interviewing for the 3–11 shift and I asked, 'Do you mind doing housekeeping?' because there is a lot of housekeeping on that shift. They need to know that. If they are coming here and they are nursing students and they want that experience and they want to do meds and vital signs, they would know that they would like to be here in the morning when the care coordinator who is a nurse is here so they can experience her direction."

A unique strategy used by one director to assess "fit" is to administer the Myers-Briggs personality test: "Well, in Myers-Briggs nothing is bad and nothing is good. It is all something. I just like to see something to see how they are going to be working with the other somethings. If I just have a whole bunch of IFTJs [personality type] in one shift in one area, there are some things that are not going to work. If I have an ISTJ and an ENFP [another personality type] working, they are complementing one another."

Staff Input and Trial Work Periods

Some administrators consider input from other staff a valuable tool for assessing "fit," as well as character. In small towns and rural areas, this information often comes from community knowledge. The director of a small home explained, "And a lot of them already know them because it's a small town. Somebody will come to me and say, 'I know her. She worked at Big Lots with me. She's so and so, she's a good worker. She never came into work, she had laid out all the time, she's dishonest, she had a drug problem.' So I do listen actually." Staff input also is gained through informal interactions with the applicant. This strategy can involve a one-on-one conversation between the applicant and a current staff member, as in this large home: "I do involve the employees a lot in the hiring process. I have sat an applicant down with a caregiver and have them tell her about the job. I want to see how they interact with each other." This strategy also serves to acquaint the applicant with the job.

Trial work experiences serve similar purposes. We found this method used on both a volunteer and paid basis. One small-home owner paid a likely candidate for a day in order to "let them work with other staff members" and "get their opinion." Two large homes in the same corporation used a volunteer job shadow to assist in decision making. One director explained, "We have even asked some people we weren't too sure about if they would come back and shadow with that care manger on a volunteer basis to see if they would really like it, the job, especially if they have never had any experience. Then we take the input from those care managers about what they thought."

A common practice, particularly in homes with employee benefits, is to hire workers on a trial basis, usually a 90-day period. Some administrators believe this practice allows them to hire workers with no experience. Other facilities hire all workers initially on a PRN (as needed) basis.

References

Although more administrators than not require and follow up on references, the attitudes toward the value of reference checks are mixed. Those who do not use this strategy feel either that past employers lie or provide little information beyond the dates of hire. Some, though, believe that even sparse information is useful. The director of a small home said, "We will check the references and when I do that they will say one of two things: they are fabulous and they were wonderful or they worked here and that is all I'm telling you. That tells me immediately if I am interested in hiring them." One director who uses this strategy despite its minimal value has found that knowing the applicant's former employer is helpful: "A lot of times you just get dates of hire, so it is a waste of time. If you know who you are talking to, they might tell you more." Another director uses guilt tactics to press for greater honesty: "Of course, we get references. Our staff coordinator is a genius on that, of saying if they say, 'We can only give you dates,' we always say, 'You are dealing with the elderly. You think about this. If this was your mother, would you want this person, would you trust them to take care of your mother or your grandmother?' We are pretty good about sorting out the folks. We may get the off-the-record, 'you would not want this person there' or 'this is a real fine person.' We try to get more than dates of hire."

One large-home director emphasized the value of sharing information about employees with other administrators because of the problem of administrator turnover: "These caregivers hop from AL to AL 'cause there seems to be a turnover with executive directors. Executive directors every couple years like move in different places, right? But I've been around long enough that I can see you used to work here, then you worked there, then you worked there and you see this hop thing going around and they'll go back to a community when there's a new management there. You should definitely share this with other administrators."

Background Checks, Physical Examinations, and Drug Screens

A criminal records check, tuberculosis test, and physical examination by a physician are required by the state of Georgia for all AL staff before employment. Typically these tests constitute the final stage of the hiring process. Facilities vary regarding who is responsible, facility or applicant, for costs. As a rule, larger facilities pay all expenses, although in one they are deducted from the trial work period pay and subsequently reimbursed if the employee becomes permanent. Sometimes costs are shared, as in one medium home: "The background check costs $5 to the sheriff's department. That's an applicant's expense. We pick up the drug test, the physical and the TB test. [It] costs us right now about $160 per person that we actually put on payroll." One large facility hires a private company to do an additional background check.

Many facilities require preemployment drug screens. In some, screens are conducted after hiring, either randomly, so that employees won't "think they are safe," or if a problem is suspected.

Recruitment Strategies

In the majority of study homes, administrators stated that active recruitment rarely is necessary. Rather, prospective employees find them. The most common avenue is through word of mouth. More than half of homes, in each size category, use this strategy, which typically depends on a home's reputation. One large-home director explained, "So far it has been word of mouth. I can't say we have had a recruitment initiative. I have met staff from other communities and I have an outgoing personality and, often when that happens, I have people come up and say they want jobs here. . . . I think they say she is a nice person and up front." A director of a medium home describes how his home's incentive practices attract quality applicants: "I think it's getting easier to find qualified staff for this community because the CNAs talk to one another and when our staff are saying, 'Oh yeah, man, I won a hundred bucks the other day at the drawing.' 'What you get that for?' 'Cause I came to work.' 'You got a $100 because you came to work?' 'Yeah, I didn't have any call-ins.' So, that word of mouth allows us to kind of pick and choose."

As noted in Chapters 4 and 6 in this volume, word often travels through the social networks of current employees. By and large, administrators like to hire friends and families of staff. A common rationale is that quality workers tend to recruit other quality workers. One director of a large corporate home shares this sentiment: "Most of the people we hire have been referred to us by the staff. I believe that if one of our good care managers refers someone to me, they are probably going to be pretty good, too. A good care manager doesn't want to work with someone who is not good. They know if they are working with someone who is not pulling their weight they will have to do it for them." Four large homes offer recruitment bonuses to staff who recommend a new staff person who stays for at least 90 days.

The large majority of facilities, including all the large homes, have found hiring workers' family members to be a successful strategy. In the words of one director, "character runs in families." Some facilities, though, do not permit family members to work on the same shift or supervise one another. In the few homes, most small, who do not hire family members, two potential problems were named. One concerns the loss of multiple workers during a crisis, as one owner explained: "In the small group we got, if the mama dies and they are all out, it will kill you." The other issue has to do with the effect on the social environment. One owner said, "It tends to polarize people and form cliques."

After word of mouth, facilities most commonly locate staff by way of "walk-ins" or individuals who call the facility on their own. Only 20 of the 45 study homes ever advertise in newspapers. For only one small home is advertisement the sole recruitment strategy. The lack of necessity for advertising is largely a factor of the local job market.

Nine facilities find workers through technical schools or colleges. Some hire people who have come to their facility from CNA schools to do their clinical training. The director of one large home, who considers herself "lucky" to have several colleges nearby, uses this resource: "We have found a lot of times those college students are very good hires because they do have the initiative and they are furthering their education. It is good experience for them, especially if they are going into the medical field. . . . Some of the girls who are in local colleges are able to be a permanent basis staff member, but we kind of flex with their school schedule."

Barriers to Finding Good-Quality Staff

In addition to asking administrators how they find staff, we also asked what they consider the greatest barriers to hiring staff with the qualities they seek. Administrators of facilities in each size category implicated low pay. The director of one small home with a starting hourly rate of $6.25 said, "Pay. The good ones, the ones that are nice looking, the ones that are professional, even though the pay is low, they would settle for $7.00 an hour, but when you say $6.25, they don't even want to talk to you. It is very hard to get a good professional type like I would like to have in the building." Others combined pay with "the nature of the beast, the kind of work they have to do" for "only $7.00–$7.25 an hour," as the biggest barrier.

The director of a large facility who requires that workers have CNA training admitted "that expectation has created a little more difficulty in finding people." Beginning pay in this home is only $7 per hour, likely too low for such a high bar. The director of a large home where staff start at $9.25 acknowledges the importance of pay levels but believes that other factors also influence the ability to recruit staff with adequate "commitment": "It is a competitive marketplace and everyone wants the best employee and this industry just doesn't pay that great. We pay our employees well. We have an excellent benefit program. It is probably better than most in the industry. Sometimes that is important, and sometimes they are looking for the hourly wage. The toughest part is finding someone with the commitment and is willing to work for the wage and not someone who is working for a pay check. Money is important but I have found it does not motivate everyone. Being treated well and giving them a good work environment is just as important as long as they have a pay check that will help them make ends meet." With few exceptions, as Chapter 11 will make clear, facilities tend to pay what the market will bear, rather than offering workers a wage that will do more than help workers "make ends meet."

Other barriers to finding desirable staff included the "physical" nature of the job and the lack of public transportation. Finally, for some administrators, the applicant pool in their area simply lacks candidates with sought-after traits (e.g., professionalism, patience, high school education). One director in a small-town locale said, "The biggest barrier, and I don't mean to be ugly, but it is kind of like the area. I would say maybe half the people in the county have not graduated high school." One owner who prefers older workers blames the inability of the industry to attract this segment of the population: "I love the older person, and when I say older person I mean 40 and up, even into their 70s . . . to get the older population to come in and apply for a job. I have run ads, which I have been told isn't proper, 'If you are a senior, please apply because we are interested in you.' . . . I think that my biggest hindrance is intimidation from the older population who do not feel they can do the job. I don't know how to relay that to them in the paper."

One director identified the facility's unselective practice of considering any applicant who comes in, rather than "casting a net" for a specific type of worker, as the biggest barrier. A few administrators indicated that they had no difficulty recruiting satisfactory staff.

Facility Training and Education

As the previous section makes clear, facilities vary in the criteria they use in hiring workers. Some want experienced workers with formal education and CNA training. Others care more about personality and attitude and take on the responsibility for teaching workers how to provide care. Most administrators believe that, given the right "nature," a person can be taught the necessary caregiving skills. In this section we explore how facilities train new hires and meet DCWs' continuing education needs. We also examine DCWs' attitudes about the adequacy and usefulness of these efforts. Finally, we consider the relationship between the hiring and training processes and discuss the implications of facility practices regarding both for workers' satisfaction and retention.

Initial Training

In almost all homes of all sizes and locations, a DCW's initial training includes a period of job "shadowing" with a more experienced employee. In the majority of facilities, this on-the-job training constitutes the sole source of initial training. About a third of facilities, most of them large and corporately owned, also include varying amounts and types of classroom instruction.

Shadowing

The length and content of this period of on-the-job training varies, depending on the skill set a worker brings to the job, the configuration of her or his particular job, administrator attitudes toward the amount and type of training required, and a facility's workload. In some cases the training lasts a specific number of days. In others it continues until someone, either the director, supervisor, or another DCW, deems the new worker sufficiently trained. As one medium-home owner said, "They will be trained for as many days the staff person who is training them feels they need." Administrators also consider the workers' comfort level regarding their ability to carry out their duties. One said, "We ask them how they are feeling."

The following examples provide administrators' descriptions of how on-the-job training happens in their facilities. They illustrate a range of training experiences. The description from one small home exemplifies a minimal approach in terms of length and depth: "Usually [they are] on the floor running. When a person first comes, they are put with an experienced person, whatever time is needed, which is not very long usually. Usually [when] somebody comes in, they pick it up real quick. It is housekeeping. That is what you do on a daily basis anyway." This administrator's stance regarding the extent of training needed is colored by her belief that workers, who mostly are female, come with the "housekeeping" skills they need. Another small-home owner puts greater emphasis on this period, essentially to ensure that workers follow her specific protocols: "I work with them for an entire shift and then I come in and spot-check them. I do that for a good two weeks. I put a lot of time myself into having people understand the way I want things done. I show them. I work with them a whole shift. I say, 'You know the way I want it done because I am showing you. I am not just telling you.' I take the time. That is why it is a pain in the neck to hire new people. It ruins my life."

A medium-home director also uses a more comprehensive and structured course: "We take staff around so that they meet the residents and we have them sit down at tables and talk with them and participate in activities. That is all part of the orientation, but it is an ongoing process. We put them on training as an RA for three days. They work with the lead RA and they train them on everything from our staff sign-off sheets. They go through everything with them in those three days and then we will give them three more days. Usually we don't train them more than six days."

Acquainting staff with residents typically is part of the initial training process. Some facilities emphasize conveying specific knowledge about residents during this period, as one small-home owner explained, "They get that one-on-one with each resident. That is the most important part of the training. It is not so much training them how to clean but to get them acquainted with the residents." In one medium home, workers are trained for all shifts for this reason: "They are trained every shift. During training, even third-shift people have to work on first and second to get to know all the residents, because on third shift, they don't see every single resident every night."

Thorough training is the ideal, but some administrators admit that often they "get them trained and working right away because you are short and you need them." The director of a large corporate home described the hit-or-miss initial training in her home: "It has been on-the-job training to date with either a mentor or a co-worker, which would be the lead person. We try to grab them up and have them read the handbook and talk about all the compliance issues. Then we buddy them up with someone and keep our fingers crossed."

Classroom Instruction

Georgia AL regulations specify completion of certain work-related training during the first 60 days of employment to include, at a minimum, first aid, CPR, emergency evacuation procedures, medical and social needs and characteristics of the resident population, residents' rights, and abuse reporting. Some facilities require completion of first aid and CPR before being "on the floor." Corporately owned facilities typically stipulate an additional initial training component. In some facilities this component precedes the on-the-job training. The director of a large corporate facility explained, "They have eight hours of orientation with me and then they meet with each department head and they do that with the department head. They are monitored for the first couple of weeks to make sure that they are comfortable with things. We work through the employee handbook and then assign them to work with someone for two days. If they are a new person that has never worked, I am going to put them in a longer orientation period and that would be like two weeks of training. But they always get at least three days."

In other cases, classroom instruction is conducted over a minimum period of time ranging from 30 to 90 days, the approach of another large corporate facility: "There are a couple of tracks we take. One is, there is a minimum 24 hours of classroom time we have the staff do within the first 30 days. As they are starting, we train the basics of what we do. There are three classes. One is called the Basics of Care. The second is Alzheimer and Dementia Care. The third is called Programs and Services. The other track we have is job shadowing. We have 24 hours of job shadowing. That is done in the beginning for everybody."

In one of the dementia-specific facilities, new hires first complete 20 hours of Alzheimer training, which includes validation therapy and redirection (common techniques used in dementia care). The director of this home believes such training is essential because "this is not handling a normal resident." If a DCW is going to be a med tech, additional formal training may be required. In the majority of homes, though, training for medication assistance is incorporated into the shadowing experience. The director of one medium home plans to increase the rigor of this type of training: "We are going to be starting to train certain people to give medication. They have to go to an eight-hour class and at the end of the eight hours they take a test just on administering medications."

Continuing Education

Georgia requires 16 hours of continuing education per year and specifies certain topics, including working with persons who are elderly and who have cognitive impairment, mental illness, and developmental disabilities; social and recreational activities; legal issues; physical maintenance and fire safety; and housekeeping. All facilities provide all or part of the required continuing education; 97 percent of staff received it at the facility. As with initial training, the quality of ongoing training varies considerably. At the most basic level, it consists only of watching videos or reading relevant materials, the strategy of the owner of a low-income medium home: "We do a video. I used to do staff meeting but now it is video. I let them take them home and look at them and then come back and write them up. I let them go through it with me. I get some magazines on how to help Alzheimer and they read that. That is what I do."

The following description of continuing education at a large corporate facility represents a higher bar: "We accomplish that through a variety of measures, like in-service training. Some organizations, like home health companies, come in and provide training. We have those often. We try to provide a lot more so that everyone can get it through the year. Hospice training is done by our hospice provider. We have a geriatric psychiatric nurse who comes in and does some of the behavioral training. We have had a physician do training for us. We have a lot of different people come in. We do training on falls, observing resident behavior, eating patterns and nutrition, ADL care, hospice, physical therapy, lifting and transferring. We train on monitoring health conditions."

Almost all homes take advantage of community resources to help with training, especially home health and hospice agencies and the Long-Term Care Ombudsman Program. Videotapes also are commonly used and allow flexibility for workers who have difficulty attending meetings. Some corporations have requirements beyond those of the state, as described by one director: "One part of our program is training along particular themes. The themes include hospitality, attitude, respect, and caring. I do first aid, disaster, fire safety, and I also use our nurse practitioner. The physical therapist, I have her to do one on lifting and transfers. We had a specialist in dementia and Alzheimer and did a two-day training seminar and there were five of us and we came back to train the staff here." As this quote indicates, corporate facilities also have access to shared resources.

Most facilities combine in-services with monthly staff meetings. Almost all administrators believe the training they provide is useful to care staff and "helps them do their job better." Some expressed certain caveats regarding usefulness, including whether "they [staff] pay attention to it" and "it is practiced and used everyday."

Some administrators acknowledged doubts about the overall quality or usefulness of the training offered. One said, "Some of them are valuable, and some are not." Others were more negative, likening the requirements to a necessary evil. One small-home owner said, "I think that is a waste of time and a waste of our money to have to pay. We have to offer it and you have to attend." The director at a medium home said, "I don't know how valuable the training is for them doing [their] job. I think CPR is important, but what they get out of a one-hour class, I don't know. I don't think they need it. It is more of a Georgia state requirement and they are trying to regulate how many certifications people get." Although most administrators are flexible about how DCWs fulfill training requirements, all are clear about the inevitability: "If they don't have their 16 hours within that first year, they are terminated."

Workers' Viewpoints about Training

We assessed DCWs' attitudes about the usefulness, accessibility, and adequacy of their training in several ways. In qualitative interviews we asked DCWs to describe the procedures in their homes for training new hires and about their perceptions of training adequacy. As a whole, the procedures in the ideal matched what administrators told us. One DCW, who considers the initial training at her large, corporately owned home "excellent," described practices similar to those described by her director: "They will work with someone for a certain amount of time. They are not just put on the floor. They get to know the residents and their routine. They are always put with someone. They may orient on both first and second shift regardless of what shift they come in on. It is a good thing the way they do it. The training I received was excellent because you are being trained by the people that know best, the people that are actually working with these residents. They can give you insight into their personalities and likes and dislikes. It is good."

Other assessments were less positive, as well as less closely matched to the administrator's version. A DCW in another large corporate home, where training as described by the director includes shadowing plus three "levels" of classroom instruction, said, "Usually it is a three-day training, but it depends on how we are short. Today she [new hire] had to work on the floor. You really need three-day training." When asked if she thought the initial training was "good," she answered, "Definitely not. A lot of people have worked in nursing homes and they know ahead of time. Some people they hire have never been to this kind of job and they don't know anything." As this passage suggests, initial training procedures vary, even within facilities and corporations, and sometimes the ideal does not match the reality.

Because DCWs come to their jobs with varying degrees of experience and knowledge, initial training needs vary as well. A DCW in the small home where the owner emphasized the importance of "showing" new workers how she wants tasks done suggested that initial training often is inadequate and does not allow for varying need: "You work one day with somebody and then you are on your own. To me, that don't work because everybody is not the same. Everybody is not going to catch on as quickly as you did." To a DCW in another small home, where residents' care needs are minimal, training is a breeze: "It is really easy to train them. Just learning the residents, what their likes and dislikes are."

Other workers indicated that a key factor in the quality of training is the quality of the trainer. A DCW in a small home where the majority of residents need help with three or more ADLs said, "It is not really hard to train somebody on assisted living, because it is not that hard. If you have got your mind set right, you can do it in a month or month and a half. I was trained by an ex-supervisor. She trained me pretty good. She taught me everything that I needed to know and I learned real quickly because she is a good trainer." This quote also suggests that three days may not suffice for novices.

In quantitative interviews we asked participants to rate the usefulness of the continuing education provided by their facilities on a 10-point scale ranging from "very useful" (1) to "not at all useful" (10). Overall, 87 percent of DCWs gave a rating from 1 to 5. Comparable ratings were offered in small (87%), medium (90%), and large (86%) facilities.

Responses to more in-depth questioning provide additional insight into attitudes. DCWs relate the usefulness of their training to its quality and to job outcomes. As with initial training, data show that quality varies across facilities and within corporations. A med tech in a large home with corporate training resources said, "It is good because it teaches a lot of people stuff that they don't know or they do know and it just helps them help the residents. That's what those in-services are for, how to help the residents, and they have some really good tips and good information. It has been helpful to me also." A DCW from another home owned by the same corporation was less positive: "Here, I don't think we have in-services here. They say we have meetings, mandatory meetings, all kinds of things, and we sign the paper, but most of them is not really in-service. It is completely different than nursing homes. That's like how to take care of residents."

DCWs' views also indicate that continuing education for them, like for some administrators, can become rote and simply a necessary means. A worker in a medium home said, "It is a lot of training, so sometimes you get tired. Sometimes you see a film over and over again, but if you don't see them you don't have a job."

Some administrators are aware that DCWs, particularly those with longer tenure, sometimes find training less than useful. The director of a medium facility said, "Sometimes I think the staff think it is not required, but there are so many new things they need to know. I think it is important but sometimes they think it is a waste of their time because they already know how to do everything." Another said, "They don't really appreciate or find the importance of it. It is just a class they have to sit through."

Although some DCWs consider that continuing education is more for newcomers, others value the opportunity to obtain refresher information. One worker said, "It is useful. Sometimes you forget and it brings your memory back." And from another: "For myself, I would like to have more training in what I have already learned, to revise it all over again." Only 5 percent of DCWs reported any difficulty obtaining the required number of hours, mostly owing to scheduling.

Two survey questions addressed attitudes about training adequacy. One asked, "Have you ever had a situation, such as an emergency, where you felt you lacked the skills you needed to do your job?" Overall, 14 percent of workers responded "yes" to this question. A similar proportion of DCWs with CNA training (14%) expressed deficiencies.

We also included an open-ended question asking DCWs to specify areas in which they wanted additional training. These responses indicate keen interest in learning new skills. A substantial majority (59%) named at least one area; 12 percent named two; and 3 percent, three. The topics named most frequently were medications (19%); basic caregiving skills (13%); dementia care (11%); and emergency response (9%).

In comparing responses across home size, differences are evident regarding the desire for medication training: only 8 percent of DCWs in small homes want additional training, compared with 27 percent in medium homes and 19 percent in large homes. This finding may relate to the fact that most workers in small homes (94%) already provide medication assistance, compared with 68 percent in medium homes and 51 percent in large homes (see Chapter 5, this volume). Moreover, in the larger homes, one person per shift typically is responsible for medication assistance for all residents, which may increase the stress level of the job and thus the perception of training needed. Twelve percent of workers who regularly assist with medications said they want additional training in that area. One of the DCWs in this group said, "There's always so much to learn about different meds." From another: "You need to know the good and bad effects of it. Sometimes [I] don't have time to read all of the information on it."

In addition, med techs tend to have higher rates of pay, which likely is an incentive for this type of training. A worker in one large home wanted additional training "to be a supervisor with the medication."

Our findings show that DCWs want additional training in basic caregiving, including knowledge related to skilled care and heavy physical care. Specific areas named include wound care, taking vital signs, cleaning catheters, caring for diabetics and those on oxygen, and lifting, turning, and transferring residents in a way that protects the resident and themselves. One DCW noted that such skills are necessary because facilities "are bringing in more residents that need more care." Dementia care needs pertain mainly to dealing with combative and resistant residents, understanding the needs of residents with dementia, and coping with the effect of Alzheimer disease on residents.

Slightly less than a tenth of DCWs felt lacking in crisis care, but such lacks cause considerable stress to staff and possible danger to residents, as indicated by the following examples: "There was an incident where a resident passed out. She had vital signs but just wouldn't wake up. Her family was here at the time. I didn't know what to do. No one else knows what to do"; "One person had a stroke. Even though I knew to call 911, I felt like there should be something I should be able to do to help"; "I get scared about choking. Residents have choked. I called 911."

For a few DCWs, training needs relate not to a particular area but to handling unfamiliar routines as a result of filling in for other workers. One explained, "Putting me on first shift without training tomorrow ticked me off, but I'm going with it. Not having a day on the floor to see the routine of the person, now that is where the stress and anxiety comes in."

Some DCWs believe that any training is helpful and useful and that "every little bit helps." In the words of a DCW in a large home: "You can always learn in all areas, nothing specific. The more you know, the better you are for any kind of situation." Others feel they have no training needs, either because they consider their work "really like doing my housework" or because they believe they are "overqualified to do this job."

Discussion

In this chapter, we examine the recruitment, hiring, and training practices used in the 45 sample homes, identify barriers administrators face in their effort to develop a quality workforce, and consider various individual, facility, and community factors that influence how facilities hire and train workers. In addition, we explore DCWs' attitudes toward the content and adequacy of their training. Hiring and training workers is integral to the ability of facilities to develop and maintain a quality workforce. The findings presented in this chapter have relevance for ALFs throughout the United States. Most states, like Georgia, specify few criteria for hiring and training DCWs (Mollica et al., 2005).

Facility hiring criteria encompass applicants' personal traits, formal education, and caregiving training and experience. Of these stated criteria, almost universally, the number one trait administrators seek is a caring and compassionate personality. Compassion, they believe, is a key indicator of a worker's potential to provide quality care to frail elders and to remain in their jobs. Other personal characteristics considered include age, gender, appearance, and the ability to "fit in." Only a minority of homes have specific formal education and training requirements, and just half state a preference for hiring individuals with caregiving experience. A fundamental rationale offered by AL employers for emphasizing personal traits over education and experience is their own ability to train DCWs to provide care (as opposed to how to "be nice").

Overall, our findings indicate that in recruiting, hiring, and training DCWs facilities engage in a process of balancing needs and resources. In essence, a facility's hiring process is based on the type of worker it hopes to attract given its available resources and the care needs of its resident population. The ideal is to hire not just good workers but workers who will stay. The reality is that facilities often make do with who they can get.

Training is linked to hiring. A variety of factors, operating at the individual, facility, and community levels, exert influence on both processes. The way in which facilities balance needs and resources in their efforts to develop and maintain a quality workforce is similar to the "risk negotiation" process described elsewhere (Ball et al., 2005; Perkins, Ball, Whittington, & Combs, 2004) to explain how facilities, both large and small, develop adaptive and risk-management strategies in order to survive economically in the competitive world of AL. Thus, although hiring workers with "heart" likely has positive outcomes for workers and residents, relying solely on this criterion represents a strategy to balance competing needs and entails some risk. The same can be said for training strategies.

On the positive side, our data show that administrators' preference for compassion mirrors the aspirations of the majority of DCWs in our sample, who view themselves as caring individuals with a strong value for helping others, particularly elders. This value, in fact, is a primary motivator of their decision to become professional caregivers (see Chapter 4, this volume). Moreover, validation of DCWs' altruistic motives, as well as other aspects of their relationships with elder care recipients, is a vital component of job satisfaction and contributes to retention (Ball et al., 2009; Bowers, Esmond, & Jacobson, 2000; Tellis-Nayak & Tellis-Nayak, 1989; Chapter 7, this volume). Because LTC residents rely on DCWs for emotional as well as physical care, continuing to attract compassionate workers is essential to care quality. Social bonds with caregivers have been identified as significant determinants of the care recipient's quality of life in AL and nursing homes (Ball et al., 2000, 2005; Eckert, Zimmerman, & Morgan, 2001; Gass, 2004; Piercy, 2000). All the outcomes mentioned above point to the value of a hiring strategy that emphasizes "heart."

Such a strategy, however, has potential adverse outcomes for residents and workers. First, DCWs chosen primarily for personal traits may lack certain skills necessary to care for AL's increasingly frail resident population (Golant, 2008; Spillman, Liu, & McGuilliard, 2002), particularly the high percentage of residents with dementia (Rosenblatt et al., 2004), complex medication regimens (Mitty & Flores, 2007), and heavy physical care needs. This hiring strategy thus increases the significance of the facility training process, yet our data show that despite administrators' confidence in postemployment training, the quality and quantity of training facilities provide to both new and long-term employees are uneven. Although only a minority of DCWs in the sample reported on here stated that they had encountered situations in which they lacked the skills necessary to do their jobs, even small numbers are worrisome given the potential consequences to residents.

In addition, a large majority of DCWs expressed a need for additional training. As noted, a number of studies point to the effect of poor training on care quality in LTC (IFAS, 2007; Meagher, 2006; Miller & Mor, 2006). Research in a variety of LTC settings in the United States also indicates the importance of adequate training in worker satisfaction and retention (Ejaz et al., 2008). Our findings regarding DCWs' relationships with residents (see Chapter 7, this volume) clearly show that taking "good" care of residents is integral to job satisfaction.

In the facilities we studied, two types of training are typical: initial training upon hire and ongoing training over the course of employment. Initial training most commonly consists of "shadowing" an experienced DCW. Many ALFs rely on such a period of "on the floor" training to prepare DCWs for their jobs, and this method seems sensible given the fundamental importance of each resident's personality and preferences to care quality outcomes (Kane, 2001).

In contrast, ongoing training tends toward more formal, abstract knowledge, imparted through classroom instruction and video viewing (Grant et al., 1996; Teri et al., 2005). The stark differences between these two processes could be eased so that each period of training is more coherent with the other. Research suggests that ongoing training at the "bedside" or "on the floor" could help workers apply the knowledge imparted through classroom instruction (Aylward et al., 2003; Pyle, Massey, & Nelson, 1998; Stolee et al., 2005).

Furthermore, the DCWs in our study called for additional training in topics such as skilled care and lifting and transferring residents, not because of abstract intellectual curiosity but because of job demands. With the increasing frailty of AL residents (Golant, 2008), these needs are likely to be more and more common in ALFs across the United States. Accordingly, it may be useful to use ongoing training strategies that take place in the actual care context, rather than in a classroom setting. Such strategies may improve the practice of knowledge imparted and help employers overcome staff shortages that arise when DCWs attend classes (Braun, Cheang, & Shigeta, 2005).

Although relationship training was almost nonexistent in study facilities, research on DCWs' relationships with residents (see Ball et al., 2009; Ejaz et al., 2008; Chapter 7, this volume), with co-workers (see Chapter 6, this volume), and with supervisors (Noelker & Ejaz, 2001) indicates a need for education about diversity and other relationship issues.

Our findings indicate that, in addition to the need to improve on-the-job training, AL prehiring training criteria should be strengthened, at least in some care situations. Requiring CNA training likely would make large numbers of current DCWs (45% of our sample) unqualified for AL employment, rendering such a strategy self-defeating, particularly in states like Georgia with only one AL licensing category. However, in states where regulation permits ALFs to provide varying levels of care, training requirements should be tied to the skill level required.

The emphasis on personality in hiring decisions also reinforces care work's "unskilled" identity, possibly making LTC employment even less attractive to workers who value skilled employment. Furthermore, focusing on an applicant's level of compassion likely contributes to the extreme gender segregation in LTC, owing to the specifically feminine qualities associated with such traits (Beutel & Marini, 1995; Gilligan, 1982).

Research regarding co-worker relationships (see Chapter 6, this volume) indicates that considering an applicant's ability to "fit in" with respect to a facility's social environment may be a productive strategy. The inability to get along with co-workers can lead to dissatisfaction and to thoughts of leaving a job. However, this tactic may result in increased gender segregation of LTC workers, as well as to decreased racial and ethnic diversity, since individuals with similar racial and ethnic identities are more likely to be perceived as fitting together (Roscigno, Garcia, & Bobbitt-Zeher, 2007). Consideration of applicants' appearance and gender, additionally, may contribute to worker homogeneity.

A number of administrators expressed a preference for older workers, which may be a productive strategy. One reason is that the group of workers most likely to be DCWs (women aged 18 to 54) is decreasing in relation to an increasing elder population (Leon et al., 2001), while at the same time growing numbers of older workers want to remain in or join the workforce (Kleyman, 2004). In addition, older workers tend to have traits LTC employers find desirable, including experience, maturity, loyalty, good judgment, dependability, and reliability (Rix, 2001). Moreover, research in nursing homes (Kiyak & Namazi, 1997) and home care (Feldman, 1990) found job satisfaction was greater among older care staff.

Our findings further show that ascertaining whether applicants possess sought-after qualities is challenging. We outline a number of creative strategies facilities use when selecting applicants who best fit the desired criteria. These data indicate that the interview process is crucial to evaluating applicants, as is creating opportunities for current staff to provide feedback. Administrators admit, though, that determining "heart" is not an easy task. Obtaining useful and valid information from past employers also is problematic, owing both to the reluctance of employers to share employee information and to the rate of administrator turnover. Other barriers to comprehensive assessment of applicants lie in the material costs associated with obtaining information about an applicant's health, possible drug use, and criminal activity. Our findings also show that a critical piece in hiring stable workers, particularly those who lack experience, is educating applicants about the nature of the job.

The facilities we studied rely heavily on word of mouth to recruit DCWs. Data from DCWs indicate they use the same tactic to locate facilities (see Chapters 4 and 6, this volume). As a result, few administrators need to actively recruit DCWs, yet current turnover rates suggest that a recruitment strategy dependent solely on informal networks may be problematic. Indeed, some administrators acknowledge that hiring friends and family can put employers at risk of higher turnover ("lose one, you lose two"). Because DCWs often leave one LTC employer for another (see, for example, Lopez, 2006), informal social networks could be as responsible for turnover as they are for recruitment.

Furthermore, recruiting from social networks likely contributes to the gender segregation of LTC, since women rely on close personal ties to find jobs more than men do (Drentea, 1998; Marx & Leicht, 1992). Consequently, including strategies aimed at specific subsets of the population, such as men and older individuals, may be useful. Encouraging current employees to search their networks for out-of-the-ordinary recruits may expand both the size and diversity of applicant pools with little cost to facilities. Research that specifically examines the pathways of such atypical groups to LTC would help guide recruitment strategies.

Additionally, developing recruitment strategies aimed at better-trained and -educated applicants, such as those few professionally motivated DCWs in our sample (see Chapter 4, this volume), may help strengthen the workforce. For example, the strategy used by some administrators of recruiting from nursing students and CNA trainees may be more widely used. Research on such collaborative relationships could help guide these strategies as well as determine their effectiveness.

Conclusion

The processes of recruiting, hiring, and training DCWs for employment in AL and across the LTC sector have important implications for the quality of care as well as for worker job satisfaction and retention. The present study indicates that care work's low pay shapes both the characteristics of workers who are attracted to these jobs—those with few other job options—and the criteria for hiring DCWs in Al and other LTC settings. With limited resources to attract skilled workers, employers emphasize applicants' personal qualities more than professional criteria. This strategy reinforces occupational gender segregation because the qualities employers seek are themselves gendered. Our findings suggest that, to attract and retain a more diverse and better-trained AL workforce, employers need to expand current recruitment and training strategies.

REFERENCES

Aylward, S., Stolee, P., Keat, N., & Johncox, V. 2003. Effectiveness of continuing education in long-term care: A literature review. *The Gerontologist* 2, 259–71.

Ball, M. M., Lepore, M. L., Perkins, M. M., Hollingsworth, C., & Sweatman, M. 2009. "They are the reason I come to work": The meaning of resident-staff relationships in assisted living. *Journal of Aging Studies* 23, 37–47.

Ball, M. M., Perkins, M. M., Whittington, F. J., Hollingsworth, C., King, S. V., & Combs, B. L. 2005. *Communities of care: Assisted living for African American elders.* Baltimore: Johns Hopkins University Press.

Ball, M. M., Whittington, F. J., Perkins, M. M., Patterson, V. L., Hollingsworth, C., King, S. V., et al. 2000. Quality of life in assisted living facilities: Viewpoints of residents. *Journal of Applied Gerontology* 19, 304–25.

Banaszak-Holl, J., & Hines, M. 1996. Factors associated with nursing home staff turnover. *The Gerontologist* 4, 512–17.

Beutel, A. M., & Marini, M. M. 1995. Gender and values. *American Sociological Review* 60, 436–48.

Bowers, B., Esmond, S., & Jacobson, N. 2000. The relationship between staffing and quality in long-term care facilities: Exploring the views of nurse aides. *Journal of Nursing Care Quality* 14, 55–64.

Braun, K. L., Cheang, M., & Shigeta, D. 2005. Increasing knowledge, skills, and empathy among direct care workers in elder care: A preliminary study of an active-learning model. *The Gerontologist* 45, 118–24.

Drentea, P. 1998. Consequences of women's formal and informal job search methods for employment in female-dominated jobs. *Gender and Society* 12, 321–38.

Eaton, S. 2001. What a difference management makes! Nursing staff turnover variation within a single labor market. In *Appropriateness of minimum nurse staffing ratios in nursing homes phase II final report.* Baltimore: Centers for Medicare and Medicaid Services. Retrieved from http://cms.hhs.gov/medicaid/reports/rp1201-5.pdf.

Eckert, J. K., Zimmerman, S., & Morgan, L. 2001. Connectedness in residential care: A qualitative perspective. In S. Zimmerman, P. D. Sloane, & J. K. Eckert (Eds.), *Assisted living: Needs, practices, and policies in residential care for the elderly* (pp. 292–313). Baltimore: Johns Hopkins University Press.

Ejaz, F. K., Noelker, L. S., Menne, H. L., & Bagaka, J. G. 2008. The impact of stress and support on direct care workers' job satisfaction. *The Gerontologist* 48, 60–70.

Feldman, P. H. 1990. *Who cares for them? Workers in the home care industry.* New York: Greenwood Press.

Gass, T. E. 2004. *Nobody's home: Candid reflections of a nursing home aide.* Ithaca, NY: Cornell University Press.

Gilligan, C. 1982. *In a different voice: Psychological theory and women's development.* Cambridge: Harvard University Press.

Golant, S. 2008. The future of assisted living residences: A response to uncertainty. In S. Golant & J. Hyde (Eds.), *The assisted living residence: A vision for the future* (pp. 3–46). Baltimore: Johns Hopkins University Press.

Grant, L. A., Kane, R. A., Potthoff, S. J., & Ryden, M. 1996. Staff training and turnover in Alzheimer's special care units: Comparisons with non-special care units. *Geriatric Nursing* 17, 278–82.

Hawes, C. 2003. *Nursing home quality: Problems, causes, and cures.* Written testimony before the U.S. Senate Committee on Finance. College Station, TX: Texas A&M University System Health Science Center.

Hawes, C., Rose, M., & Phillips, C. D. 1999. *A national study of assisted living for the frail elderly: Results of a national survey of facilities.* Beachwood, OH: Myers Research Institute.

Howes, C. 2008. Love, money, or flexibility: What motivates people to work in consumer-directed home care? *The Gerontologist* 48 (Special Issue 1), 46–60.

Institute for the Future of Aging Services. 2007. *The long-term care workforce: Can the crisis be fixed?* Report prepared for the National Commission for Quality Long-Term Care. Washington, DC: IFAS.

Kane, R. A. 2001. Long-term care and a good quality of life: Bringing them closer together. *The Gerontologist* 41, 293–304.

Kiyak, H., & Namazi, K. 1997. Job commitment and turnover among women working in facilities serving older persons. *Research on Aging* 19, 223–46.

Kleyman, P. 2004. Boomers to redefine workplace. *Aging Today* 25, 7–10.

Leon, J., Marainen, J., & Marcotte, J. 2001. *Pennsylvania's frontline workers in long-term care: The provider organization perspective.* A Report to the Intergovernmental Council on Long-Term Care. Philadelphia: Polisher Research Institute at the Philadelphia Geriatric Center.

Lopez, S. H. 2006. Culture change management in long-term care: A shop-floor view. *Politics and Society* 1, 55–79.

Marx, J., & Leicht, K. T. 1992. Formality of recruitment to 229 jobs: Variations by race, sex, and job characteristics. *Sociology and Social Research* 76, 190–96.

Meagher, G. 2006. What can we expect from paid careers? *Politics and Society* 1, 33–54.

Miller, E. A., & Mor, V. 2006. *Out of the shadows: Envisioning a brighter future for long-term care in America.* A Brown University Report for the National Commission for Quality Long-Term Care. Providence, RI: Brown University.

Mitty, E., & Flores, S. 2007. Assisted living nursing practice: Medication management: Part 1. Assessing the resident for self-medication ability. *Geriatric Nursing* 26, 83–89.

Mollica, R., Johnson-Lamarche, H., & O'Keeffe, J. 2005. *State residential care and assisted living policy, 2004.* Prepared for the U.S. Department of Health and Human Services. Washington, DC: National Academy of State Health Policy.

Mollica, R., Sims-Kastelein, K., & O'Keeffe, J. 2007. *Residential care and assisted living compendium.* Prepared for the U.S. Department of Health and Human Services. Washington, DC: National Academy of State Health Policy.

Noelker, L. S., & Ejaz, F. K. 2001. *Improving work settings and job outcomes for nursing assistants in skilled nursing facilities. Final report.* Cleveland: Benjamin Rose Institute.

Perkins, M. M., Ball, M. M., Whittington, F. J., & Combs, B. L. 2004. Managing the care needs of low- income board-and-care home residents: A process of negotiating risks. *Qualitative Health Research* 14, 478–95.

Piercy, K. 2000. When it is more than a job: Close relationships between home health aides and older clients. *Journal of Aging and Health* 3, 362–87.

Pyle, M., Massey, M., & Nelson, S. 1998. A pilot study on improving oral care in long-term care settings. Part II: Procedures and outcomes. *Journal of Gerontological Nursing* 24 (10), 35–38.

Rix, S. E. 2001. The role of older workers in caring for older people in the future. *Generations* 25 (1), 29–34.

Roscigno, V. J., Garcia, L. M., & Bobbitt-Zeher, D. 2007. Social closure and processes of race/sex employment discrimination. *The ANNALS of the American Academy of Political and Social Science* 609, 16–48.

Rosenblatt, A., Samus, Q. M., Steele, C. D., Baker, A., Harper, M., Brandt, J., et al. 2004. The Maryland assisted living study: Prevalence, recognition and treatment of dementia and other psychiatric disorders in the assisted living population of central Maryland. *Journal of the American Geriatrics Society* 52, 1618–25.

Seavey, D. 2004. *The cost of frontline turnover in long-term care.* A Better Jobs Better Care practice and policy report. Washington, DC.

Spillman, B. C., Liu, K., & McGuilliard, C. 2002. *Trends in residential long-term care: Use of nursing homes and assisted living and characteristics of facilities and residents,* #HHS-100-97-0010. Washington, DC: Urban Institute.

Stolee, P., Esbaugh, J., Aylward, S., Cathers, T., Harvey, D., Hillier, L., et al. 2005. Factors associated with the effectiveness of continuing education in long-term care. *The Gerontologist* 45, 399–405.

Stone, R., & Wiener, J. 2001. *Who will care for us? Addressing the long-term care workforce crisis.* Washington, DC: Urban Institute and the American Association of Homes and Services for the Aging.

Strauss, A. L., & Corbin, J. 1998. *The basics of qualitative research: Grounded theory procedures and techniques.* Newbury Park, CA: Sage Publications.

Tellis-Nayak, V., & Tellis-Nayak, M. 1989. Quality of care and the burden of two cultures: When the world of the nurse's aide enters the world of the nursing home. *The Gerontologist* 29, 307–13.

Teri, L., Huda, P., Gibbons, L., Young, H., & Van Leynseele, J. 2005. STAR: A dementia-specific training program for staff in assisted living residences. *The Gerontologist* 45, 686–93.

Wright, B. 2005. *Direct care workers in long-term care.* Washington, DC: AARP Public Policy Institute.

CHAPTER ELEVEN

Rewarding Workers

Mary M. Ball, Ph.D.
Carole Hollingsworth, M.A.
Candace L. Kemp, Ph.D.

Frontline workers in long-term care (LTC), including those who work in nursing home, assisted living (AL), and home care settings, are among the nation's most unrewarded workers (National Center for Assisted Living, 2004; Paraprofessional Healthcare Institute, 2006). Low wages result in high poverty levels among this group, and many also lack health insurance coverage (National Clearinghouse on the Direct Care Workforce, 2006). In addition, the large majority of these direct care workers (DCWs) are women and increasingly have minority status and are foreign-born (Institute for the Future of Aging Services, 2007; Redfoot & Houser, 2005). Compared with the workforce in general, DCWs are more likely to be unmarried African American or Hispanic women who are supporting children under the age of 18 (Harris-Kojetin et al., 2004). Almost half (45%) of DCWs have only a high school education (National Clearinghouse on the Direct Care Workforce, 2006).

Workers such as these tend to have low employment options, and although other motivations may be present, as pointed out in Chapter 4 of this volume, the need for money both draws DCWs to LTC and keeps them in the field. Yet evidence exists that the low extrinsic rewards of the job also contribute to both the acute shortages and the high turnover rates among these workers (Close, Estes, Linkins, & Binney, 1994; Foner, 1994) and to their low job satisfaction (Grieshaber, Parker, & Deering, 1995; Helmer, Olson, & Heim, 1993).

In this chapter we address the reward systems for DCWs found in AL, including salaries, benefits, and less formal recognition programs. Specifically, we ask (1) How are facility reward systems structured? (2) How are these reward systems perceived by DCWs? and (3) What factors influence the development and maintenance of reward systems and the meanings they have for DCWs?

Methods

This chapter is based on data from all 45 homes involved in the study, "Job Satisfaction and Retention of Direct Care Staff in Assisted Living," described in detail in Chapter 3. Specifically, we use data from in-depth interviews with 44 administrators and 41 DCWs and from surveys of 370 DCWs. We asked administrators to describe the reward systems in their facilities, including salary structures, benefit programs, and other ways they reward and recognize DCWs. DCW surveys included questions about their pay rates, work schedules, participation in benefit programs and access to health care, other jobs, and their attitudes toward the various components of the facility's reward systems. Qualitative DCW interviews explored survey topics in greater depth and also included questions about family life and work history.

We analyzed qualitative data from in-depth interviews and open-ended survey questions following the principles of grounded theory methods (Strauss & Corbin, 1998; see Chapter 3, this volume, for study details.) This analysis reveals the multilevel factors that influence the structure, development, and maintenance of facility reward systems and the meaning these systems have for DCWs and their ultimate effect on job satisfaction and retention. In addition, we used descriptive statistics (e.g., frequencies, measures of central tendency and variability, and bivariate correlational analyses) to summarize relevant survey data.

Reward Systems

Facility reward systems include employee salaries, health insurance, retirement benefits, leave programs, and assorted employee recognition programs. Administrators must consider multiple competing demands when planning reward systems, namely, resident services, facility maintenance, capital improvements, and often unforeseen expenses. How these systems are structured and what they encompass depend primarily on each facility's resources but also on such factors as corporate policies, administrator attitudes and values, and the economics of the geographic area in which the facility is located. Below we describe the rewards systems of the 45 facilities we studied and examine various factors that influence them and the outcomes they have for DCW satisfaction and retention.

Salaries and Opportunities for Advancement

Table 11.1 shows the mean, median, and range of beginning hourly pay rates and the rates that were current during the time of our study for the total sample of 370 DCWs and according to facility size and location. These figures are revealing. First, overall salaries are low, with a mean hourly rate of $8.30. It is also clear that smaller facilities and those in more rural areas pay less well. The mean pay rate for small facilities is $7.30, compared with $8.10 for medium and $8.90 for large facilities. Area-1 facilities (the majority of which are large and all urban) and urban facilities have the highest pay rates. No large homes are in rural areas, whereas 3 (of 13) medium and 8 (of 18) small homes are in such locales. Four of the small homes are in completely rural places or areas with populations less than 25,000. In addition, the range of salaries within size and location categories shows considerable variation across facilities and within groups.

The pay rates shown in Table 11.1 reflect how facilities determine starting salaries as well as whether and how they provide for salary increases. Below we examine the effect of facility size and fees on DCW salaries, as well as the influence of other factors at the individual, facility, and community levels.

Table 11.1 Starting and Current Hourly Pay Rates, by Facility Size and Area

	Starting			Current		
	M	MD	Range	M	MD	Range
Small	6.6	6.5	5.0–10.0	7.3	7.3	5.0–10.3
Medium	7.1	7.0	3.4–11.0	8.1	7.8	5.5–15.0
Large	8.1	8.0	4.5–16.5	8.9	8.7	6.3–17.5
Rural	6.8	7.0	5.3–10.0	7.5	7.4	5.3–10.0
Urban	7.7	7.5	3.4–16.5	8.6	8.3	5.0–17.5
Total	7.5	7.4	3.4–16.5	8.3	8.0	5.0–17.5

Fees, Census, and Other Facility Influences

The importance of facility size largely has to do with resident fees and census. As shown in Chapter 3 (Table 3.1), mean fees increase with size: $1,498–$1,983 in small homes, $1,772–$2,803 in medium, and $2,097–$4,037 in large homes. Administrators of facilities in all size categories struggle with balancing the competing needs of staff and residents. In the words of one small-home owner: "Their salary comes from residents." The director of a medium home expanded on this dilemma: "It's in direct proportion to what the residents are paying. So, it's like if I'm going to pay my staff in the $9 to $10 area, then my residents are going to need to be paying more for those services, and so costwise if we're going up 3 to 5 percent on our residents fees, then I think we should reflect that in our personnel salary, but I think I'm in the minority as far as that feeling. The business is still very competitive."

In some homes, particularly small homes, increasing resident fees is rarely an option because of residents' own financial limitations. One owner of a small home with a top hourly pay rate of $8.50 wants "to pay them more," but 80 percent of her residents participate in the Medicaid waiver program, making further salary increases almost impossible.

A facility's resident census, as well as capacity, is a key factor affecting overall resources and a significant determinant of staff salaries in general and of raises in particular, especially in smaller homes. The owner of a home with only 15 residents (8 under capacity) said, "Being a little small business, it is hard to go higher. I wish I could hire them for what they are worth, but if I did I couldn't pay the bills." Another owner revealed the tenuous nature of salary increases tied to census: "I normally look at everybody at least once a year. If we are able to, we give a raise, and if we don't have the money, we don't. Again it goes back to census."

The majority of homes have some mechanism for raising pay with increased tenure. Most are merit-based. Only three homes provide annual cost-of-living raises. Size and resources influence the availability and rate of increase and, if present, the level of salary caps and the overall stability of the salary structure. Only one large home provides no regular raises, whereas three medium and twelve small provide either no or only minimal increases. Corporate ownership tends to add stability to an individual facility's resources.

In facilities where regular raises are standard, increases of from 1 to 4 percent are typical. Even when structures are corporately determined, administrators have some leeway, depending on their facility's financial situation and personal strategies. The director of a large, corporately owned home explained her practice: "The company has a minimum percentage and we do merit-based on that percentage. Three percent is the top. Now, that doesn't mean if we have an exceptional employee we couldn't give them above that, but we would have to get approval from higher above, which we have done for several people."

Some administrators make an effort to push salaries up across the board. The director of a large corporate home explained: "We have annual raises. The budget says 3 percent, but I am not known for giving 3 percent raises, more like 5 and 6. It depends on the individual. I am trying to get our budget a little higher." Administrators understand that their pay rates affect their ability to recruit and retain workers. The director of a large urban home with a corporately set merit increase of 4 percent explained: "I go to salaries.com and try to look at the long-term care salaries to see what people are paying. Midpoint right now is under $11 by a bit. If I am going to keep them, then I am going to pay them the max merit I can give them. I think mine [salaries] are getting the reputation of being good because I am having a lot more people come and want jobs."

Decisions about pay rate increases, though, are complex. One administrator voiced the need to balance multiple demands while watching the all-important bottom line: "When it is time for their raises, as long as we can afford their raises we do it. I tell them [staff] that there is a bottom line, that we have to be profitable. If our census goes down, we still have bills we have to pay. It always seems when it is annual time, that is when we don't have the money to go to raises and when things get torn up and we are having to replace things and repair things. That comes off our bottom line."

In one medium home a consistently low census has prevented pay increases and led to a reduction in DCW work hours. The director explained: "What we did when the census started dropping, we would cut someone back a day, whoever was the last one hired. No one has gotten a pay raise but no one has lost their job." The director of a small home located in a small town simply adjusted salaries up or down depending on inevitable census fluctuations. A common practice is to provide a minimal raise ($0.25 to $0.50) after a probationary period, generally from 30 to 90 days. In many of the smaller homes, these initial raises are the only opportunities for rate increases.

Even when corporations dictate periodic raises, continuing to reward long-term workers can be problematic for administrators. The director of a large home where caregivers start at $7.00 and the current highest rate is $8.75

explained: "It has to get to a stopping point because almost all my caregivers who've been here since the beginning have reached their maximum amount and are getting ready to get raises again, and I mean how much are we going to go? Because these girls will be probably with us for 10 years, but it might [be that] my home office say that they get a 4 percent raise, because it doesn't matter how long they've been with us, because of the cost of living." The majority of facilities maintain a salary cap, whatever the level.

Whether or not a facility has multiple, distinct DCW positions affects salary increases and opportunities for advancement. As noted in Chapter 5 of this volume, the complexity of a facility's organizational structure tends to increase with size. Thus it is mostly large and, less frequently, medium facilities with such positions that typically include, in addition to care aide, shift supervisor and med tech or some combination of the two. Our findings show that mean hourly pay rates for care aides tend to be lower ($8.11) than those for shift supervisors ($9.41) and med techs ($9.76). DCWs in the better-paid positions, however, account for only 16 percent of the total sample, indicating that only a minority of DCWs have the option of occupying a more advanced and better-paid position.

Hierarchical pay differentials generally are aimed at encouraging workers to stay. The director of a large home with only two levels explained: "What we found is that when you have people that are coming in as a caregiver, there has to be another step, there has to be something that they strive for." Lack of resources is the primary reason given by administrators for not having position-related advancement opportunities. The owner of a small home where DCWs start at $7.50 and cap at $8.00 described a typical situation in small homes: "Everybody starts out the same, and we keep everybody on the same level because they do the same work."

Administrators, even those who strive to increase rewards, employ a variety of strategies to minimize their employment costs. All avoid overtime payments, commonly accomplished through routinely scheduling fewer work hours, using PRN (i.e., as-needed) workers, and encouraging DCWs to take a day off after working extra hours. The success of this strategy is reflected in the mean (12) and median (8) monthly overtime hours reported by our sample. But even when circumventing overtime is not the goal, many administrators regularly limit work hours. This strategy is used more often in medium and large homes where DCWs work on average 37 hours per week, compared with 40 for small-home workers.

A strategy used by several homes with a med tech position is to have DCWs clock in and out when performing these duties. Facilities then pay the higher rate only for a portion of the workday. Another tactic is to rotate the shift supervisor position to avoid a permanent position and an accompanying rate increase.

As noted above, administrators commonly tie DCW wages, as well as resident fees, to the local market. Most think DCWs should be paid more, but many also believe they are paying a "fair" wage. The following quote from the director of a large home illustrates a common attitude among administrators, as well as the reality of many service jobs, especially in the LTC sector: "I think it's fair. Like I said, if you're paying people based on their value, they'd be making $30 an hour, because of what they provide to society, but, unfortunately, our society doesn't do that. It's based on what the market will bear."

Staff Influences

DCWs' personal traits, including LTC training and experience, also drive salaries and advancement opportunities. Certified nursing assistants (CNAs) in some homes automatically garner higher rates, ranging from $0.25 to $1.00 more. In one large home, this payment strategy is designed also to encourage future training. The director explained: "If you're coming in here off the street, $7.00, but if you're coming in here and you have one to three years' experience, it's $7.25 and if you have three to five, then it's like $7.50 and it's a staggered wage so you can get those more seasoned caregivers, because if you have a caregiver with 10 years experience and they have their CNA, then you're going to want to pay them $8.00 or $9.00 an hour. Okay, so that's so it encourages them to want to be able to get that CNA training to learn more." Not all homes, though, pay for training. At one home, located in a small metro area, that hires only CNAs, the starting pay for all workers is $6.50. Some homes waive or reduce the probationary period for more skilled workers.

A worker's job performance and attitude also are considered in determining salaries, as indicated by the use of merit-based increases. Such raises as a rule mean doing more than expected. One director explained her criteria: "Well, good attitude, initiative, drive, faithfulness, coming in when you're called, even if you're not on the schedule. I've got one or two that will only work their schedule, and you just don't call them. They won't answer the phone. They are good when they are here, but they're not going to ever really go very far as far as advancement."

Most DCWs who stay in a job receive higher pay over time. Correlation analysis demonstrates a significant relationship between pay rate and tenure in all size homes ($p < .0001$ in small and large homes and $p < .05$ in medium homes). These findings suggest that staying put pays off.

Staff Attitudes: "Very poor pay"

Findings for the 72-item Job Descriptive Index (JDI) reflecting DCWs' satisfaction with their salaries indicate pervasive dissatisfaction with this job component (see Chapter 3, this volume, for description of this measure). Scores for all workers range from 0 to 54, with a mean of 24. We found some variation in scores according to facility size (22.7 for small, 23.4 for medium, and 24.9 for large) and location (21.7 in rural and 24.4 in urban), indicating that DCWs who work in large homes and homes in urban areas are somewhat more satisfied with pay, although all scores are indicative of dissatisfaction.

In our survey of 370 DCWs we asked several open-ended questions related to job satisfaction and retention. Three questions elicited responses relevant to this section: (1) What do you like best and least about working in this facility? (2) What do you find most satisfying and frustrating about your job overall? and (3) What would make you stay or leave this job? Only negative responses related to salary: 20 percent of DCWs named their pay as what they like least; 11 percent reported pay as most frustrating; and 29 percent said that their pay would cause them to leave. These responses reflect attitudes toward current salaries as well as opportunities for raises.

In qualitative interviews we explored in greater depth DCWs' attitudes toward pay. Despite some variation in attitudes, one worker captured in colloquial terms a representative viewpoint of most DCWs regardless of pay level: "It sucks." Elaborating on this general negative attitude, a common theme voiced by workers is that salaries are not "fair" and they "deserve" more for what they do and how they do it. As one DCW with two-year tenure in a small home with a top hourly rate of $8 said, "I feel like I am better." She went on to say that $9 would be a "fair" starting rate and she "should be making at least $11." A long-term caregiver supervisor whose rate is $13 said, "I think it is fair, but I know I am worth more than that. A lot of these ladies, for what we do, no, we are not getting paid enough. I know they all say that." A med tech working in a large home making $10 admits salaries there are better than in most facilities in the area but still believes she deserves to be "paid more" because "there's a lot [of responsibility] to what I do."

Our analysis reveals that DCWs' views of their salaries are influenced by factors other than pay rates. Some relate to the facility, some to the DCW, and some to the surrounding community. The attitude of unfairness often is tied to absence of raises. Again, negative attitudes are represented among lower- and higher-paid workers. A DCW who works in the corporately owned medium home operating at half capacity said, "I think they could give us a little more money. Everything is going up and we are just making $6.25. That is not right. I have been here three years and have not had a raise. They say they are going to check into it, and then they turn around and give their own people [management] a raise and there is nothing we could do about it." A higher-paid DCW with six years in her facility and no salary increase in five feels similar frustration: "I have talked to her [the director] about it and all she says is, 'Well, for what you make an hour,' I make $10.50, which is not a lot of money, 'the number of residents, blah, blah, blah, blah.' She has an explanation for everything. She doesn't listen, she dictates. I have a lot of training behind me, I have been doing this for 33 years now, I'm a CNA, I'm not a nurse but I have taken different classes and different things, you know, to help it, and I just feel like that if you have an employee that has been with you for that long, you could do a little something, if you care." Her dissatisfaction is heightened by the level of her training and experience.

Another worker expressed outrage when the annual raises at her medium facility converted to performance bonuses and ultimately disappeared, resulting in a pay decrease (from $8.00 to $7.50): "No, it is not fair! I am highly upset about it, which is why I want another job! . . . The only reason I haven't raved about it is because I need the money." Other negative attitudes stem from employers' failure to follow through on promised raises, as expressed by a DCW in a medium home: "An employee works and works and works and you tell them in so many days they will get a raise and they don't get that raise, are they happy? No, because they are expecting what you told them but it never happens." Embedded in each of these examples is both a sense of powerlessness and a sense of feeling unappreciated by administrators.

A minority of DCWs expressed more positive views of pay rates. Some of these views were voiced by workers whose salaries are in fact in the higher range. One, who has moved up to a supervisory position and is paid $10.50 in a facility with a starting rate of $6.50, thinks her pay is "pretty good, considering I am not an LPN or RN." A part-time DCW at an independently owned small-town facility where salaries are higher than at others in the area is "happy" with her rate of $9.75. This worker also is married, with a husband who is the primary breadwinner. For a small number of DCWs like her, salary is less critical because of their personal economic situations. Another example is an older woman who receives Social Security benefits and because of government regulations "can make only so much."

For some workers, dissatisfaction with pay is offset by satisfaction with other job aspects. Workload is one. DCWs who feel less job stress tend to feel less underpaid. One who works in a home with low capacity and is paid $7.05 assesses her hourly rate as "fine for me, because we really don't do anything. But as of the place getting fuller, they should compensate me a little bit more, not a lot, because you're doing more now than you were doing."

Often it is the care of residents that is the principal compensating factor, as expressed by a DCW in a small home with a top rate of $7.50: "If I quit, who would take care of my residents? . . . I mean, eventually I will get a raise. I could use it, but I'm not going to sweat it because, like I said, they [the residents] hardly even have anyone come and see them. They are my family." Another offsetting factor is convenient facility location. An example is provided by a worker who remains in her rural facility, where she is paid $8.00, rather than drive to "the other side of the mountain" to make $9.65.

A common view is that "some money is better than none at all." This attitude typically was expressed by DCWs with fewer job options because of their personal traits (e.g., age) or geographic location (e.g., rural). The words from an older worker in a large rural home are representative: "My poor salary, I wish it could be better, but it was either that or not work at all, so I just deal with it." Another older worker expressed a similar view: "The money pays my bills and I don't want to have to go on welfare." She went on to verbalize another common attitude—that care work is more satisfying than other low-paying options: "I know you could go down the road and flip hamburgers and probably make more than what I am making, but this is my home. This is where I need to be."

Although 81 percent of DCWs work full-time in their facilities, almost half (48%) would like to work more hours than they do. Percentages are higher for workers in large (54%) and medium (45%) homes, compared with those in small homes (36%). These figures likely reflect the number of hours DCWs typically work as well as their economic situation. Only 7 percent of DCWs would like to work fewer hours.

Hours worked, together with pay rates, contribute to the need for DCWs to have second and even third jobs. One-fourth of workers have at least one other job. The proportion is higher in large homes (30%) compared with small (22%) and medium (19%) homes. The lower percentage in small homes likely relates to the greater number of facility hours worked as well as the lack of employment opportunities in rural locales.

A "Dead End" Job

Scores from the JDI reflecting DCWs' satisfaction with opportunities for advancement also indicate dissatisfaction. Scores for all workers range from 6 to 54, with a mean of 23. Scores of rural workers are somewhat higher (24.9) compared with those in urban areas (22.8). In addition, 8 percent of DCWs reported that lack of opportunities to advance to higher positions would make them leave their current jobs.

Qualitative data reveal that DCWs in general feel they have no opportunity to advance to a higher position. This view is found among workers in all size homes. The following quote from a worker in a small home is representative: "Where I am at right now, I don't know if there is anybody that moves up. To me it is like a dead end." This attitude is typical even in homes with multiple DCW positions, as expressed by a DCW in a large corporate home: "I don't have much of an opportunity because where are you going to go? I mean there is not much further you can go unless you become the nurse, or one of the managers." Only a few DCWs in our sample advanced to higher levels, such as unit supervisor or activity director.

Qualitative data show also that some DCWs do not want to move to positions with greater responsibility or that entail supervision or more "paperwork." One preferred not to move up and "sit around and give orders." Another said, "I don't care about being no chief; a little Indian is fine with me." Some DCWs feel they lack the ability or training to perform other jobs. One worker in a large home illustrates this view: "You can become med tech, but I wouldn't want to do med tech. I don't think I'm smart enough to do that, really." An older worker with less than a high school education also feels unprepared: "I am not educated to work in the office. I wouldn't have an office job anyway. I don't want to be the boss. I just want to be a caregiver, a good caregiver." These types of workers may account for the higher JDI scores found in rural areas.

Benefit Programs

Benefits offered by the facilities in our sample include medical and dental insurance, vacation and sick leave, and retirement and tuition reimbursement programs. Below we describe these different types of programs and examine the factors that influence their existence and structure, as well as the outcomes for DCWs.

Medical and Dental Insurance

The majority of facilities (62%) offer medical insurance, and slightly over half (51%) offer dental, although variation exists across size categories. All large and the majority of medium facilities offer both kinds of insurance, but only 4 of the 18 small homes offer medical and only 2 have dental. The facility factors affecting benefit programs are similar to those that influence salary and include fees, census, and ownership. For example, all the small homes with medical benefits are corporately owned and among the higher-fee homes in this category. The cost of health insurance obviously also is a contributing factor. The director of an independently owned home with 44 residents explained her situation: "The worst thing is I don't have health insurance on them. I have retirement for them, but that is one thing I have not been able to find anything I can afford. That is one of the big reasons we went on and did those two wings so maybe I could help them get some health insurance."

In addition to the existence of health insurance programs, facilities vary also in the employee costs for these benefits. Only one facility, a religiously affiliated and not-for-profit one, pays the full cost of medical insurance. Employee costs range from a low of $9.23 per two-week pay period in a small, corporately owned facility to a high of $112 in a large, independently owned home. Most employee cost shares are in the higher range.

Although a majority of all DCWs (58%) have medical insurance, less than half (47%) of workers in small homes do, compared with 61 percent in medium and 62 percent in large facilities. Only a minority (34%) of all workers (30% in small homes, 37% in medium, and 31% in large) have dental insurance.

Data regarding DCWs' source of medical insurance indicate that presence of a benefit program does not necessarily reflect workers' true access to this benefit. Only 9 percent of DCWs in small homes, 30 percent in medium homes, and 34 percent in large homes receive medical insurance from their facility.

Almost one-fifth (18%) of workers overall receive medical insurance through their families, and 5 percent are poor enough to be insured through the federal Medicaid program. Other DCWs have children who are eligible for Medicaid but are themselves ineligible. Four percent of DCWs in small homes and 2 percent in medium homes receive medical insurance through the Medicare program; no workers in large homes have insurance from this source.

When we asked DCWs their reasons for not participating in their facilities' medical insurance programs, half of all workers said that the cost share for participation was too expensive for them to afford. The words of a worker in a large home illustrate a common theme: "The health [insurance] for our pay rate and what we make as RAs, most people cannot afford it. That is the bottom line. This is the only place I have worked where I could not afford the health insurance. If I took the health insurance, it would take such a big chunk out of my check."

The next most common reason offered for nonparticipation is lack of eligibility (28% of DCWs). These responses reflect mostly part-time workers and those who are still in trial work periods. In most homes, DCWs must work full-time (32 hours) to be eligible, although one large corporation, which includes four sample homes, only requires 20 hours. A small minority of DCWs (6%) cited the poor quality of the policy (typically lack of comprehensiveness or large co-pays) as the reason for nonparticipation.

Qualitative interviews reveal the hardship that lack of health insurance causes these workers. One DCW in a small home explained, "There is no insurance here, none whatsoever. If you have insurance, it is because you go outside and get it. That is not something that is established here and it makes for a hard life but it is something you have to deal with." Another said, "I tough it out. I go buy Tylenol and, you know, just whatever I can get over the counter that might help." One DCW expressed the anxiety that accompanies being uninsured: "Well, I got to have it. I mean, I need to have it. I know this because anything could happen, anything. I could walk out there now and just accidentally get hit by a car or something. My family would be in terrible shape because I have no life insurance and no medical insurance." One worker who does participate acknowledged the difficulty of both choices: "I do and it is costing me a fortune, but I will not work anywhere without insurance. Some of my personal things, I just cut out so I can afford insurance. A lot of women here can't afford it, like the girl [another DCW] having a baby. It is terrible and you are stuck with all of those bills."

Vacation and Sick Leave

All small and large and the majority (85%) of medium homes offer paid vacation leave. In most of these facilities, DCWs receive one week of vacation, beginning after one year. In a few homes, workers accrue a certain number of hours per month from the beginning or after the trial work period. In the majority of homes, vacation hours increase with tenure up to a maximum amount.

Paid sick leave is available in all large, 62 percent of medium homes, and half of small homes. This benefit generally is available either immediately in a worker's tenure or after the trial work period. The typical pattern is the accrual of a certain number of hours per month, usually four hours. In six homes, the vacation and sick leave are combined.

One worker in a medium home commented positively about receiving these benefits: "We get enough days for sick and vacation. One year I had about three. I like that. My girlfriend went almost two years before she got a week. It adds up, it is good." Not having access to any type of paid leave is another factor that "makes for a hard life" for these low-wage workers, especially those with children at home.

Retirement and Tuition-Reimbursement Programs

Only one-third of all homes offer any kind of retirement program for DCWs. These include 64 percent of large homes, 38 percent of medium, and only one small home. Available data show that the employer match for the 401(k)-type programs ranges from 3 to 25 percent. Although our DCW survey did not ask about participation in this benefit, administrators indicated that almost none did because of the cost.

Less than a fifth of homes (18%) offer tuition reimbursement to DCWs— six large homes and one medium and one small, all corporately owned. The amount of reimbursement varies, and eligibility depends typically on coursework relevance and grade maintained. One director described his home's program: "We have tuition reimbursement, which I took advantage of when I was going to grad school. It is up to $1,000 a year and you just have to be taking something that has to do with it, like business to nursing. Since I took advantage of it, I passed it along so we now have about four people taking advantage of that. It doesn't help the budget but it is great thing. It was something that was in their team member handbook but they don't read it so I try to let them know it is there." As indicated, this director's promotion of the program is encouraged by his own former benefit. The quote below from a DCW who is enrolled in nursing school and works in his home suggests that this type of benefit is well received but, as the director points out, not well advertised or used: "This semester is going to be the first time I take advantage of that. I never really knew about it until last year. They never said anything about it. But this semester I already gave a copy to Alex [the director]. At the end of the semester they just want to see my grades so they can put in the reimbursement. I think if you have been here over a year it is 50 percent of tuition and books. I am hoping I will get something this semester."

Other Ways of Rewarding Workers

Almost all the facilities in our sample reward DCWs in tangible ways that supplement their paychecks and benefit programs. In this section we examine these supplementary rewards from the standpoint of the administrators who implement them and from that of the DCWs who are the recipients. Reward programs include recurring awards for consistent good work, less formalized recognition of special efforts "beyond the call of duty," and assorted types of bonuses and appreciation events. Through these programs, administrators aim to both *acknowledge* and *encourage* good work. Overall, the goal is to keep DCWs happy and in their jobs while providing quality care to residents. The director of a large corporate home with multiple recognition efforts explained: "You know everyone feels good when they are recognized and acknowledged for the work that they have done so it is definitely a plus; it never hurts. We want them to feel good about what they do because we definitely want them to be happy when they are at work."

As the previous section indicates, most administrators also believe that DCWs are underpaid, and these supplementary rewards are intended in part to compensate for the low wages. They understand the difficult nature of the DCW job, as well as the crucial role DCWs play in the operation of their facilities. A common refrain voiced was "We can't do it on our own." The range and extent of acclamation efforts vary across facilities, but most "try to share" as best they can. One director of a not-for-profit home said, "We give every perk we can find to give. I totally value my caregivers. Someone asked me how I keep such caregivers, and my answer is that at four o'clock everyday I kiss their feet, and that is about the size of it. They know how valued they are."

Below we describe the reward programs found in the sample homes and examine barriers administrators experience in implementing certain efforts.

Table 11.2 shows the program types found in each size facility. We also examine DCWs' perceptions regarding the various ways that facilities recognize their work. Table 11.3 summarizes their responses to the open-ended survey question "What type of facility recognition do you most value?"

Recurring Awards

As shown in Table 11.2, more than a third (36%) of sample homes (all medium and large homes, with the exception of one small, corporately owned home) have some type of recurring award to recognize good work. Typically, tributes are monthly, with one DCW designated Employee of the Month, although a few facilities have quarterly or annual awards or use different labels. In one large corporate home, DCWs compete quarterly within the community and annually across all company sites.

With the exception of two medium homes, these recurring awards include a monetary component, either cash or some type of gift card. Most have a value of $25, but a few facilities give more. In one large home, two DCWs receive $100 each month. In another, workers recommended by the director compete companywide for 25 $500 awards. One medium home gives the monthly winner a day off with pay. Typically monetary awards are accompanied by public recognition, such as an announcement in a staff meeting or newsletter and display of names on a plaque. In one home, recipients wear a special flower on their name tags. Several facilities provide recipients with designated parking spaces for the award month.

Most administrators who implement recurring awards believe they have positive outcomes for both DCWs and the facility. One director said, "I definitely think it makes them take more pride in their work. They know they are going to be recognized for doing something and will be appreciated for it." Others expressed the view that they help staff "feel better about their job," "want to do a better job," and "do a little bit more each day."

Some administrators, though, believe this type of recognition has little meaning. The director of a large home said, "I don't believe in that kind of thing because in my opinion you've been doing it for a year and you end up being the employee of the month, and [in] December, what does that mean? that I'm the twelfth best employee here? And what kind of satisfaction or prestige is there in being the twelfth best employee of the year?"

Employees are selected for these awards by management, co-workers, or residents or a combination of these groups. In one large home, residents

Table 11.2   Facilities with Reward Programs, by Facility Size

Type of Reward	Small (N=18)	Medium (N=13)	Large (N=14)	Total (N=45)
Recurring awards	1	7	8	16 (36%)
Awards for special effort	7	2	7	16 (36)
Performance incentive	0	5	4	9 (20)
Holiday bonuses/gifts	13	10	6	29 (64)
Birthday bonuses/gifts	2	4	2	8 (18)
Recruitment bonus	1	3	2	6 (13)
100% occupancy bonus	0	0	4	4 (9)
Appreciation events	6	8	12	26 (58)

choose two recipients each month, and department heads choose one. According to administrators, each method can be problematic. Issues noted with the resident selection system include lack of resident follow-through and the tendency of residents to select the same individuals repeatedly. In one facility where the resident system is used successfully, residents receive a "ballot" in the monthly newsletter.

A key concern of any method is the potential for staff conflict. One administrator described her Employee of the Month attempt as "the biggest disaster" because staff "were resenting" the recipient. Another reported that when staff voted "it got to be a personality contest." The director of one large home said, "We don't do employee of the month. That gets to be a game. It just doesn't work, especially with this small amount of people." Administrators who employ this strategy make an effort to implement it fairly. One said, "We try to be fair. We won't let the same person get employee of the month three months in a row. We try to make it evenly distributed." The goal of even distribution, however, could possibly result in an award that does not reflect performance.

Table 11.3 shows that 11 percent of DCWs value this type of recurring award. These include workers in homes with and without the award. Qualitative data indicate that some DCWs share administrators' views of positive outcomes. One DCW in a medium home said, "They started it this year, and I was the first one. I got Employee of the Quarter. They gave me $25, and they gave all the employees a little dinner at two o'clock. They had snacks and cake and stuff. It was nice. They put your picture on the board so everybody can see. . . . It makes you feel good that they think about you." A DCW in a large home described receiving an annual recognition as "an honor." One in a small home

Table 11.3 DCWs' Reward Preferences, by Facility Size (in percentages)

Type of Reward	Small (N=79)	Medium (N=103)	Large (N=187)	Total (N=370)
Cash bonus	21	35	19	24
Gift certificate	1	1	7	4
Salary increase	14	17	27	22
Paid time off	6	2	4	4
Employee of month	8	14	12	11
Plaque/pin	3	3	5	4
Verbal praise	44	24	22	27
Other	3	5	4	4

with no reward program feels such recognition "makes you try harder" and "gives people initiative to do better." Another DCW feels the *lack* of a monthly award means that administrators do not appreciate "what everybody does to keep this building running."

Other DCWs are more negative about recurring awards. In some cases, negative attitudes stem from the method of selection, and their words mirror those of administrators. Fairness in implementing the award is a key concern. A DCW in a large home said, "You have someone who has been working here less than two months and they are Employee of the Month. Everybody got upset. You need three months' trial period. She should be doing everything she could for her job because that is a probation period. That is nothing extra. I feel like that is wrong. They did that twice. The second one, she was so upset, she felt like everyone was going to come after her." Another worker described the process as "a joke" because "they pick people that are not even good." A night-shift worker finds the resident selection "one-sided" because she works at night and "no residents' family members visit at night to nominate us."

Other negative viewpoints have to do with the nature of the award, specifically the lack of monetary value, the opinion of a DCW in a large home: "They give you, what is it, a plaque? Also they put your name, we have a little plaque that they put your name on and it's right out in the hall there by the front desk. Yeah, but the other jobs that I have worked at also they give a $25 gift certificate." Table 11.3 indicates that only 4 percent of workers favor receiving a plaque or pin as an award. One worker dislikes public recognition: "I am a shy person and I can't stand the reward system they have here, where they call you up in front of everybody. I would rather for them to walk up to me and tell me I am doing good."

Although little variation is seen across home size, workers' preferences for recurring awards vary across facilities. For example, in the large facility that awards two $100 prizes monthly, 9 of the 11 staff interviewed prefer this award type. In another large home where the Employee of the Month receives a $25 gift certificate, only 1 of the 14 employees interviewed values this type of recognition. The others named either a cash bonus or salary increase. Such findings also indicate that how the award is structured influences staff outcomes.

Periodic Recognition for Special Efforts

Facilities also reward individuals for efforts "above and beyond" in less formalized ways. Such recognition tends to be at management's discretion and more on the spot. The following description from the director of a large home is typical: "The other things we do in terms of bonuses, if you will, if a staff person has really done something very special, I might give them $50. If someone has done something really nice for a resident, Ted [a DCW supervisor] might give them $5. We try to find ways to recognize people who have really done something that should be recognized and rewarded." DCWs generally are positive about this type of recognition. A worker in a small home where only this method is used said, "A lot of places don't do that. That makes up, that makes you feel like you did a good job. It really makes you feel good."

A number of corporate homes pass out fake "money" to DCWs when, in the words of one director, "we catch them doing something fabulous." This "money" then can be redeemed for various items a home has purchased. One director who is "into instant gratification" prefers just to give real money, one reason being that the fake versions are easily misplaced. A DCW in this home believes that such cash rewards encourage employees to "work harder."

The majority of small and medium homes provide a Christmas bonus (either cash or gift certificate); six large homes employ this strategy. The amount ranges from $25 to $200 (in one home). In most cases, DCWs receive equal amounts, but some administrators vary the amount based on staff effort, to encourage as well as reward. In one large home, med techs and shift supervisors receive a little more. The director of a medium home described her allocation method: "I give them a bonus at Christmas time, and that is based on their hours worked, five cents for every hour worked. That came out to say $150 to $200 per person. That was an incentive to get them to work full-time and work as many hours as they could. I gave a ham, I gave Christmas cookies. Every year I try to do something to let our employees know that we do appreciate them. We can't do it on our own." A DCW in a small home with this type of award said, "You get a Christmas bonus here, which I look forward to coming up next month. We get ours in November. At the nursing home I put in double shifts. My little girl was in the hospital and I missed one day and they took my Christmas bonus. Here it wouldn't be an issue. . . . This is like a second home to me."

A few homes give gifts instead of cash. A number have holiday parties or dinners. The director of one large home holds a special event at the facility:

> I'll tell you one of the things that we do that make staff happy is every year at Christmas we have a staff party and rather than taking everybody out to Appleby's and spending a ton of money on food, what we do is we have it here. I save the money in the budget, and we go out and I buy DVDs and televisions and stereos and all kinds of cool stuff that you really want for Christmas. Everybody brings a present and we do that fun gift exchange, that throughout the night we draw names out of a hat to see who gets what present, and they look forward to that, they start talking about that. And you can go to Walmart and get a television for a couple of hundred bucks. You know it's something that they might not have been able to afford. And so I set aside $1,000 for those type things and we go shopping and buy it and we display it out in the activities room so they can see the gifts and get excited about the party.

A few small and medium homes also recognize DCWs on their birthdays. In one small home, workers receive $50. The owner of a medium home who gives $50 to $100, depending on hours worked, said: "They [staff] all tell me no one ever recognized their birthday on their job before. I think it is the little personal things [that matter]." The director of a large home gives all DCWs a cake on their birthday, which they select and take home to share with their families. In addition, she has a "birthday drawing" each month where DCWs receive "an Applebee's gift certificate if it was their birthday and their name was drawn." This director believes that her rewards, though "not much," do "add up." Her strategy is an example of how administrators cobble together small efforts with the hope of overall providing meaningful recognition.

Performance Incentives

Some homes, mostly medium and large, offer rewards aimed more at encouraging than rewarding good work. Typically these rewards have to do with showing up regularly and on time. In one home, DCWs who are 100 percent on time and present as scheduled for two consecutive pay periods receive a bonus of 10 percent of their earnings for the two previous pay periods. In one large home, DCWs receive a $10 gift certificate for each month they have perfect, on-time attendance. In another, staff members with perfect attendance are eligible for a monthly drawing of $100. At the end of the year, the prize is increased to $1,200, and each person's name is placed "in a pot" one or more times, according to the number of months that she or he achieved perfect attendance.

A few homes reward employee safety. One large home has monthly drawings for $100 if no on-the-job injuries have occurred. In another, workers play "safety poker" with a jackpot that is based on the numbers of days with no work-related injuries.

Our findings indicate that such performance bonuses are effective and important to staff. A DCW in a medium home where the practice was discontinued said, "She used to have an incentive program to make the employees come to work because there would be so many employees that would call in at least once or twice a week or some of them a couple of times a month so she started this incentive program if you're not late and you come to work every day you get a bonus. If you're full-time you get a $50 bonus, if you're part-time you get $25, and that worked fine. I mean a lot of employees were coming in on time and they were staying but we had to have 32 residents or more before she could do that and we kept dropping down and so the incentive program kind of faded out." A DCW in a large home indicated that even small rewards would be meaningful: "Or say if you are on time you get a bonus of $10 in your check, or if you are early, you get your check the day before pay day, you get a star or a pin on your shirt, even a little card or little inspiration saying keep up the good spirit, it would show something. It would make you feel that management really does care."

The owner of a medium home has a unique way of rewarding DCWs for increasing their housekeeping efforts: "To get people to do more, like picking up trash in the hallways or organizing someone's closet, hanging up people's clothes, put away old towels, we'll hide envelopes with money or little food vouchers to Chick-Fil-A around the building. You have to look underneath the curtains in the living room." DCWs in this home reacted positively to this strategy.

A few of the larger homes give bonuses for recruiting residents or staff, and a number reward staff, in amounts ranging from $25 to $100, when 100 percent occupancy is achieved. One director of a large corporate home believes these bonuses provide "an incentive to give good care, incentive to keep our residents healthy and happy." These rewards generally are funded by the corporation. As one director said, "When we are full our owners come down and they hand $100 bills to every employee."

Appreciation Events

The majority of homes (58%) hold parties or other group events to recognize staff. These include pizza parties, potluck dinners, and cookouts at the facility, as well as meals at restaurants. A few facilities hold week- or even month-long appreciation events. The director of a medium home described her facility's annual employee appreciation week: "In that week we put everybody's name in a pot and I accumulate nice little gifts and prizes. We do drawings and it ends up that every employee gets something. Each shift designates a day and a time and a restaurant and they are taken out for a lunch for appreciation of them. Each day there is a little treat of some sort along with the drawings. Then on Saturday, to end the week, we have a barbeque for all of the employees to attend. We try."

The primary reasons given by administrators for not having group events are lack of time or interest on the part of staff and the difficulty of getting staff together at any one time because, as one said, "This place is open 24-7 and they're busy." The way one administrator solved the problem was to hire PRN staff to cover during the event. An employee at a large home without such events said: "When I worked at the nursing home, they have Nurse's Day and would have ice cream and make you feel important. We don't do that here."

Verbal Acclaim

Three homes have no formal recognition program. The primary reason given for this lack is inadequate resources. As the owner of one home said, "No, I don't have no money to give no bonus." All three homes serve low-income residents. What these three homes do offer is verbal acclaim. The owner of one said, "I always take the time to thank them for what they are doing." Most administrators emphasize the value of ongoing verbal praise. Many offer this praise in public, such as in staff or family meetings. One director described his strategy: "I'm a one-minute manager mind-set: I try to catch people doing something right. So whether it's answering the telephone, whether its interacting with the resident, if a family member comes and tells me that a staff person did something right, I go to them right away and give them the feedback and the praise in front of their peers and in front of other residents or family members." Another said, "I usually just sing with praises, let everybody hear it." A DCW in this home reported that she would not leave "unless somebody paid her double because it is nice here."

Close to a third (27%) of DCWs named verbal praise as the type of recognition they most value from management. This choice, though, is mentioned almost twice as often by workers in small homes (44%) compared with those in medium (24%) and large (22%) homes. Possibly this difference relates to the greater interaction possibilities between administrators and DCWs in the small homes or simply is a realistic appraisal of facility resources. Qualitative data provide further evidence of the value of verbal appreciation, whether the sole form of recognition or not. A worker in a large home with multiple reward efforts said, "If someone tells you did a good job, that is worth $100. That is what is important to me." A DCW in a medium home voiced a similar value: "Basically she is always telling us she is proud of her staff. I don't think you can be recognized any more than the person telling you that you are a good worker."

Material Rewards

Although verbal praise clearly is valued by DCWs, our findings indicate that the majority of staff also desire material reward. Survey data show that 24 percent of DCWs prefer to be rewarded with cash bonuses; 22 percent want a salary increase. Combining these responses with those that indicate preferences for paid time off and gift certificates shows that over half (54%) of DCWs favor material compensation. Given the generally low wages DCWs receive and the tenuous economic situation of many, the choice of monetary rewards is not surprising. Qualitative data also point out that even small amounts are valued. One older DCW who regularly experiences financial difficulty because of health problems said, "If it is just a $10 certificate to Ingles, that would buy a gallon of milk and a loaf of bread."

The Importance of Recognition

A few workers told us they needed no recognition for this work. One said, "I come in here and deal with the residents and if I get recognized, if I don't, fine." Overall, though, our findings show that demonstrating to workers they are valued is essential. Although across-the-board bonuses of various types are clearly important to workers, our data also indicate that most DCWs want to be recognized for their individual efforts, whether verbal or monetary. One DCW in a home that offers Christmas bonuses, appreciation events, and sporadic awards for effort still feels unrecognized: "Any kind of recognition would be better than nothing. We don't get anything here." Another worker emphasized the importance of multiple, ongoing demonstrations of appreciation: "holidays, Mother's Day, for example. I know these ladies [residents] all out here are mothers. They get recognized with a flower, but the employees are mothers also. I think they should be recognized. Why can't they have a flower or something showing the fact that, hey, you are recognized too as a parent? That is just an example, little stuff like that, stuff to make you feel good, make you want to come to work, instead of just, it is like you get talked to when you do something wrong. Just recognize both of it, you know, instead of just the bad. Recognize the good too, and let them know you are highly appreciated. And I know sometimes they say, 'You know I sure appreciate what you do.' Well, show me, tell me all the time."

What comes through loud and clear in this last quote and throughout our findings is the importance of *affirmation*. DCWs want and need regular affirmation for their contribution to resident care and to overall facility operation. If structured appropriately, facility reward programs contribute to this affirmation. Our findings also indicate that no one type of recognition works for all workers or forever. Administrators must strive constantly to develop recognition strategies that have meaning for all workers.

Discussion

In the preceding sections we laid out the reward systems found in the 45 facilities we studied, including salaries, advancement opportunities, benefits, and other reward programs. We also explained how a variety of individual-, facility-, and community-level factors influence whether and how the different components of these systems are developed and maintained, and we explored the meaning of reward systems for DCWs and ultimately their significance for job satisfaction and retention. Figure 11.1 depicts these processes, which have implications for frontline workers in AL and other LTC settings across the United States.

Individual factors that influence reward systems include DCWs' job performance and attitudes, as well as the number of hours they work and their LTC

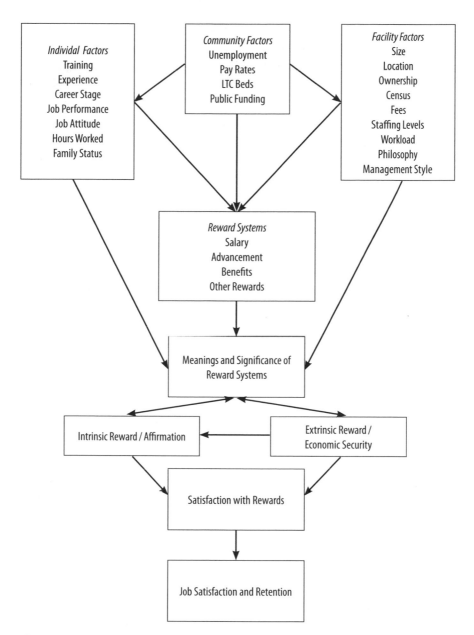

Figure 11.1. The Development, Maintenance, and Meaning of Facility Reward Systems

employment history and training. Other individual factors, such as a DCW's family status or career, also contribute to reward meaning.

Facility factors affecting reward systems include capacity, census, fees, ownership, geographic location, and administrators' philosophy and management styles. Those that affect a facility's "bottom line" have the greatest influence. Other facility factors, such as staffing levels and workload, have direct bearing on the meaning of rewards.

Community factors, including local wage structures, unemployment rates, public LTC funding, and number of LTC beds, affect reward systems directly and indirectly, through individual and facility factors. Community factors also have a direct and indirect effect (through rewards systems) on the meaning and significance of rewards.

As illustrated in Figure 11.1, our findings indicate that the meaning and significance of reward systems is twofold, representing intrinsic and extrinsic components. Intrinsic reward is derived principally from *affirmation*. Facility rewards, whether tangible or intangible, have meaning for DCWs when they demonstrate that management appreciates their contribution to the care of residents and to the overall running of the facility. Thus they operate in a way that is similar to DCWs' relationships with residents in that they affirm the moral and professional worth of DCWs (see Chapter 7, this volume). Higher salaries, performance bonuses, and verbal acclaim all can provide affirmation.

Extrinsic reward comes mainly from the contribution that reward systems make to a worker's economic security. Having a regular paycheck, albeit a small one; having access to health insurance and paid leave during illness; and receiving a holiday bonus all play a part in overall economic security. The degree of extrinsic reward experienced and economic security achieved depends on the level of the material reward as well as on a DCW's personal situation and the economy of the locale.

Conclusion

The findings presented here clearly indicate that the large majority of workers are not satisfied with their extrinsic rewards—not with their wages nor with their opportunities for pay increases, position advances, or health care. This lack of extrinsic reward makes for a "hard life." Our findings also indicate that these Georgia AL workers are worse off than DCWs nationwide in their level of extrinsic reward. Their median hourly wage is $8.00, lower than the

$8.61 reported for all U.S. AL workers in 2003 (National Center for Assisted Living, 2004) and the $9.51 of nursing home DCWs in 2005 (Paraprofessional Healthcare Institute, 2006).

Our data also show that almost no DCWs are able to achieve true career advancement in AL, and only a minority are able to make small position increments. Although our data suggest that some workers do not want increased responsibility or supervisory roles, the majority would welcome some type of advancement, accompanied by a salary increase.

Our sample of Georgia DCWs also has lower rates of health insurance coverage, 58 percent compared with the 75 percent reported for nursing home workers (Lipson & Regan, 2004). In addition to the fact that less than two-thirds (62%) of facilities offer medical insurance, our data show that, similar to AL in other states (Michigan Assisted Living Association, 2001), high insurance co-pays make the insurance unaffordable for the majority of workers in the facilities where coverage is an option.

We found that although a few facilities pay relatively high hourly rates and utilize a consistent means of rate increases, the almost universal strategy is to adjust DCW wages to local AL markets. Facilities have additional strategies aimed at minimizing the effect of reward systems on the all-important bottom line, including limiting workers' hours to reduce overtime payments and avoid providing benefits and curtailing salary increases. DCWs express considerable frustration when they fail to receive raises, particularly when promised and, in their view, warranted, and with their lack of medical coverage. In addition, almost half of DCWs want to work extra hours, one possibility for increasing their low wages. Another indicator that facilities do not provide sufficient extrinsic reward is found in the supplemental jobs held by one-fourth of our sample. Overall the findings presented here indicate that life is "hard" for Georgia AL workers, the majority of whom are unmarried (61%), have children living at home (54%), and provide some material support to others who live either in or outside their homes (81%).

The tenuous economic situation of the majority of DCWs accounts in part for their appreciation of the smaller and less steady material rewards they receive through the various facility recognition programs. Some facilities use these programs in lieu of regular, or any, pay raises. Obviously an outlay of $25 or $100 per month to recognize one or two employees is less taxing to the bottom line than even a minimal hourly wage increase. Such extrinsic rewards generally are valued by DCWs. A performance bonus of $10 will buy a gallon of milk and a loaf of bread, but such awards on the whole contribute little to workers' overall economic security.

As Figure 11.1 indicates, extrinsic rewards are also intrinsically rewarding. Whether DCWs receive a salary increase, a Christmas bonus, or a gift certificate for outstanding work, the material recognition also provides affirmation. It lets them know administrators "care" and appreciate their efforts.

DCWs on the whole, though, believe they deserve more than their current reward systems offer. The majority of administrators share this viewpoint. Our data indicate that some administrators provide the best rewards they can for their workers. Some facilities clearly are experiencing economic insecurity too, mostly the smaller ones and those operating under capacity and depending on fees from low-income residents and Medicaid reimbursement. No doubt all facilities have multiple competing needs for limited resources, but since many administrators admit that they cannot "do it without" DCWs, they need to put them higher up on their list of priorities. After all, if residents are their number one priority, then those who take care of them should be at least number two. But if the "economic imperative" put forth by Stone (Chapter 1 of this volume) is not enough, the "moral imperative" should be. These workers deserve to be treated better, and increasing their rewards, both intrinsic and extrinsic, would be a good way to start.

REFERENCES

Close, L., Estes, C. L., Linkins, K. W., & Binney, E. A. 1994. Political economy perspective on frontline workers in long-term care. *Generations* 18 (3), 23–28.
Foner, N. 1994. *The caregiving dilemma*. Berkeley: University of California Press.
Grieshaber, L., Parker, P., & Deering, J. 1995. Job satisfaction of nursing assistants in long-term care. *Health Care Supervisor* 13 (4), 18–28.
Harris-Kojetin, L., Lipson, D., Fielding, J., Kiefer, K., & Stone, R. 2004. *Recent findings on frontline long-term care workers: A research synthesis, 1999–2003*. Washington, DC: American Association of Homes and Services for the Aged, Institute for the Future of Aging Services.
Helmer, F., Olson, S., & Heim, R. 1993. Strategies for nurse aide job satisfaction. *Journal of Long Term Care Administration* 21, 10–14.
Institute for the Future of Aging Services. 2007. *The long-term care workforce: Can the crisis be fixed?* Report prepared for the National Commission for Quality Long-Term Care. Washington, DC: IFAS.
Lipson, D., & Regan, C. 2004. *Health insurance coverage for direct care workers: Riding out the storm* (Issue Brief no. 3). Washington, DC: Better Jobs Better Care National Program Office.

Michigan Assisted Living Association. 2001. *Mental health provider 2001 wage and benefit survey.* Lansing, MI.

National Center for Assisted Living. 2004. *Facts and trends: Assisted living sourcebook.* Washington, DC.

National Clearinghouse on the Direct Care Workforce. 2006. *Who are direct-care workers?* New York: Paraprofessional Healthcare Institute.

Paraprofessional Healthcare Institute. 2006. *Who are direct care workers?* Fact Sheet, November 2006, of the PHI National Clearinghouse on the Direct Care Workforce. Retrieved from www.directcareclearinghouse.org.

Redfoot, D. L., & Houser, A. N. 2005. "We shall travel on": Quality of care, economic development, and the international migration of long-term care workers. Washington, DC: AARP Public Policy Institute.

Strauss, A., & Corbin, J. 1998. *The basics of qualitative research: Grounded theory procedures and techniques.* Thousand Oaks, CA: Sage Publications.

Informing Policy and Practice

Mary M. Ball, Ph.D.
Molly M. Perkins, Ph.D.
Carole Hollingsworth, M.A.
Candace L. Kemp, Ph.D.

In the first chapter of this book, Robyn Stone makes a strong case for a "more long-term, systemic approach to developing and sustaining a qualified and committed direct care workforce." The need to improve the workforce is driven by three key issues: quality of care, economic development, and moral concerns for the status of workers. In Chapter 2, Larry Polivka lays out the need to regulate the assisted (AL) environment in ways that enhance the quality of care and life of residents and make it affordable to a more diverse group of elders. These two experts on long-term care (LTC) make evident the sometimes contradictory goals involved in caring for frail elders. Although we leave many questions unanswered, we hope in this volume we make a credible contribution toward understanding these multifaceted issues. In Chapters 4 through 11 we address key topics regarding the AL workforce. In each we discuss implications for policy and practice in light of our own findings and those of other researchers. In this concluding chapter, we highlight our principal findings and offer recommendations for maximizing the satisfaction and retention of direct care workers (DCWs) in AL while acknowledging the difficulty of quick fixes. Many of our findings will be relevant for the diverse settings found throughout the AL industry, as well as for other LTC setting that rely on frontline workers. In each chapter we make explicit the parallels between the experiences of Georgia DCWs and those who work throughout LTC.

Key Themes of Our Research

Becoming a Caregiver

As seen in Chapter 4, the complexity of addressing job satisfaction and retention problems in AL becomes apparent with individuals' initial decisions to become frontline workers. Decision making regarding this choice is guided by a combination of moral, material, and professional motives, which are influenced by multiple, multilevel "push" and "pull" factors (see Reed, Cook, Sullivan, & Burridge, 2003). The majority of DCWs act on their strong value for altruism, particularly regarding elders, and many have cared for elderly family members. Many also are pulled to LTC by family members who are themselves caregivers. Most also are pushed to care work by their need for a job to support themselves and their families and by a lack of human capital (e.g., education and training) that would qualify them for more skilled and higher-paying jobs. The forces pulling and pushing these Georgia workers to their jobs are similar to those experienced by other frontline workers in AL as well as in nursing home and home care settings.

The LTC environment, particularly AL, offers the promise of a work setting in which DCWs can realize their values for elder care and receive a paycheck to help meet their basic needs, even with limited skills. A minority of individuals also are drawn to an environment where they can gain relevant experience for future, higher-level care jobs. We find that the extent to which DCWs' motives for pursuing employment in a given facility match with the reality of their job experiences has significant bearing on job satisfaction and retention.

Caring for Residents

The findings presented throughout this book definitively show that, for the majority of DCWs, how they relate to and care for residents is central to job satisfaction and contributes to job commitment and retention in each facility, in AL, and in the field of LTC as a whole. As seen in Chapter 7, DCWs attribute three key intersecting dimensions of meaning to their relationships with residents and care work: (1) the quality of the relationship and interactions with residents; (2) the professional affirmation derived from providing care; and (3) the moral affirmation of their caregiving values. Satisfying social relations and high levels of professional and moral affirmation typically result in higher overall job satisfaction and retention.

Throughout the book, note is made of the individual-, facility-, and community-level factors that have bearing on how DCWs relate to and care for residents. Some of the more important considerations include the racial and cultural commonality of residents and staff; the attitudes and personality of staff and residents; DCWs' experience and training; co-worker solidarity and teamwork; facility size and design; resident impairment and staffing levels; policies regarding resident-staff relationships; and practices for hiring and training DCWs.

Universal Workers

Findings presented in Chapter 5 confirm the universal nature of the DCW job, regardless of position, across a range of AL settings and have relevance for frontline workers in the multiple manifestations of AL found throughout the United States. The primary complaint from workers regarding this component of the job relates to the effect that multiple task performance has on their ability to "care" for residents. The required handling of too many tasks, including those that do not involve interacting with residents, leaves them with limited time to spend with residents, a primary value of the job. For some DCWs, tasks ancillary to hands-on care do not reinforce their professional caregiver identity and thus are not in their view an appropriate component of the DCW job. The universal role then sometimes impedes the realization of the three key dimensions of meaning derived from caring for and relating to residents. However, a more universal job can foster contact between DCWs and more independent residents who require no hands-on care.

This chapter and others point out that workload, rather than task configuration, has the greater potential to influence job satisfaction. As Chapter 4 indicates, the expectation for less and lighter care loads pulls DCWs to AL. The multivariate analyses reported on in Chapter 8 reveal that workers who feel more pressed to complete their work are less satisfied. Workload levels also influence co-worker relationships and the significance of teamwork in caring for residents. The key factors affecting workload are a facility's resident profile and staffing ratios. Our findings regarding the effect of workload on job satisfaction have bearing on the entire LTC sector.

Being a universal worker also means having universal skills. Although some of the tasks require little skill, others, such as medication management, transferring residents, and providing nursing-type care, call for greater competence. Findings in Chapter 10 show that some DCWs feel they lack the requisite training and skills to care for residents in a way that is morally and professionally affirming and that does not create undue psychological and physical stress. The experiences of these workers likely parallel those in assisted living facilities (ALFs) throughout the United States that house residents with increasing functional impairment. Chapter 10 also points out that administrators' criteria for hiring DCWs tend to emphasize "heart" (that is, moral motivation) over LTC skills and credentials. Such practices, while tapping key motives of many workers, help to perpetuate the low status of all frontline workers.

Affirmation

Multiple findings establish the role of affirmation in job satisfaction. DCWs want to feel appreciated for the work they do and want to believe that their contribution matters—to the residents and their families, to facility owners and administrators, and to society. Without doubt, the moral and professional affirmation that comes from residents is of utmost importance, but other sources and forms of affirmation have the potential to affect satisfaction. Multivariate analyses demonstrate that DCWs who feel valued by management are more satisfied. Qualitative analysis also reveals the importance of administrators and co-workers showing their appreciation for workers' efforts in both tangible and intangible ways.

Material Rewards

We present evidence in Chapter 11 that the level of material reward received by DCWs in Georgia ALFs is comparable to that of other DCWs in other LTC settings in other states. On the whole, wages are low, health insurance is either not offered or unaffordable, and not all DCWs have access to paid time off from the job.

Material rewards influence job satisfaction and retention primarily through their capacity to provide affirmation and economic security. DCWs do not feel affirmed when their pay is low, when they are paid less than they believe they deserve, and when they lack opportunities for pay increases—the situation of most workers. Clearly, such conditions do not afford economic security. Like DCWs nationwide, most of these workers are poor, support children and other relatives, and subsist from one paycheck to the next. Rural workers and those in small facilities are paid less and have less access to health benefits compared with workers in urban areas and may represent an especially vulnerable segment of the low-wage AL workforce.

Although multivariate analyses show no significant relationship between pay rates and overall job satisfaction, our qualitative data show that the lack of statistical association between pay and overall satisfaction may relate to DCWs' realistic appraisal of the limits on opportunities for material rewards. Although some DCWs have no aspiration to "move up" in their jobs, many are dissatisfied with their opportunities for advancement and believe that their jobs are "dead end."

Our findings also demonstrate clearly that facility administrators face considerable challenge in balancing the economic needs of DCWs with competing facility demands. Of primary concern for most is keeping resident fees affordable while maintaining good-quality care in a safe, comfortable, and attractive physical environment, all key factors in holding on to and attracting residents. Industry competition is fierce, more so in some areas than others. Local economic indicators, as well as the number of LTC consumers and providers, influence the manner in which facilities reward their workers.

Race and Culture

A key theme throughout this book is the effect of race and, to a lesser degree, culture on DCWs' work experience and their job satisfaction. The majority of ALFs in Georgia are racially diverse, similar to ALFs nationwide. This diversity stems largely from the coexistence of nonwhite DCWs and white residents. Statistical analyses presented in Chapter 8 make clear that racism from residents toward DCWs has a significant negative impact on job satisfaction. Qualitative analysis also confirms the existence of racist behavior of white residents directed toward nonwhite DCWs. Although data indicate that some DCWs rationalize such behavior and not all white residents behave in a racist way, racism on the part of residents creates problems in the majority of ALFs.

Racism, though, is not restricted to resident-staff relationships. We find evidence of racism on the part of white administrators and DCWs directed at nonwhite DCWs, of nonwhite administrators and DCWs directed at white DCWs, and of native-born blacks directed at non-native-born blacks. Such differences influence the culture of a home, and when they cause discord, they influence job satisfaction. Conflicts between co-workers also interfere with DCWs' ability to care for residents and thus to realize moral and professional affirmation.

The Connection between Job Satisfaction and Retention

Although on average DCWs in this study were fairly satisfied with their jobs and expressed relatively low levels of intent to leave, 42 percent did leave within the year following their interview. This finding is consistent with national trends showing a high level of turnover across LTC settings. Multilevel analyses presented in Chapter 9 show that facility-level factors explain little, if any, variation in DCW turnover, which suggests that decision making regarding turnover is highly individualized and may be influenced by additional individual-level factors not included in the present analysis. Our analysis does offer insight into macro-level influences on turnover in that the county unemployment rate has an important influence on employee tenure, which emerges as the most important determinant of the decision to leave. Additionally, a DCW's intent to leave the job has a significant direct effect on turnover.

Other factors indirectly influence turnover through their effect on intent to leave. Facility location, another indicator of local economic conditions, is one. The finding that DCWs who reside in rural areas are less likely to say they will leave further implicates the role of opportunity in turnover decisions. Although our analyses reveal little direct association between job satisfaction and turnover, they do show a significant influence of satisfaction on intent to leave, indicating a strong indirect effect. Obviously, job satisfaction is important in and of itself, but we also believe it plays a key role in retention.

Our Model for Job Satisfaction and Retention

Figure 12.1 encapsulates what we believe to be the key elements and outcomes of the process of maximizing the satisfaction and retention of DCWs. We have made clear throughout this book the complexity of this process and have laid out the multiple, multilevel factors that influence DCWs' motives for entering the field of caregiving and the rewards they receive from their jobs. Both motives and rewards have moral, material, and professional meanings that affect DCWs' job satisfaction and retention. These outcomes in turn have bearing on Stone's broader outcomes for care recipients, DCWs, and communities: quality of care; economic development; and DCWs' position in the labor market and in society at large. We believe that our model captures the situation of frontline workers throughout the LTC spectrum.

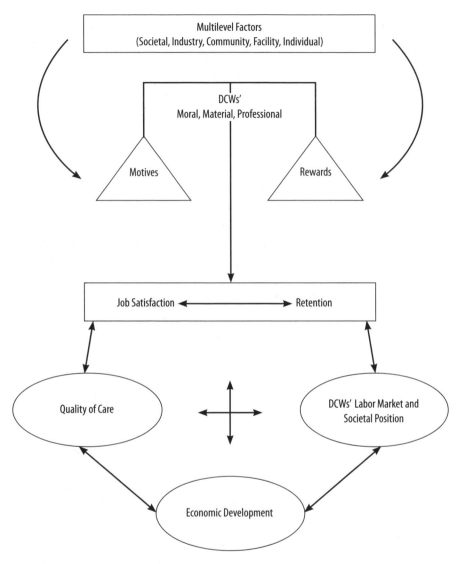

Figure 12.1. Elements and Outcomes of Direct Care Workers' Satisfaction and Retention in Assisted Living

Recommendations for Policy and Practice

The recommendations below are organized around four key facility work-force concerns: (1) recruitment; (2) hiring and training; (3) job design; and (4) reward systems. In making these recommendations, we are guided by DCWs' need for moral, material, and professional affirmation. They incorporate successful strategies used by administrators in our study, as well as some we developed ourselves, using our own findings as well as those of other researchers. In particular we draw on the body of work generated by the Better Jobs Better Care program (Yallowitz & Hofland, 2008), a broad initiative aimed at improving the satisfaction and retention of high-quality DCWs in nursing homes and community-based LTC settings.

All our recommendations are grounded in the perceptions of DCWs. They are directed primarily at facility administrators and owners and point toward change at the facility level. Our findings without doubt have implications for policy and practice recommendations directed at residents, DCWs, the state of Georgia, and beyond, but here we focus on AL providers. We are confident that these recommendations can be adapted to the diverse AL industry found in the United States.

Many of our suggestions may appear obvious. Some are guiding principles, rather than specific directions. Additional recommendations and ideas for policy and practice can be found at the end of each chapter. Our hope is that both our research and our conclusions inspire ideas for additional strategies. Each AL setting both here in Georgia and throughout the United States is different, and administrators everywhere must tailor their satisfaction and retention strategies to their unique workers and environments. Our findings in AL lend support to those of Pillemer and colleagues (2008), who propose that nursing homes have *intervention teams* composed of administrative and direct care staff and charged with *customizing* retention strategies to suit a facility's particular needs and resources.

Recruitment

Although our findings indicate that facilities exert little effort in recruitment because DCWs largely rely on contacts through their social networks to find employment, we do have some suggestions for targeting workers with potential for satisfaction and retention and for expanding the would-be pool of DCWs.

- Continue to draw from families and friends of current high-quality workers. This strategy has proved successful among most of the sample ALFs.
- Reach out to local technical schools, colleges, and even high schools. In addition to expanding the worker pool, this strategy allows facilities to target individuals with professional aspirations. Provider associations can visit these venues to educate students about the true nature of direct care work, as well as use this opportunity to recruit prospective staff into the field. Long-term care ombudsman programs also should assume the role of developing and educating new workforce resources as one of their advocacy roles.
- Target places of worship, senior centers, and other community organizations as potential sources of new workers. These places may attract older persons, who are a largely untapped but promising resource. Our findings indicate that facility administrators value older workers and that older workers value direct care work. Other research (Hwalek, Straub, & Kosniewski, 2008) lends support to this idea.
- Make use of the Internet. This strategy is a fruitful avenue for recruiting people who are relocating. Web pages are a convenient source of information about facility characteristics, the nature of the DCW job, and job vacancies.

Hiring and Training

The hiring process is instrumental in screening potential employees to find DCWs who are most likely to be satisfied and stay. Hiring is linked to training through the belief administrators have in their own ability to train workers as well as through the skill level a worker brings to the job. Both the hiring and training processes are fundamental to DCWs' ability to achieve moral and professional affirmation. They also can affect material affirmation, such as when DCWs receive training to advance to higher-paid positions.

- Consider applicants' personal qualities. Using "heart" as a key criterion for hiring makes sense given the key role of DCWs' relationships with residents in their job satisfaction and retention. Based on our findings, some practical strategies that may be used to determine "heart" during the interview process include observing how applicants interact with residents and asking about family relationships and past caregiving experiences. Compassion, though, should not be administrators' sole criterion unless they are prepared to provide DCWs with adequate training to do their jobs.

- Take into account experience and training, especially with the increasing frailty level of residents in most AL settings. Requiring CNA training likely may not be a productive or realistic strategy for all DCWs, particularly in states like Georgia with only one AL licensing category, but this tactic may be fruitful for some positions and in some facilities.
- Use the hiring process to tell applicants about the nature of direct care work in general and in the specific facility. Administrators can provide this information during the interview; they also can allow applicants to speak with and observe DCWs at work, which provides the additional advantage of observing how applicants might "fit in" with co-workers.
- Use the interview to ask applicants about their own goals and preferences for care work and the particular job. This type of questioning helps administrators, when they have options, to match the individual to the most appropriate shift and position.
- Ask DCWs at hiring and at regular intervals about their perceptions of needed training; to the degree possible, tailor training to specific needs, depending on DCWs' skills and abilities and the job configuration. We learned that training must be relevant to be meaningful and effective. DCWs with adequate training tend to experience less job-related stress and be more satisfied.
- Vary the type of training to avoid boredom and reach DCWs with different learning styles. One-on-one training and mentoring relationships with experienced workers can help DCWs apply knowledge imparted through classroom or DVD/video–type instruction.
- Enlist the help of local health care providers in staff training. Many welcome the opportunity to improve patient care, and DCWs indicate the need for greater knowledge regarding residents' health conditions and the associated signs and symptoms.
- Encourage and support DCW participation in educational programs outside the facility (e.g., conferences, workshops). This strategy will foster professionalism among DCWs and allow contact with their counterparts in other settings.

- Provide DCWs with information about residents' histories, needs, and preferences to facilitate caregiving and relationship development, particularly for residents unable to communicate this information themselves.

- Provide information to DCWs about death and the dying process, as well as counseling for DCWs who grieve the loss of residents. Local hospice organizations are a good resource.

- Provide training in developing and negotiating workplace relationships, including those between DCWs and residents and between DCWs and co-workers, direct supervisors, and administrators. These training efforts should include residents and their families as well as administrative and other types of staff. Some staff in supervisory positions, both DCWs and management personnel, have had little or no leadership training. Other research suggests that supervisor training can lead to increased DCW retention in nursing homes (Morgan & Konrad, 2008).

- Make improving the cultural competence of all employees and residents and their families an integral part of relationship training. This training should be ongoing and incorporate all facets of facility life. Facility activity programs, for example, can play a role in this process. One ALF in our sample with a large number of non-native-born DCWs held an "international day," during which staff had an opportunity to teach residents about their own countries and cultural backgrounds. The dinner served that day reflected DCWs' native food.

Job Design

Both job configuration and workload have direct bearing on moral and professional affirmation. These job design components also affect how DCWs view the material rewards of their job.

- Attempt to match task configuration to DCWs' preferences and abilities and avoid the one-size-fits-all approach. This task allocation strategy will require administrators to communicate with DCWs on a regular basis and to negotiate co-worker conflicts if they feel task distribution is unfair.

- Give DCWs leeway in how they carry out their tasks. Our findings show that DCWs value even small amounts of autonomy. Each has a particular work style, and catering to residents' individual preferences is important for their moral and professional affirmation.

- Keep DCWs' workload to a level that allows them a reasonable amount of time to complete assigned care tasks and to develop and maintain relationships with residents. Fair distribution of tasks across shifts helps alleviate stress for some workers and lessens co-worker conflicts. Pay special attention to workers assigned to dementia care units, where workloads tend to be the heaviest.
- Encourage and facilitate teamwork among DCWs. Sharing tasks with co-workers can reduce stress, particularly for heavy-care residents and those who resist care efforts.
- Expand the direct supervisor role to include mentoring, teaching, and soliciting input from DCWs. This strategy must operate in tandem with increased supervisor training.
- To improve resident care and ensure staff safety, provide DCWs with the necessary equipment to carry out their jobs.

Reward Systems

Reward systems have both intrinsic and extrinsic meaning for job satisfaction and retention. Thus both intrinsic and extrinsic rewards are important. Overall DCWs want and need better pay. They also need increased access to health care. These material rewards may be the most difficult to provide, but they hold the greatest promise for improving the economic situation of DCWs. While not retreating from the larger goal, below we offer suggestions for smaller and more short-term rewards, which our findings show that staff also value.

- Express appreciation to DCWs on a regular basis. Tell them daily, weekly, privately, publicly, verbally, and materially how much they are valued. DCWs want and deserve recognition for the vital job they do. Some feel administrators do not appreciate their merit.
- Use a range of strategies to reward DCWs as a means of appealing to a larger group and providing rewards that all workers will value.
- Find ways to recognize individual efforts in addition to across-the-board rewards.
- Involve residents in recognition programs for DCWs, given the importance of residents to DCWs.
- Provide DCWs with a dependable number of weekly work hours; al-

low a full, 40-hour workweek for DCWs who desire the maximum number of hours. Extra hours and a reliable salary often are necessary to meet DCWs' needs.

- Provide resources when possible for DCWs to improve their education and training. Be sure that DCWs are aware of current opportunities for tuition reimbursement and other benefits and be willing to adjust schedules to meet the needs of those who attend school.
- Find ways to materially reward DCWs who improve their knowledge and skills.
- Make every effort to provide regular salary increases, especially if raises have been promised. DCWs value this reward above all others. Although dissatisfaction with advancement opportunity is widespread, moving to a higher position is valued more for money than status.
- Provide some opportunity for paid time off. Although this group of low-wage workers generally are unaccustomed to "taking vacations," everyone needs at least occasional respite from job-related stress, and DCWs need to be paid when they must be away from work because of illness or when a family member needs their attention.
- Develop specialist positions, similar to the medication tech position, in other areas, such as dementia care and activities. This would require increased training and should come with a salary increase.
- Work toward improving the professional status of DCWs. As low-wage workers, DCWs reflect a marginalized group. Professionalizing the job in even small ways may improve society's perceptions of these critical workers.

A Final Word

The culture of each AL community depends to a large degree on the administrator. Administrators influence who lives and work there, when they come, and how long stay. Their personalities and administrative style infuse the social environment. One could say they "set the tone" of a facility. One also could say that they set the stage for job satisfaction and retention of frontline workers. In their key role, administrators should be visible and available to these workers, and they should listen with respect to what they think and how they feel. This should be a guiding principle for all people who lead.

Confronting the Future

Developing and maintaining a good-quality direct care workforce is a tough challenge and will only grow more difficult in the future. No one needs to be reminded of the worsening fiscal conditions currently affecting the U.S. and world economy as the first decade of the twenty-first century ends. Few communities have escaped the effects of these economic downturns, which have obvious impact on LTC facilities and their residents and employees. The DCWs and the facilities who participated in our study are likely a little worse off as we write this book than they were a few years ago when we first met them. But, as Stone powerfully advocates, we cannot afford to abandon the challenge. As conditions worsen, the need for workforce improvement will only increase. Significant future improvement for frontline workers throughout LTC will depend on structural change beyond the facility level.

REFERENCES

Hwalek, M., Straub, V., & Kosniewski, K. 2008. Older workers: An opportunity to expand the long-term care/direct care labor force. *The Gerontologist* 48 (Special Issue 1), 90–103.

Morgan, J. C., & Konrad, T. 2008. A mixed-method evaluation of a workforce development intervention for nursing assistants in nursing homes: The Case of WIN A STEP UP. *The Gerontologist* 48 (Special Issue 1), 71–79.

Pillemer, K., Meador, R., Henderson, C., Robison, J., Hegeman, C., Graham, E., et al. 2008. A facility specialist model for improving retention of nursing home staff: Results from a randomized, controlled study. *The Gerontologist* 48 (Special Issue 1), 80–89.

Reed, J., Cook, G., Sullivan, A., & Burridge, C. 2003. Making a move: Care-home residents' experiences of relocation. *Ageing and Society* 23, 225–41.

Yallowitz, Y., & Hofland, B. 2008. Better jobs better care: A foundation initiative focusing on direct care workers. *The Gerontologist* 48 (Special Issue 1), 17–25.

INDEX

activities, 102, 105, 106, 107, 153, 296. *See also* task configuration

activities of daily living (ADLs): bathing, 13, 95, 106, 107, 117, 233; and dementia care units, 107; dressing, 13, 95, 106, 107, 117; eating, 13, 101, 113, 114, 117, 242; and job satisfaction, 115; and resident functional status, 107, 117; and shift, 106–7; toileting, 13, 32, 95, 113; and workload, 11, 107, 113, 115. *See also* task configuration

administrator: attitudes toward staff, 127; backgrounds of, 136; boundaries with staff, 139–40; and DCW training and education, 238–43, 244; definition of, 52, 103; direct supervision by, 134; disciplining of staff by, 129; educational level of, 136; and hiring process, 138, 226–36, 237–38, 247; as mirroring staff backgrounds, 135; and money-saving strategies, 137; personal characteristics of, 62, 64, 162; and race of staff, 130–31; and racial issues, 168–69, 288; relationships with staff, 126, 135; and staff-resident relationships, 154; and staff shifts, 132; support of staff by, 137–38, 142, 155; turnover of, 128, 139, 143n1, 216n4, 235, 250; unequal treatment of staff by, 128. *See also* director; executive director; reward systems

advancement, 265; and job satisfaction, 3, 4, 265; lack of opportunities for, 21, 32, 265, 281, 288; and personal traits, 261; recommendations for, 296; and work assignments, 117, 260

affirmation: from administrator and co-workers, 142; from family members, 142; and hands-on care, 119; and identity, 119, 142, 164; and job satisfaction, 287; moral, 119, 151, 164–65, 285–86; professional, 119, 151, 163–64, 285–86; and recommendations,

291; from residents, 142, 151, 162–65; and rewards, 278, 279, 280, 282

African American workers, 5, 14, 255; and co-worker relationships, 130, 131; perception of racism by, 187. *See also* black workers; race

African workers, 5, 61, 62, 63, 130. *See also* black workers; race

age: and hiring criteria, 228, 247, 250; of home care aides, 14; and job content and design, 81; and job satisfaction, 173, 174, 177, 180; and motivations, 78; and national averages, 136, 141; of nursing home aides, 14, 81; and race and job satisfaction, 5, 181, 182; and recruitment, 292; regulations concerning, 50; in research sample, 53, 56, 62; of staff in Georgia vs. national facilities, 65; and staff-resident relationships, 159; and turnover, 197, 199, 205, 207, 210, 212, 214. *See also* older workers

aging: demographics of, 78; knowledge of, 32; process of, 24

aging in place, 33, 42, 92, 112; ability to afford, 152; conditions aiding, 38–39; issues involved in, 35–36; and regulation, 42

alienation, 127, 130, 132

Alzheimer disease, 65, 230, 241, 246. *See also* dementia

American Indian workers, 131

Asian workers, 130. *See also* race

assisted living, 23–24; choice of work environment, 79–86; definition of, 28–29, 31, 36; in Georgia vs. nationally, 63–66; minimum staffing requirements in, 16; racial composition of, 171–72; range of difference within, 28–29; resident quality of life in, 33–37, 41–42; residents' characteristics, 40, 50, 178. *See also* quality of care; quality of life; regulation

and literacy, 229; regulation of, 24, 50; skills needed for, 286–87; and stress, 113, 115–16; training for, 241, 245–46, 248; and universal worker, 102, 106

medication manager (med tech), 99, 100; responsibility of, 116–17; role of, 104, 105, 106; and staff-resident relationships, 160; wage for, 246, 260, 261

men: as administrators, 64, 127; as DCWs, 80, 91, 98, 156, 228, 251; as residents, 98, 113; in sample, 61, 62, 74. *See also* gender

motivation: altruism as, 74, 80, 89, 215, 248, 285; for care work, 69–70, 159; compassion as, 248; and culture and group social norms, 69–70; for employment in assisted living, 79–85; for employment in long-term care, 74–93; extrinsic and intrinsic, 2, 3, 69–70; material, 74, 77–78, 90, 91, 92, 215, 285; moral, 74, 75–77, 89–90, 91, 92, 93, 285; professional, 74, 78, 89, 90, 91–92, 285; and social networks, 74, 78–79, 128, 129

nativity, 14, 15, 53, 181, 182, 183; and co-worker relationships, 130, 141, 143; and hiring, 231; and job satisfaction, 180, 184; in research sample, 61, 62, 63; of staff in Georgia vs. national facilities, 65; and staff-resident relationships, 152, 168. *See also* immigrant workers

non-white workers. *See* African American workers; black workers; race

nurse: as administrator, 64; in assisted living, 31, 32, 34, 38, 66, 105; LPN, 34, 105; and motivation, 90; opportunities for training as, 92; oversight by, 17; and professional motivation, 78; in research sample, 60, 62; RN, 31, 32, 34, 38, 105; role of, 24, 38; as staff in Georgia vs. national facilities, 66

nurse aide, 16, 177

nurse delegation, 24, 39

nursing home, 3, 14, 17, 33; and assisted living, 28, 59; DCW choice of assisted living over, 79–84, 89, 91, 92, 120; demand for, 19; discharge to, 31, 32; expenditures for, 37; job design in, 95, 96; neglect and abuse in, 83; preference for alternatives to, 37, 38; racism in, 177; resident characteristics in, 32–33,

38, 96; resident numbers in, 22; and staff-resident relationships, 96, 147; training for, 16; transition from assisted living to, 92; and worker stress, 96

older workers, 14, 20, 62, 136, 174, 228, 250; care experience of, 159; hiring of, 228, 229, 238, 250, 251, 292; and immigrants, 23; and job satisfaction, 174, 177; and material rewards, 277; and other low-wage workers, 136, 141; in rural areas, 214; and technology, 23; and training, 265; and wage, 264. *See also* age

poverty: and health insurance, 267; and low wages, 255; and material rewards, 287; and motivation, 20–21, 90; risk of falling into, 135, 140, 141; in rural South, 214. *See also* socioeconomic status

privacy, resident, 32, 34, 37, 40, 41, 42

quality of care, 32 33, 89, 92, 137, 284; and compassion, 248; concern about, 83; enhancement of, 39; and hiring, 225; and job satisfaction, 249; model for, 289, 290; and motivation, 82, 83, 87; and regulation, 42; regulations for, 30; and staff-resident relationships, 147, 148; and staff socioeconomic status, 136; and training, 225; and workforce improvement, 16–19, 23

quality of life, 23, 33–37; and DCW job design, 121; and regulation, 39–40; and staff-resident relationships, 147, 148, 161, 167, 248; studies of, 1

race: and administrators, 64, 168–69; and co-worker relationships, 127, 128, 129–31, 133–34, 141, 142, 143; of direct care workers, 14, 32, 65, 71, 159, 178, 255; and emotional work, 186; and job satisfaction, 5, 174–75, 183–84, 288; and motivation, 76; in research sample, 52, 53, 56, 62, 63; and residents, 50, 155–56, 172, 178, 288; and segregation, 214; and staff-resident relationships, 151, 152, 155–56, 159, 161, 167–69; and turnover, 199, 205–6, 207. *See also* African American workers; ethnicity; white workers